Biocontamination Control for Pharmaceuticals and Healthcare

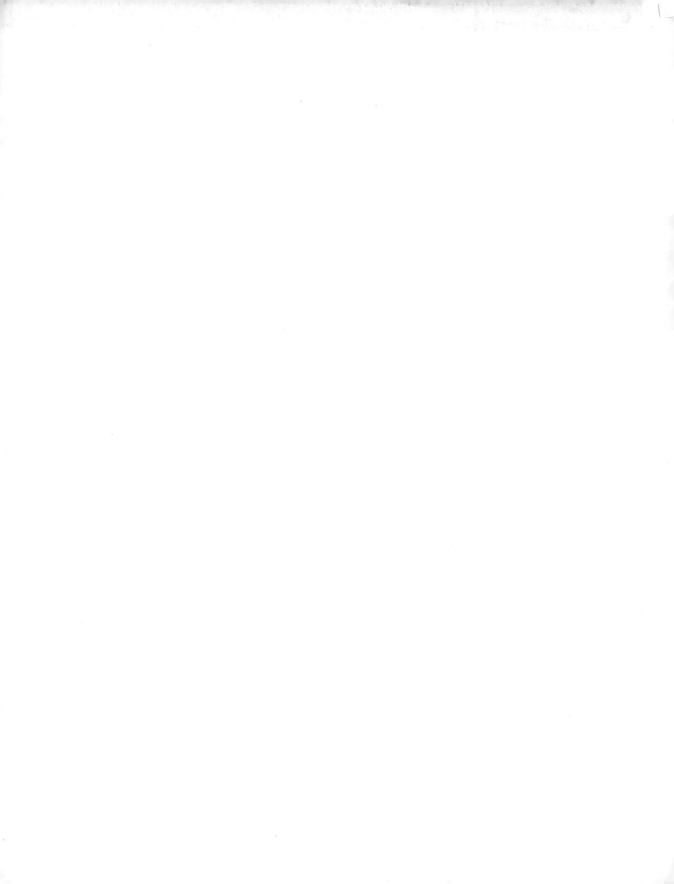

Biocontamination Control for Pharmaceuticals and Healthcare

Tim Sandle

Head of Microbiology, Bio Products Laboratory,
Elstree, UK and Visiting Tutor,
School of Pharmacy and Pharmaceutical Sciences,
Manchester University, UK

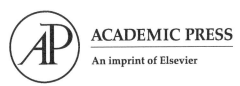

ELSEVIER

ACADEMIC PRESS

An imprint of Elsevier

Academic Press is an imprint of Elsevier
125 London Wall, London EC2Y 5AS, United Kingdom
525 B Street, Suite 1650, San Diego, CA 92101, United States
50 Hampshire Street, 5th Floor, Cambridge, MA 02139, United States
The Boulevard, Langford Lane, Kidlington, Oxford OX5 1GB, United Kingdom

Notices

Knowledge and best practice in this field are constantly changing. As new research and experience broaden our understanding, changes in research methods, professional practices, or medical treatment may become necessary.

Practitioners and researchers must always rely on their own experience and knowledge in evaluating and using any information, methods, compounds, or experiments described herein. In using such information or methods they should be mindful of their own safety and the safety of others, including parties for whom they have a professional responsibility.

To the fullest extent of the law, neither the Publisher nor the authors, contributors, or editors, assume any liability for any injury and/or damage to persons or property as a matter of products liability, negligence or otherwise, or from any use or operation of any methods, products, instructions, or ideas contained in the material herein.

Library of Congress Cataloging-in-Publication Data
A catalog record for this book is available from the Library of Congress

British Library Cataloguing-in-Publication Data
A catalogue record for this book is available from the British Library

ISBN 978-0-12-814911-9

For information on all Academic Press publications visit our
website at https://www.elsevier.com/books-and-journals

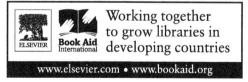

Working together
to grow libraries in
developing countries

www.elsevier.com • www.bookaid.org

Publisher: Andre Wolff
Acquisition Editor: Glyn Jones
Editorial Project Manager: Carlos Rodriguez
Production Project Manager: Maria Bernard
Designer: Matthew Limbert

Typeset by SPi Global, India

Contents

CHAPTER 1 Introduction to Biocontamination and Biocontamination Control 1

  Introduction 1

  Conclusion 9

  References 9

CHAPTER 2 Sources of Microbial Contamination and Risk Profiling 11

  Introduction 11

  Types of Microorganisms 12

  Assessing Product Risks 13

  Sources of Microbial Contamination 15

    Air 15

    Water 17

    Materials and Surfaces 18

    People 20

  Weaknesses With Environmental Controls 21

  Facility Repairs and Maintenance 22

  Remediation Actives 22

  Effective Cleaning and Disinfection 23

  Environmental Monitoring 24

  Summary 24

  References 25

CHAPTER 3 GMP, Regulations and Standards 27

  Introduction 27

  Cleanrooms and Classification 28

  European Regulations 29

  North American 30

  Synergy of US and European Regulations 31

  International 32

    ISO 14644 32

    Particle Sizes to be Measured 34

    Number of Locations to be Measured Within the Cleanroom 35

    Location of Particle Counters Within the Cleanroom 36

Volume of Air to be Sampled 36

Assessing Results...37

ISO 14698 Biocontamination Control and Microbiological Monitoring

Methods..39

cGMP 40

The Issue of Limits: Competing Standards 40

Common GMP Deficiencies 44

Documentation and Record Keeping 45

Summary 45

References...45

CHAPTER 4 **Biocontamination Control Strategy** 47

Introduction..47

Regulatory Expectations..49

Biocontamination Control Strategy..50

Understanding the Design of Both the Plant and Process.....................50

Detail of Equipment and Facilities 50

Training and Control of Personnel..51

Control of Utilities..51

Raw Materials Control 52

Product Development 53

In-Process Controls...53

Product Containers and Closures 54

Vendor Approval 54

Outsourced Services 54

Process Risk Assessment..55

Process Validation 57

Preventative Maintenance 58

Cleaning and Disinfection 58

Monitoring Systems..58

Prevention 60

Data Recording and Handling...61

Continuous Improvement 61

Summary 62

References...62

CHAPTER 5 **Cleanrooms and Environmental Monitoring** 65

Introduction..65

Cleanrooms and Clean Air Devices...66

Isolators, Gloveboxes, and Hatches 67

Contamination Control 68

Particles..73
Cleanroom Classification 74
    Assessing Results..77
Ongoing Environmental Monitoring 79
Summary 81
References...81

CHAPTER 6 Viable Environmental Monitoring Methods 83
Introduction...83
Application of Environmental Monitoring Methods 84
Settle Plates...85
    Assessing Suitability of Settle Plates..87
Active (Volumetric) Air Samplers 88
    Air Sampler Efficiency..92
    Practical Use of Air Samplers...94
    Compressed Gas Sampling...94
Surface Sampling...95
    Swabs 96
    Qualification Criteria for Swabs 97
    Contact Plates 98
    Selection of Contact Plates and Sampling Methods...............99
Personnel Monitoring 99
Summary 99
References...100

CHAPTER 7 Selection and Application of Culture Media 103
Introduction...104
Defining Culture Media..104
Supply of Culture Media 105
Types of Culture Media Used for Biocontamination Control.................105
    Tryptone Soy Agar 106
    Nutrient Agar...107
    Sabouraud Dextrose Agar..108
    Blood Agar..109
Quality Control Testing..109
Incubation Strategies for Environmental Monitoring.....................110
Temperatures of Incubation and Microbial Recovery 111
General-Purpose Culture Media..112
Incubation Strategies 112
    Studies to Evaluate Two-Tiered Incubation 114
    Marshall's Study..114

Sandle's Study 115

Gordon' Study 117

Sage's Study 117

Symonds' Study 118

Guinet's Study 119

Summary of Studies 119

Incubation Time 120

Summary 121

References 122

CHAPTER 8 Particle Counting 125

Introduction 125

Particle Counts and Contamination Risk 126

Particle Counters: Operation Basics 128

Limitations of Particle Counters 130

Operational Issues With Particle Counters 131

Limits Setting 133

Frequency of Particle Counting 134

Cleanroom Classification 135

Particle Sizes 135

Number of Locations 135

Location of Particle Counters 136

Air Volumes to be Sampled 136

Results Assessment 137

Summary 137

References 138

CHAPTER 9 Rapid and Alterative Microbiological Methods 141

Introduction 141

Developments With Pharmaceutical Microbiology 142

Benefits of Rapid and Alternative Microbiological Methods 144

Regulatory Acceptance of Rapid Methods 145

Classes of Rapid Microbiological Methods 146

Growth-Based Methods 146

Direct Measurement 146

Cell Component Analysis 147

Optical Spectroscopy 147

Nucleic Acid Amplification 147

Micro-Electrical-Mechanical Systems 147

Guidance for Selecting Rapid Microbiological Methods 148

    Key Considerations.. 149

    Internal Company Obstacles 150

    Validation.. 151

    Method Transfer 154

    Training... 154

    Expectations From the Vendor.. 155

Summary 155

References.. 156

CHAPTER 10 Designing and Implementing an Environmental Monitoring Program 159

Introduction.. 159

Frequency of Monitoring... 161

    A Risk-Based Approach 163

Time of Monitoring 167

Duration of Monitoring 168

Locations for Monitoring 169

Monitoring Methods 171

Cleanrooms in Different Operating States 172

    Newly Built Cleanrooms 172

    In-use Cleanrooms 172

    Other Considerations 173

Assessing Cleaning and Disinfection Effectiveness 174

Data Review 174

Monitoring for Particulates 175

Staff Training.. 176

Written Program 176

Summary... 177

References.. 177

CHAPTER 11 Special Types of Environmental Monitoring 179

Introduction.. 179

Monitoring to Support Parametric Release 180

The Need for Anaerobic Monitoring?... 182

The Need for Psychrophilic Monitoring? 183

The Need for Thermophilic Monitoring? 186

Compressed Gas Monitoring.. 187

    Microbial Survival in Compressed Gases................................. 189

Microbiological Requirements 190
Bacterial Endotoxin and Compressed Gases 192
Monitoring Sterility Test Environments 192
Monitoring Microbiology Laboratories...194
Test Controls...194
Summary 196
References...197

CHAPTER 12 Cleanroom Microbiota 199
Introduction..199
Growth Requirements of Microorganisms...200
Strategies for Microbial Survival in the Cleanroom Environment 201
Effect of Survival Strategy on Microbial Identification.........................202
Types of Microorganisms Found in Cleanrooms
and Their Origins..203
Personnel.. 203
Air 204
Surfaces (Equipment, Walls and Ceilings) 205
Raw Materials... 205
Packaging Materials 206
Water... 207
Details of Cleanroom Microbiota...207
Viruses 210
Conclusion 210
References...211

CHAPTER 13 Assessment of Pharmaceutical Water Systems..................... 213
Introduction..213
Use of Water in Pharmaceutical Manufacturing 214
Potable Water 214
Purified Water... 215
Water for Injections.. 215
Sterile and Nonsterile Products 216
Endotoxin Risks and WFI 216
Controlling Endotoxin Risks in WFI 217
Controlling Other Microbial Risks to
Water Systems 218
Addressing Water System Contamination 219

Water System Monitoring: Sampling, Testing, and Reporting 220
   Total Aerobic Viable Counts 220
   Undesirable ("Objectionable")
   Microorganisms 222
   Test for Bacterial Endotoxin 222
   Sample-Related Contamination.. 223
Summary 223
References..223

CHAPTER 14 Data Handling and Trend Analysis..225
Introduction..225
Microbial Data Variations 226
   Distribution of Microbial Data 227
Trending Microbial Data 229
   Histograms 229
   Control Charts.. 230
   What Control Charts Can Indicate 230
   Common Causes 231
   Special Causes 231
   Setting Up Control Charts 233
   Shewhart Charts... 233
   Cumulative Sum Charts... 237
   Other Charts 239
Frequency of Trending 239
Investigating Out of Trend 241
Tracking Microorganisms..242
Alert and Action Levels 244
   Setting Alert and Action Levels... 244
Data Integrity 245
Summary 246
References..246

CHAPTER 15 Bioburden and Endotoxin Control in
Pharmaceutical Processing 249
Introduction..249
Gathering Information About Microbial Control 250
Microbial Risks During Manufacturing 251
Process Factors Affecting Contamination...............................253
Process Hold Times and Process Validation 254

Sterile Products Manufacturing...255
Testing Regimes 256
    Sampling 256
    Test Methods 257
    Monitoring Plan 258
Investigating Data Deviations 258
Summary...258
References...259

CHAPTER 16 Risk Assessment and Investigation for
Environmental Monitoring.. 261
Introduction..261
Introducing Quality Risk Management 263
Applying Risk Assessment to Environmental Monitoring 265
    Intrinsic Hazards.. 266
    Extrinsic Hazards.. 266
Using Risk to Construct the Environmental
Monitoring Program 267
    Frequencies of Monitoring 267
Risk Assessment Tools..268
Hazard Analysis Critical Control Points
(HACCP)...270
Failure Modes and Effects Analysis 273
    The FMEA Exercise 274
Numerical Approaches to Risk Assessment 275
Risks Associated With Conducting
Environmental Monitoring 280
Out-of-Limits Investigations 281
Root Causes 283
Summary...284
References...284

CHAPTER 17 Assessing, Controlling, and Removing
Contamination Risks From the Process...................... 287
Introduction..288
Quality by Design..288
Cleanroom Design 289
Equipment Design and Use 291
Cleaning and Disinfection 292
    Cleaning 292

Disinfectants 292

Types of Disinfectant and Activity 293

Selection of Disinfectants.. 296

Disinfectant Qualification 298

Control of Personnel and Contamination Transfer Risks......................299

Cleaning Validation...301

Process Hold Times..302

Sterilization and Biodecontamination 302

Moist Heat 303

Dry Heat.. 304

Radiation 304

Gas 305

Sterilizing Grade Filtration... 305

PUPSIT 306

Biodecontamination 306

Sterile Products: Aseptic Processing and Terminal Sterilization...........307

Single-Use Sterile Disposable Technology...................................... 308

Nonsterile Products: Preservative Efficacy...309

Primary and Secondary Packaging..311

Risk Assessment 311

Conclusion 311

References..312

CHAPTER 18 The Human Factor and Biocontamination

Control 315

Introduction..315

The Human Risk Factor 316

The Human Microbiome 316

Implications for Biocontamination Control 321

Importance of Clothing 321

Cleanroom Garments 322

Cleanroom Personnel Behavior..326

Training...331

Changing Into Cleanroom Garments 332

Materials Access..333

Personal Hygiene 334

Summary 336

References..337

CHAPTER 19 Biocontamination Deviation Management..339
Introduction...339
Assessing Data Deviations: Terminology and Categories.....................341
Structuring the Investigation 342
Investigation of Laboratory Error 346
    Laboratory Controls...347
Assessing the Evidence 347
Impact Assessment 348
Concluding Investigations 352
Summary..353
References..354

Index 355

Introduction to Biocontamination and Biocontamination Control

CHAPTER OUTLINE

Introduction   1
Conclusion   9
References   9

INTRODUCTION

Biocontamination refers to biological contamination of products by bacteria and/or fungi, as well as the toxic by-products of these microorganisms, such as endotoxin and mycotoxins from Gram-negative bacteria and fungi, respectively. This book considers biocontamination within the context of pharmaceuticals and healthcare, with the focus of developing medicinal products that are safe. This level of safety cannot simply be achieved through putting individual protective measures in place and it certainly cannot be achieved through simply monitoring. To achieve the aim of biocontamination control each element needs to be looked at in the connected sense and fitted into a biocontamination control strategy (Sandle, 2015). Such a strategy is a fundamental element of the pharmaceutical quality system. The core points are relevant, to different degrees, to both sterile and nonsterile pharmaceuticals, as well as medical devices and biotechnology products (Sandle, 2013a).

When designing a biocontamination control strategy there are three components that need to be taken into account, and each of which needs to be risk based, drawing on the principles of quality risk management. First, processes need to be designed to avoid contamination. This demands the application of quality by design principles, which will vary according to different types of manufacturing and facilities. Important here is the selection of appropriate technologies, their design, and consideration of how they can best be implemented to minimize contamination and to lower the possibility

Biocontamination Control for Pharmaceuticals and Healthcare. https://doi.org/10.1016/B978-0-12-814911-9.00001-8

of cross-contamination occurring. Second, there needs to be a sound monitoring process to detect contamination. Third, there need to be a rapid response to contamination events and for putting proactive measures in place. When considering contamination events, the data from monitoring programs needs to be considered holistically. A breakdown of control downstream or in lower graded cleanrooms can signal later deterioration of control in relation to the product or the environment where the product undergoes final formulation or filling. Of these different elements it is the design of process where maximal effort needs to be placed (Sandle, 2013b).

There is, of course, a role for monitoring, especially once good design principles are in place. Environmental monitoring program should be designed in order to provide information about the state of control of the facility. Yet it remains important that an environmental monitoring does not replace good environmental control (the design of cleanrooms and operational practices); environmental monitoring only provides a "snapshot" of time. Individually counts are rarely significant, but it is the trends over time that are important: as counts, as frequency of incidents, and as microflora. The presence of microflora, such as waterborne bacteria or organisms that are hard to kill with disinfectants, may indicate the breakdown of control (Sandle, 2011).

The requirements for maintaining biocontamination control, together with the core elements of a robust strategy, are presented in the chapters that make up this book. Chapter 2 opens the substantive part of this book with discussion of microbial sources within pharmaceutical and healthcare processing environments. This is important since identification of these sources helps to identify where control is most required.

Contamination within healthcare and pharmaceutical facilities can arise from a number of sources. These may vary depending upon the type of cleanroom, its geographic location, the types of products processed, and so on. Nevertheless, these sources can generally be divided into the following groups: people, water, air and ventilation, surfaces, the transport of items in and out of clean areas. These sources are illustrated in Fig. 1.

Most contamination within the pharmaceutical facility can be traced to humans working in cleanrooms.

Chapter 3 assesses the regulatory framework, looking at the regulations that are applicable to contamination control (and the differences between them) and the gaps between regulations, identifying the aspects of a control strategy that are not so clear-cut. What the regulations share is that products are

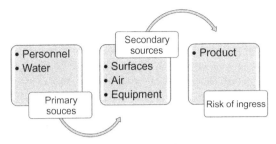

■ **FIG. 1** Microbial contamination sources and routes of transfer.

developed and manufactured in areas which minimize the potential for contamination. This is through the control of environmental cleanliness and in minimizing the opportunities for personnel to introduce contamination into the process.

Chapter 4 presents the main elements for a biocontamination control strategy. The aim here is to present the key aspects of the strategy and allow those who need to develop such a strategy to mirror the requirements and for those who have a strategy in place to benchmark their practices against. The strategy set out here is risk based (including risk profiling); proactive (in that identified risks need to be addressed); holistic (in seeing each part of the process as interrelated); and which highlights the importance of communication, in that the importance of risk escalation is emphasized.

Chapter 5 considers cleanrooms and the physical and microbiological measurements that can be used to assess cleanroom operations. With cleanrooms, there are a number of physical parameters which require examination on a regular basis. These parameters generally relate to the operation of HVAC systems and the associated air handling system. Air handler, or air handling unit (AHU) relates to the blower, heating and cooling elements, filter racks or chamber, dampers, humidifier, and other central equipment in direct contact with the airflow. Weaknesses or exceptions with any of these areas should be risk assessed and the outcome might lead to variations in the environmental monitoring program (Whyte & Eaton, 2004).

The chapter also assesses the classification and recertification of cleanrooms. The qualification of cleanroom classification is sometimes run as a separate activity to the environmental monitoring program and sometimes it is integral to it. Whichever management model is used, those tasked with routine and batch specific environmental monitoring need to be aware of the outcome of cleanroom classification exercises, including any variations in data and any design issues that are raised.

Chapter 6 looks at viable microbiological monitoring methods, with a focus on environmental monitoring. While these methods are commonly described in text books the limitations with the methods and their variabilities are too often overlooked. Understanding the weaknesses with the methods helps to lower expectations of what can be discerned from the data and helps focus the mind on the importance of environmental control. The methods can be strengthened through assessment and qualification, and the chapter provides some guidance over how each of the core methods can be evaluated.

Following on from Chapter 6, the seventh chapter looks at culture media. This is relatively ill defined in terms of assessing pharmaceutical environments. Here the key questions are Which culture media to use? Should one or two culture media be used? What is the incubation time? What is the appropriate temperature? The chapter assesses key studies that attempt to answer these questions, some of which are better designed than others, and puts together a framework for the optimal use of culture media. Growth promotion requirements are also covered in the chapter.

The nature of particle counting is based upon either light scattering, light obscuration, or direct imaging, and variations inform about control breakdowns. Chapter 8 addresses particle counting, as required for cleanroom classification and ongoing monitoring. The chapter considers the selection criteria for particle counters and some of the specifications which need to be evaluated, such as sensitivity (the smallest size particle that can be detected); false count rates; counting efficiency (the ratio of the measured particle concentration to the true particle concentration, which is typically at 50%); channels, in relation to differential and cumulative counting; and flow rate (the amount of air that passes through the particle counter).

Chapter 9 considers rapid and alternative microbiological methods and what these can offer biocontamination control, especially in relation to faster and more accurate responses, as well as reacting to events in real time. There are an array of different rapid microbiological methods, each with their own technologies and testing protocols, at different levels of maturity. The test methods are grouped in the chapter into the following three categories according to their uses: qualitative, quantitative, and identification.

When assessing alternative methods, data integrity is an important requirement. Data integrity concerns arise at the design, validation, and operation stages. Taking validation, samples need to be representative of what will be tested using the instrument and tested multiple times and by different technicians in order to build in repeatability and robustness. Aspects that give validity to the result, such as limit of detection and limit of quantification (either directly in relation to microorganisms or indirectly through monitoring biological events) need to be introduced.

In terms of operations, data integrity extends to data capture, retention, archiving, and processing. Most rapid methods use computerized systems and here systems should be designed in a way that encourages compliance with the principles of data integrity. Examples include multilevel password control, user access rights which prevent (or audit trail) data amendments, measures to prevent user access to clocks, having automated data capture, ensuring systems have data backup.

Chapter 10 puts together some of the elements of the previous chapters to present the detailed requirements for a risk-based environmental monitoring program. As a minimum, the program should address the following elements:

- Types of monitoring methods,
- Culture media and incubation conditions,
- Frequency of environmental monitoring,
- Selection of sample sites (where monitoring will take place),
- Maps showing sample locations,
- Duration of monitoring,
- When and where the samples are taken (i.e., during or at the conclusion of operations),
- Method statements describing how samples are taken and methods describing how samples are handled,
- Clear responsibilities describing who can take the samples,
- Chain of custody for samples,
- Processing and incubation of samples,
- Alert and action levels,
- Data integrity,
- Data analysis, including trending,
- Investigative responses to action level excursions,
- Appropriate corrective and preventative actions for action level excursions,
- Consideration if special types of environmental monitoring are required (such as the use of selective agars for objectionable microorganisms or anaerobic monitoring).

These important elements of the environmental monitoring program are examined in the chapter, together with the practical aspects.

There are other dimensions for environmental monitoring, required for specific processes or facilities. For example, some facilities may have identified a need for anaerobic monitoring; for other facilities, there is a need to monitor compressed gases. These disparate areas are pulled together in Chapter 11.

Characterizing the types of microorganisms found in the pharmaceutical environment is important for trending and for assessing control. A rise in spore-forming organisms, for example, may signal a breakdown of cleaning and disinfection practices or a weakness with material transfer. Chapter 12 provides details on research into the cleanroom microbiota, offering a benchmark for other facilities to compare against; discusses the significance of the findings; and provides tools for undertaking such assessments. The reasons for the selection of the most common strains for application in media growth promotion studies and disinfectant efficacy studies are setout.

Pharmaceutical water systems are the subject of Chapter 13. Here different types of water, generation methods, and testing requirements are outlined. The chapter also considers good design principles that can prevent contamination of water systems and the measures that need to be undertaken following water system modification. The chapter extends to a discussion of biofilms, which are microbial communities common to badly maintained water systems. Biofilms are difficult to remove, and some methods to do so are offered here.

Chapter 14 looks at microbial data. Data collection can relate to numbers of microorganisms or to the incidence of detection, or to both (against predefined monitoring levels). As well as incidents, some of the microorganisms recovered should be characterized and trended (La Duc et al., 2007). In order to identify patterns and possible reasons for a given trend, it is useful to include appropriate information with tables and graphs. Such information includes locations, dates, times, identification results, changes to room design, operation of new equipment, shift or personnel changes, seasons, and HVAC problems (e.g., an increase in temperature).

When action levels are exceeded or adverse trends spotted appropriate investigations must be performed, using documented procedures, to determine the contamination source and any impact upon the product and process. This should be followed by corrective and preventative actions. Such data also informs about the effectiveness of the cleaning and disinfection regime. Additional information can be obtained about the performance of people and equipment, and of operating protocols. The chapter presents the appropriate techniques and tools that can be deployed for data assessment.

Although microbiology tests represent only a small portion of a pharmaceutical quality testing program, their importance is critical to product safety. Chapter 15 is about in-process control, in terms of bioburden and endotoxin levels. This is central to a quality control strategy, which should take into account manufacturing risks to select samples and to determine risks, and to use the sample results generated as Critical Quality Attributes (CQAs). Controlling these microbial attributes, whether downstream or upstream, is fundamental to product protection. The chapter looks at methods, sampling regimes, and important aspects of control, such as process hold times.

Chapter 16 draws together some of the conversations on risk and considers more fully how risk assessments can inform about biocontamination control. Given the variety of contamination sources, consideration should be given to risk control. That is, where contamination risks are identified the risk should be minimized as part of the strategy of bringing the cleanroom under tighter control. Where a risk cannot be minimized adequately then this should be encompassed into the environmental monitoring program, with the data reviewed and studied for trends. This requires selecting locations for monitoring that are meaningful and by monitoring at frequencies that allow trends to be discerned.

There are two groups of approaches to the risk analysis process. These are qualitative and quantitative methods. Perhaps the most suitable for environmental monitoring is Hazard Analysis Critical Control Points (HACCP), although the merits of Failure Modes and Effects Analysis (FMEA), which can assist with equipment reviews, are also presented. These tools allow process within a cleanroom (or across several cleanrooms) to be mapped, for hazards to be identified, and for risks to be evaluated.

Chapter 17 considers the different ways through which contamination can be minimized in pharmaceutical processes. The chapter looks at this from the both the perspective of sterile and nonsterile pharmaceuticals. With nonsterile products, factors like objectionable microorganisms need to be considered in relation to the use of preservatives.

With sterile pharmaceuticals, a fundamental concern is with people. To minimize contamination from people, proper gowning is essential to curtail the amount of shedding of skin matter and microorganisms that a person can deposit within a cleanroom. Localized protection, such as isolators and unidirectional airflow cabinets, should also be established around the product to minimize contact with people. Good cleanroom design includes high-efficiency particulate air filters (HEPA), pressure cascade, and air distribution. Cleanrooms must also be cleaned and disinfected regularly, and transfer of items in and out of the cleanroom must be controlled (Sandle, 2017).

Chapter 18 considers people, how they contaminate, and how much of this is a product of how people behave and how they are trained. Training links to gowning as well as behaviors within the cleanroom.

The final chapter of the book, Chapter 19, looks at deviation management: how to respond when things go wrong, and microbial excursions and/or upward trends occur. Certain factors will lead to contamination risks being more likely. These factors include poorly designed cleanrooms; water remaining on surfaces for prolonged periods; inadequate cleaning and sanitization; inadequate personnel gowning; poor aseptic practices such as direct surface-to-surface transfer (such as by personnel directly touching the product or contaminated water entering the process, or a failure to sanitize trolley wheels); and airborne transfer, often arising from personnel shedding microorganisms. Here shedding increases with increased personnel movement and fast movement also increases the potential for microbial dispersion. The chapter looks at some of these types of contamination events and provides guidance on undertaking investigations. Prior launching into certain investigations it is important to verify that the results are valid; hence the chapter discusses "out of specification/limits" investigations to assess the likelihood of laboratory error, before commencing an investigation, root cause analysis, and proposals for corrective and preventative actions. Cutting across both sterile and nonsterile pharmaceuticals, cleaning and disinfection features strongly in the text.

Putting each of the chapters together the basis of a holistic biocontamination control strategy is presented, considering:

- Why microbial contamination is a problem;
- The primary contamination sources;
- The importance of contamination control and its relationship to design;
- Cleanrooms and process controls;
- Having a robust environmental monitoring, including an emphasis upon risk assessment and trend analysis;
- The importance of investigation, setting corrective and preventive actions, and feeding the lessons learned back into design and control improvements.

This feeds into the importance of product protection and the safety of the patient. Failure to adequately abrogate any microbial challenge associated within process or product will result in contaminated marketed product, essentially regarded as adulterated. The administration of microbially contaminated pharmaceuticals or medical devices could have an acute impact upon the individual recipient patient and the broad recipient patient population. Hence, this is why biocontamination control matters.

CONCLUSION

In capturing the necessary elements of biocontamination control, this book complements two others written by the author for the publisher. The first looks at sterile products and sterilization, assessing these control measures in more detail ("Sterility, Sterilisation and Sterility Assurance for Pharmaceuticals: Technology, Validation and Current Regulations"). The second looks at the wider role that pharmaceutical microbiologists play in designing laboratory testing, assessing data, and helping with new product development ("Pharmaceutical Microbiology: Essentials for Quality Assurance and Quality Control").

REFERENCES

La Duc, M. T., Dekas, A., Osman, S., Moissl, C., Newcombe, D., & Venkateswaran, K. (2007). Isolation and characterization of bacteria capable of tolerating the extreme conditions of clean room environments. *Applied and Environmental Microbiology, 73*(8), 2600–2611.

Sandle, T. (2011). Environmental monitoring. In M. R. Saghee, T. Sandle, & E. C. Tidswell (Eds.), *Microbiology and Sterility Assurance in Pharmaceuticals and Medical Devices* (pp. 293–326). New Delhi: Business Horizons.

Sandle, T. (2013a). Biocontamination control—moves toward a better standard. *Cleanroom Technology, 21*(4), 14–15.

Sandle, T. (2013b). Revision of ISO 14698—Biocontamination control: personal reflections on what might be desirable. *Clean Air and Containment Review*, (14), 20–21.

Sandle, T. (2015). Development of a biocontamination control strategy. *Cleanroom Technology, 23*(11), 25–30.

Sandle, T. (2017). Establishing a contamination control strategy for aseptic processing. *American Pharmaceutical Review, 20*(3), 22–28.

Whyte, W., & Eaton, T. (2004). Microbiological contamination models for use in risk assessment during pharmaceutical production. *European Journal of Parenteral and Pharmaceutical Sciences, 9*(1), 1–8.

Chapter 2

Sources of Microbial Contamination and Risk Profiling

CHAPTER OUTLINE
Introduction   11
Types of Microorganisms   12
Assessing Product Risks   13
Sources of Microbial Contamination   15
   Air   15
   Water   17
   Materials and Surfaces   18
   People   20
Weaknesses With Environmental Controls   21
Facility Repairs and Maintenance   22
Remediation Actives   22
Effective Cleaning and Disinfection   23
Environmental Monitoring   24
Summary   24
References   25

INTRODUCTION

All pharmaceutical manufacturing areas will have some form of microbiological contamination (including, at times, EU GMP Grade A/ISO Class 5 areas). Microbiological contamination, in general, is not necessarily a problem—for all people who come into contact with microorganisms each day. What matters is the context. Where contamination occurs during pharmaceutical manufacturing: the location and nature of the contamination to the "critical area" is of significance. Even then there are complex variables to consider. These include, especially in relation to nonsterile products:

- The function of the product;
- What the product is intended to be used for;

Biocontamination Control for Pharmaceuticals and Healthcare. https://doi.org/10.1016/B978-0-12-814911-9.00002-X

- The type of contamination;
- The numbers of microorganisms present.

This is because at one extreme the contamination in an injectable can lead to death; at the other an aroma in a tablet that may be simply off-putting. Therefore there are different contamination concerns for sterile and nonsterile products and with regard to where in the process they occur. With sterile products even low-level contamination on a filling needle could result in direct harm to a patient, particularly if there is no preservative in the product or no subsequent pretreatment steps (such as, freeze-drying or heat treatment). With sterile products the aim is to manufacture a product free from viable life forms (here "sterility" is an absolute term) and thus even low numbers of microorganisms at critical areas poses a potential problem.

Understanding the origins of microbial contamination and vectors for contamination are important to the biocontamination program, in terms of seeking and designing appropriate environmental controls and for developing effective remediation strategies.

TYPES OF MICROORGANISMS

For nonsterile products the more direct concern is often the type of pathogens rather than absolute numbers. For example, some microorganisms of concern for different products are as follows:

Staphylococcus aureus	Topical preparations
Pseudomonas aeruginosa	Topical preparations
Escherichia coli	Oral products
Salmonella spp.	Oral products

The above are "indicator organisms"; where the species themselves may not be present, they signify other organisms that present an equivalent risk. In this context it is incumbent upon the manufacturer to develop their own list of organisms of concern.

Regulations require pharmaceutical manufacturers to prevent objectionable organisms contaminating products (USA: CFR 211.113 and 21 CFR 211.165; Europe: Ph Eur. 5.1.4). Some objectionable organisms are specified in the pharmacopeias but these are not exclusive and other organisms may be objectionable depending on the nature of the product, route of administration, and intended patient population. There is an expectation that the significance of other microorganisms is evaluated (as per the main pharmacopeia) (Sutton & Jimenez, 2012).

Most information relating to "objectionables" is provided in the FDA CFRSs, which state:

- 21 CFR 211.84(d) (6) "Each lot of a component, drug product container, or closure with potential for microbiological contamination that is objectionable in view of its intended use shall be subjected to microbiological tests before use."
- 21 CFR 211.113(a) "Appropriate written procedures, designed to prevent objectionable microorganisms in drug products not required to be sterile, shall be established and followed."
- 21 CFR 211.165(b) "There shall be appropriate laboratory testing, as necessary, of each batch of drug product required to be free of objectionable microorganisms."

To identify objectionable microorganisms and to respond to contamination events, a risk-based assessment should be conducted, including personnel with specialized training in microbiology and data interpretation. In addition to dealing with isolates as they arise, it is advisable that an assessment is done proactively to generate a documented list of objectionable microorganisms which should be incorporated into procedures and internal specifications as appropriate.

With nonsterile products other significant types of contamination must also be evaluated. There are other factors to consider which may increase or decrease the risk, such as the water activity of the product. As the remit of this module is environmental monitoring the risk factors associated with the actual product are not discussed in great detail.

ASSESSING PRODUCT RISKS

Different types of pharmaceutical products will be at a greater or lesser risk to microbial contamination than others (and the extent to which this becomes a serious risk requires an assessment of the organism as objectionable, as discussed before). While taking care not to overgeneralize, in a manufacturing facility dealing with dry powder mixing, granulation and drying, and final sacheting or tabletting, contamination risks to the product from the environment will predominantly be bacterial and fungal spores. Such contamination arises from the environment dust, together with anything shed by the operators. With such processes, good handling and ventilation control can keep cross-contamination to a minimum (Würtz, Sigsgaard, Valbjørn, Doekes, & Meyer, 2005).

Risks to dry products, such as tablets, can be re-presented at later manufacturing stages. Aqueous granulation and drying can become a problem if drying is not carried out immediately or if temperature tray drying is carried out over an extended time. Proliferation of microbiota originating from the raw materials can occur during the tray drying stage. These microorganisms may die through the process of drying as the available water activity is reduced.

Further in terms of considering points of risk, it should be noted that the mechanical forces, together with the application of heat, involved in pressing tablets are often sufficient for the destruction of fungal spores and vegetative bacteria. However, the concern is that bacterial spores can survive this process.

Contamination of microorganisms in products from the environment does not necessarily mean that the product will harm the patient or that the environment is at a permanent risk. There are several scenarios that can happen with regard to microbial contamination. These are as follows:

- The microorganisms may die;
- The microorganisms may survive without proliferating;
- The microorganisms may metabolize, grow, and multiply;
- The microorganisms may be transferred.

Further to risk, several factors that should be considered include (Sutton, 2012):

- The nature of the product—Can the product support microbial growth? Does it contain an effective concentration of antimicrobial preservatives? Is the product liquid based or anhydrous?
- Whether the microorganism is likely to survive for long periods of time in the product.
- The nature of the microorganism—Is the organism an opportunistic pathogen? Will the addition of this microbial species at the administration site adversely affect the patient? Is the microorganism itself an indicator of other pathogenic species that might be present but not detected on this occasion? Keep in mind that some microorganisms should be regarded as indicator strains, that is, they may indicate a concern with contamination from undesirable species. For example, the presence of Enterobacteriaceae may suggest a risk from *Escherichia coli* even if *E. coli* is not detected.
- The absolute numbers of the microorganism recovered.
- Microbial toxins—Is the microorganism likely to release a toxin (exotoxin, enterotoxin, or endotoxin) that could cause patient harm even if the microorganism is no longer viable?
- The route of product administration—What are the hazards associated with the route of administration? Is the target site normally sterile?

- The intended recipient—Will the product be used in immunocompromised patients? Is the patient currently suffering from any diseases or open wounds?
- The use of other medications—Is the patient currently using other medications that may result in diminished immunity?

Therefore much environmental monitoring is an assessment of risk. Risk is commonly assessed by severity of the risk x the probability that the risk will occur. The risk can be mitigated if there is a good system of detection in place. A good system of detection relates to a robust environmental monitoring program. Risk is compounded by the fact that very little of the product is actually tested given the small sampling sizes involved. This limitation is particularly apparent for the sterility test, which will only detect gross contamination.

When risk assessments are used, for sterile products in particular, it is important that no distinction is be made between microorganisms that can cause disease and those considered to be benign, as any microorganism can potentially cause infection in an immunocompromised individual. What matters is the trend of the environment and probability of product contamination.

SOURCES OF MICROBIAL CONTAMINATION

There are various sources of microbial contamination. These can typically be divided into four generic groups (Sandle & Vijayakumar, 2014):

- Air,
- Water,
- Manufacturing equipment; surfaces and consumables,
- Personnel.

Often contamination occurs in combinations. In a cleanroom, for instance, contamination could potentially arise from air, personnel, and from equipment at different proportions during the same event.

These different sources of contamination are examined:

Air

The air in most manufacturing areas is microbiologically "contaminated" (contains microorganisms), although the level will vary: a cubic meter of air in an office will have considerably more microorganisms per cubic meter than an equivalent volume of air in an EU GMP Grade B/ISO Class 7 (dynamic) cleanroom. While air is a vector of microorganisms, it is not a nutritive environment. Therefore many microorganisms in the air die from desiccation or photosensitivity. Many other microorganisms are anaerobic and thus will not survive or be unable to multiply.

While bacteria do not increase in number, some bacteria can survive in the air. Typically these are spore-forming bacteria like *Bacillus* spp. Other Gram-positive bacteria, such as *Micrococcus* spp., and some fungi, can also survive in airstreams.

Bacteria in air are normally present in association with dust particles and skin flakes, rather than as individual microorganisms. A skin flake is typically 33–44 μm. Flakes of skin often break down to typically between 20 and 10 μm (which is important for when airborne particle counts are assessed, as discussed later). What is important, when considering the contamination risk from bacteria in the air, is the potential for deposition onto critical surfaces. Much of the risk centers on air velocities and airflows.

The contamination risk from air in cleanrooms is overcome by air filtering (the effectiveness of this is typically measured by standards for different grades of air filter and their ability to capture different levels and sizes of airborne particles). Other preventative measures include the airflow and room pressure design (where air from the cleanest room moves out into a room of a lower cleanliness level), which prevents recontamination for microorganisms cannot move against an air current.

Further in relation to air is the ease of dispersal of fungal spores. Fungal spores are produced by all fungi—yeast (single-celled or unicellular fungi), filamentous fungi, and dimorphic genus. With filamentous fungi the process of growth is through the production of hyphae (tubular branches), which expand as a mass (called the mycelium) in multiple directions. Some of the hyphal branches grow into the air and spores form on these aerial branches (Nazaroff, 2004).

Fungal spores are either unicellular or multicellular, developing into a number of different phases through the complex life cycles of the fungi. The objective of most fungal spores is reproduction. Fungi are often classified according to their spore-producing structures, for example, spores produced by an ascus are characteristic of ascomycetes. This class of fungus typically produces between four and eight spores in an ascus. The ascus resembles a "pea pod" like structure which holds the spores until environmental conditions are optimal at which point the spores are released.

Fungal spores can spread over considerable distances. Unlike bacterial spores, fungal spores are more likely to be carried in airstreams and can therefore be spread over wide areas; within an enclosed space like a cleanroom this could readily be all parts of the cleanroom. Hence fungal spores can travel long distances, depending on the fungus, spore size (aerodynamic diameters are important because dynamics of particles are known to vary depending on their size, and the prevailing conditions). The distance traveled and direction taken are dependent upon the force of dispersal and whether any further vectors are at play, for example, carried in airstreams or by water droplets. A concern in the as-built environment is that most spores will germinate when conditions are optimal (and here fungal spores are more likely to germinate than bacterial spores).

The purpose of these fungal spores is to allow fungi to reproduce; they serve a similar purpose to that of seeds in the plant world (although the mechanisms are different). Some fungi also produce a second type of spore. These are called chlamydospores and they are thick-walled resting spores, able to survive unfavorable conditions (such as hot and dry environmental conditions, lack of nutrients, alterations to osmolarity, and hostile pH levels and chemicals). These fungal spores are thick walled, dark-colored, spherical, microscopic biological particles. The spores are typically the result of asexual reproduction. These spores are equipped to survive in environments like cleanrooms.

Ingress of spores into cleanrooms can lead to some bacterial or fungal spores germinating and many of the fungal spores will remain in the spore state waiting for favorable conditions. Damage to parts of the cleanroom due to the water leaks (e.g., seals) can lead to reservoirs for spore survival. At the same time, the presence of water underneath vinyl would have led to conditions that would encourage the growth of fungi and lead to proliferation. Research suggests that fungi grow best and survive for longer where water is available (certainly there is no evidence that fungi grow when carried in air or can utilize air to promote growth). There is also an association with fungal presence and dust; with survival enhanced where water is present with dust particles. These add up to fungal spores being a particular problem in cleanrooms when fungi settle onto surfaces (Sandle, 2014).

Water

The second contamination source in cleanrooms is water. Water is both a vector and a source of contamination. Water therefore poses more of a problem than air as it not only allows microorganisms to remain present within a cleanroom but it also can increase the numbers of microorganisms present (through the microorganisms replicating). The time interval required for a bacterial cell to divide or for a population of bacterial cells to double is called the generation time. Generation times for bacterial species growing in nature may be as short as 15 min (especially for Gram-negative bacteria). Typically, water is unavoidable in pharmaceutical processing as it is needed as an ingredient, as a cleaning agent, a dilute for disinfectants, and is used as steam.

Water is ubiquitous in pharmaceutical industry. It is the most common raw materials in pharmaceutical formulations and processes. It is also used in different processes for the cleaning and rinsing of equipment. Water is a major source of microbial contamination when GMP standards are not followed. During processing, validation, and production, water samples are analyzed to determine the microbial quality of the facilities water. There are three types of water commonly used in pharmaceutical facilities. These are as follows:

- Potable water: For example, used for cleaning and hand washing;
- Purified water: For example, used for clean-in-place systems;
- Water for injection: For example, used for final rinsing of equipment and product formulations.

Water can be a serious source of contamination, Gram-negative rods, in particular, can grow and multiply even in low nutrient states. Therefore, small deposits of water or damp areas can become reservoirs for contamination. For example, typical Gram-negative bacteria can include *Acinetobacter* spp., *E. coli*, and *Pseudomonas* spp. Some Gram-negative rods, such as *Pseudomonas* spp., need only very low concentrations of organic nutrients to grow and multiply. Such microorganisms are invariably found in all residues of water and areas that have recently been wetted.

Materials and Surfaces

Surfaces in cleanrooms become contaminated through deposition (e.g., settling from the air) and from direct contact. There is some variation in the risk from microorganisms depositing onto surfaces because there are some physicochemical forces that can remove microorganisms from the surface. Therefore in considering the possibility of surface contamination, it is sometimes likely that the microorganism may not remain in contact for a long period of time. Aside from surfaces, there is also a risk from the materials and equipment transferred into a cleanroom.

The condition of the cleanroom has a bearing on the possibility of a vector (like air or water) breaching the cleanroom and with the ability of a facility to respond to an incident with an effective cleaning and disinfection program (since damaged surfaces are more difficult to clean and disinfectant). The probability of this comes down to how well a particular facility is maintained, although the success of maintaining a facility becomes more difficult with aging facilities (an indefinable time, although, in the pharmaceutical context a facility over 25 years old might reasonably be defined as aging) (Sandle, 2016).

"Materials" is an all-encompassing term for things that are introduced into the pharmaceutical environment. The areas of greatest risk arise from the transfer of materials in and out of a clean room. Transfers should always be controlled and risk assessed (and transfers of equipment like environmental monitoring apparel should not be neglected as possible sources of contamination).

Materials located in cleanrooms should be of a design that can be easily cleaned and disinfected. Factors for consideration include having smooth finishes. It is important to ensure that all aspects of materials and equipment operation come under an appropriate cleaning regime.

Incoming raw materials can sometimes contain bacterial spores, especially with drier substances. In general, synthetic materials have a low bacterial count; however, they can contain spores. Dry powders of natural origin are more likely to carry high numbers of spore-forming organisms. Hence purchasing such materials from an approved supplier and carrying out appropriate indicator organism testing (for certain risk materials, it may be appropriate to add a *Bacillus* species to complement the standard USP specified microorganisms).

In addition to chemicals, packaging—especially cardboard, can contain *Bacillus* species. The introduction of cardboard into cleanroom facilities should be avoided. In contrast, laminates, metal foils, and blister-pack materials all have smooth impervious surfaces with a high-temperature stage employed in their manufacture and, therefore, have low surface microbial counts (Tang, Kuehn, & Simcik, 2015).

Controls should be introduced where incoming materials for pharmaceutical processing are held before transfer to the process areas. One key aspect is with storage, and in ensuring that sufficient air can circulate around the storage containers. Air movement will allow outer packaging to dry out if it has become damp. On movement into core production, a risk of cross-contamination from the outer packaging remains a possibility. This can be minimized through effective air handling systems (Payne, 2007).

A further area of concern is with poorly maintained machinery. This can also be a source of fungi and bacterial spores, in particular. Repairing damage should form part of a facilities biocontamination remediation strategy. An example is with worn or damaged filters, which can blow air around a facility. A second area is following maintenance activity, such as the opening of panels on machines. The inner areas of equipment, especially those not typically intended to be exposed to the cleanroom environment, can be a source of contamination.

People

It is arguable if people or water represents the most critical source of contamination in cleanrooms. Certainly, people are a very significant source of contamination for all people carry microorganisms and even the most "embracing" gowning procedure will not avoid the risk of microbial contamination. People also represent a highly variable and unpredictable source, in that one individual may behave in a way that increases a contamination risk one day but not the next.

The microbial ecology of the human body is complex and many of the species of microorganisms which form the microbiota are unknown. There is considerable diversity of species and variation between different locations on the body and across individuals over time. Nevertheless, there are some genera of bacteria which are generally represented. When research of the bacteria biota of human skin is compared with published work of cleanroom microorganisms, there is an association between the microorganisms commonly found in cleanrooms and those which are transient to, short- or long-term resident on, human skin.

Typical microbial contamination arising from people includes *Propionibacterium* spp., *Staphylococcus* spp., *Streptococcus* spp., and *Micrococcus* spp. Such microorganisms shed from hair, skin, and eyes and other mucus membranes. Typically, these microorganisms are shed into the air although transfer via hands is also a common risk area (Sandle, 2012a).

Our understanding of the microorganisms found on and in the human body has been advanced through the work of the Human Microbiome Project (2008–13). The Human Microbiome Project (HMP) began in 2008 as a United States National Institutes of Health initiative. The core objective of this continuing project is to identify and characterize microorganisms associated with both healthy and diseased humans (the human microbiome) using a combination of culture techniques, metagenomics, and whole genome sequencing. As the Human Microbiome Project continues to improve our ability to characterize and understand the human microbiome, it has become evident that there are many implications to pharmaceutical microbiology that must be taken into consideration regarding the development, production, and use of therapeutic products, as well as the controlled environments within which medicinal products are produced.

An element of personnel control is achieved by protection of critical activities through unidirectional airflow and isolators and by the use of correct cleanroom grade clothing and discipline. Cleanroom disciplines including correct aseptic technique and ensuring personnel are trained in appropriate behavior, that is, behavior related to both movements and actions. The shedding of microorganisms increases with increased movement. Fast movement also increases potential for wider dispersion through airflow disruptions. In EU GMP Grade A/ISO Class 5 environments, such disciplines are very important and include slow movement, minimizing talking, and well-practiced operations (such as activities supported through media trials). Therefore an important emphasis should be placed on operator training.

WEAKNESSES WITH ENVIRONMENTAL CONTROLS

Control of the pharmaceutical environment is important in relation to microbiological control in general. With *Bacillus* and fungal spores in particular, control should be centered on good cleanroom design, with a focus on minimizing airborne contamination. Airborne contaminants are mainly spore formers, in addition to other organisms shed by individuals via the deposition of skin flakes. Air control is achieved through having air filtration and ensuring good turbulent airflow within cleanrooms (and unidirectional airflow as required in cabinets). Rooms of different cleanliness classes should be at different pressure differentials in order to prevent air from the "dirtier" area trailing into the "cleaner" area.

Spores can also be carried into cleanrooms by staff via their clothing. Adequate changing facilities should be provided to enable staff to change effectively on entry into the cleanroom and to change quickly at the end of working sessions. Where cleanroom clothing may be reworn (such as with nonsterile manufacturing) changing practices should be defined so that personnel do not contaminate their factory clothing.

With control of spore formers, inadequate facility design can lead to areas where spore formers remain undiscovered, presenting a contamination risk in the future. Of particular concern here is damage to surfaces which can create niches in which spores can settle and remain. Surfaces should be designed to minimize contamination and to enable them to be easily cleaned and disinfected. For example, the use of coving and designing chemically resistant surfaces.

Repair and maintenance should extend to all areas of the facility, including cold areas. All species of *Bacillus* will survive in cold temperatures and some are capable of growth. For example, psychrotrophic *B. cereus* strains can grow at commercial refrigeration temperatures (2–8°C) (Daelman, Vermeulen, Willemyns, et al., 2013).

FACILITY REPAIRS AND MAINTENANCE

Bacterial and fungal spores are often introduced into pharmaceutical areas through dust contamination. Based on this, any structural alterations to buildings or uncontrolled sweeping may give rise to these contaminants remaining in the vicinity. One area of concern is with damages to cleanroom fabric, such as torn vinyl. Thus strict controls should be in place during facility downtime.

Within cleanrooms and controlled environments, risk areas where spores can occur include:

- Door kick back plates
- Bags
- Incubators
- Boxes
- Cart wheels
- Ceiling tiles
- Poor flooring
- Vibrations from construction
- Light fixtures
- Faulty HVAC systems (a fungus like *Cladosporium* spp. can reside within blower wheel fan blades, ductwork, and cooling coil fins; other fungi have been found with drip pans, as well as air humidifiers and cooling towers).

REMEDIATION ACTIVES

There are broadly two remediation activities. The first is with addressing the point of origin and correcting it. The second is with recovering the area, which involves making repairs and running an effective cleaning and disinfection regime. The latter involves selecting the optimal type of disinfectant—often one that is sporicidal and which has demonstrated surface efficacy against fungal spores (Lopolito, Bartnett, & Polarine, 2007).

In terms of reacting to problems, one common concern is with wet areas or areas that become damaged through water leakage. Cleanroom personnel should react quickly to water damage within a facility and treat or replace damaged walls and ceilings quickly.

EFFECTIVE CLEANING AND DISINFECTION

Even with other control measures in place, microbial contamination remains a risk. To guard against this, cleaning and disinfection practices need to be robust. Some organisms are resistant to hostile physical and chemical conditions; this means that they can be difficult to remove if a sanitization regime is not effective (Haberer, 2008).

This leads to some points that are worth considering in relation to cleaning and disinfection (Sandle, 2012b):

1. The importance of detergents: are detergents used prior to the application of a disinfectant? This is a necessary step since many disinfectants have poor penetrative ability and require the removal of the soil barrier in order to reach microorganisms.
2. The efficacy of cleaning practices is important. Both detergents and disinfectants need to be wiped onto surfaces in order for them to be effective.
3. The preparation of detergents and disinfectants. It is important to check if "clean" water is being used as not to add a high bioburden to the cleaning solution. Furthermore, the mops and buckets should be suitable for cleanroom use (and with an aseptic facility, the cleanroom items should be sterile).
4. Arguably the most important point when considering the risks posed by spore-forming microorganisms is whether a sporicidal disinfectant is being used routinely. The periodic use of a sporicide is important because standard disinfectants, such as alcohols, quaternary ammonium compounds, phenols, and amphoteric surfactants, while effective against bacteria in their vegetative state, are ineffective against spores. Although the spore state itself is not capable of causing infection, under suitable conditions, germination of *Bacillus* spores may take place within minutes (the rate and the extent of spore germination is dependent on strains, treatments, and environmental factors).
5. Biocides that have sporicidal activity include hypochlorites and hydrogen peroxide/peracetic acid blends.
6. The disinfectants used for the routine sanitization program need to be qualified to show that they can reduce a known population of microorganisms from a surface. Such an evaluation should be undertaken using an appropriate method.

The robust adherence to good cleaning and disinfection practices is important, for many microbial spores, especially spores of *Bacillus* species, are very adhesive to surfaces of equipment due to three characteristics: (1) their relatively high hydrophobicity, (2) low spore surface charge, and (3) unique morphology (Ronner & Husmark, 1992).

ENVIRONMENTAL MONITORING

The adequacy of controls in place in manufacturing environment is assessed through environmental monitoring. Here the importance is not only with undertaking monitoring at a sufficiently high frequency and with orientating monitoring locations to points of risk toward the product. There is also a need to understand and to characterize the microorganisms recovered.

In relation to the types of microorganisms recovered, environmental contamination of dry surfaces such as floors and walls comprise mainly Gram-positive rods, cocci, and fungal spores. Here species of *Bacillus* will be found (these organisms are less common in "wet areas" like wash bays, where Gram-negative bacteria will predominate). In establishing an environmental monitoring regime, the agars used must demonstrate that they can recover a wide range of microorganisms. Chapter 10 considers the environmental monitoring program in greater detail.

SUMMARY

This chapter has looked at microbial risks in cleanrooms and controlled environments, discussing different contamination vectors and factors that promote microbial survival. While many factors are important, microbial contamination of pharmaceutical products is mainly caused by human interventions or environmental factors. Microbial contamination in the pharmaceutical production facilities continues to be a difficult challenge for the industry and can provide significant health hazard to human safety when pathogens get into nonsterile products (and potentially fatal should sterile products be compromised). The human factor is explored further in Chapter 18.

The assessment of any contamination event should be addressed through an investigation and root cause analysis. There are different techniques available for such reviews. When approaching an investigation it is important to define and describe properly the event or problem ("the five whys" technique can be useful here). This should be followed by establishing a time line from normal situation until the point of concern. Risk tools like failure modes and effects analysis (FEMA) and hazard analysis critical control points (HACCP) are often useful. Information should then be collected and challenged, using methods like "is/is not" tables and contradiction matrices, which help to distinguish between root causes and causal factors. These approaches help shape the method of problem prediction.

When investigating fungal contamination in pharmaceutical facilities, a number of different areas should be considered. These include:

1. The association between the organism and the environments (is it dry or wet?),
2. Room conditions,
3. Maintenance and machine conditions,
4. Personnel activities,
5. The types of organisms recovered,
6. The numbers of organisms recovered.

Chapter 19 considers approaches to investigating microbial numbers and organisms further. The key message here is about good design and risk assessment in attempting to avoid contamination arising and, where it does arise, by minimizing the opportunities for survival or distribution.

REFERENCES

Daelman, J., Vermeulen, A., Willemyns, T., et al. (2013). Growth/no growth models for heat-treated psychrotrophic *Bacillus cereus* spores under cold storage. *International Journal of Food Microbiology, 161*(1), 7–15.

Haberer, K. (2008). Cleaning and disinfection in the control of pharmaceutical cleanrooms. In J. P. Agalloco, & F. J. Carleton (Eds.), *Validation of pharmaceutical processes* (3rd ed., pp. 303–337): Informa Healthcare.

Lopolito, P., Bartnett, C., & Polarine, J. (2007). Control strategies for fungal contamination in clean rooms. *Control Environment, 372*, 1–5.

Nazaroff, W. W. (2004). Indoor particle dynamics. *Indoor Air, 14*, 175–183.

Payne, D.N. Microbial ecology of the production process. In Denyer, S. and Baird, R.M. (Eds.) Microbiological control in pharmaceuticals and medical devices, CRC Press, Boca Raton, FL, 2007: 60–61.

Ronner, U., & Husmark, U. (1992). Adhesion of *Bacillus cereus* spores—a hazard to the dairy industry. In L. F. Melo (Ed.), *Biofilms* (pp. 403–406). The Netherlands: Kluwer Academic Publishers.

Sandle, T. (2012a). A review of cleanroom microflora: types, trends, and patterns. *PDA Journal of Pharmaceutical Science and Technology, 65*(4), 392–403.

Sandle, T. (2012b). Cleaning and disinfection. In T. Sandle (Ed.), *The CDC handbook: A guide to cleaning and disinfecting cleanrooms* (pp. 1–31). Surrey: Grosvenor House Publishing.

Sandle, T. (2014). Fungal contamination of pharmaceutical products: the growing menace. *European Pharmaceutical Review, 19*(1), 68–71.

Sandle, T. (2016). Risk consideration for aging pharmaceutical facilities. *Journal of Validation Technology, 22*(2), 11–20.

Sandle, T., & Vijayakumar, R. (2014). Microbiological environmental monitoring of cleanrooms, Part 1: Contamination sources and methods. In *Cleanroom microbiology* (pp. 83–114). River Grove, IL: PDA/DHI Publishing.

Sutton, S., & Jimenez, L. (2012). A review of reported results involving microbiological control 2004–2011 with emphasis on FDA consideration of "objectionable organisms" *American Pharmaceutical Review*, *15*(1), 42–57.

Sutton, S. V. M. (2012). What is an "objectionable organism"? *American Pharmaceutical Review*, *15*(6), 36–42.

Tang, W., Kuehn, T. H., & Simcik, M. F. (2015). Effects of temperature, humidity and air flow on fungal growth rate on loaded ventilation filters. *Journal of Occupational and Environmental Hygiene*, *12*(8), 525–537.

Würtz, H., Sigsgaard, T., Valbjørn, O., Doekes, G., & Meyer, H. W. (2005). The dustfall collector—A simple passive tool for long-term collection of airborne dust: a project under the Danish Mould in buildings program (DAMIB). *Indoor Air*, *15*, 33–40.

Chapter 3

GMP, Regulations and Standards

CHAPTER OUTLINE
Introduction   27
Cleanrooms and Classification   28
European Regulations   29
North American   30
Synergy of US and European Regulations   31
International   32
   ISO 14644   32
   Particle Sizes to be Measured   34
   Number of Locations to be Measured Within the Cleanroom   35
   Location of Particle Counters Within the Cleanroom   36
   Volume of Air to be Sampled   36
   Assessing Results   37
   ISO 14698 Biocontamination Control and Microbiological
   Monitoring Methods   39
cGMP   40
The Issue of Limits: Competing Standards   40
Common GMP Deficiencies   44
Documentation and Record Keeping   45
Summary   45
References   45

INTRODUCTION

There is an array of regulations and standards that outline a general approach for the biocontamination control of sterile facilities and minimal guidance for nonsterile areas. Many of these standards focus on cleanroom design and operations. The key importance of these standards is where the text states that it is the activity in a cleanroom that *determines* its classification or grade. The determination of this influences the environmental monitoring regime employed (including limits, locations for monitoring, frequency of monitoring, and so on). These factors are normally determined by risk assessment tools, which are explored in subsequent units in this module.

Biocontamination Control for Pharmaceuticals and Healthcare. https://doi.org/10.1016/B978-0-12-814911-9.00003-1

The problem is that different standards sometimes compete, and they are often lacking in information or detail (hence one of the requirements for this book). The general importance of regulations is that they give an indication of applicable limits and some of the sample types to be used; this impacts upon the development of the biocontamination control program. Limits relate to different *methods* for environmental monitoring and to different cleanroom *classifications*.

CLEANROOMS AND CLASSIFICATION

Before exploring different GMP requirements, it is useful to assess the differences for global requirements in terms of grading cleanrooms and controlled environments. For both sterile and nonsterile manufacturing, cleanrooms are the areas in which manufacturing takes place and toward which the environmental monitoring program is directed. A clean room (or "cleanroom") or zone is, simply, a room that is clean. Here it will be:

- A room with control of particulates and set environmental parameters.
- Construction and use of the room is designed in a manner to minimize the generation and retention of particles.
- The classification is set by the cleanliness of the air.

By prescribing a grade or class, the areas are regarded as controlled environments.

Within Europe, the EU GMP guidance for aseptically filled products is used to define different cleanrooms and the EU GMP alphabetic notations are adopted. These grades are set out, as per Table 1.

Room classifications according to Grades A, B, C, and D are approximately equivalent to classes adopted by ISO 14644-1, which is examined later.

Table 1 EU GMP cleanroom grades	
Grade	**Room use**
A	Aseptic preparation and filling (critical zones under unidirectional flow)
B	A room containing a EU GMP Grade A/ISO Class 5 zone (the background environment for filling) and the area demarcated as the "Aseptic Filling Suite" (including final stage changing rooms)
C	Preparation of solutions to be filtered and production processing
D	Handling of components after washing; plasma stripping
U	Freezers, computer conduits, store rooms, electrical cupboards, other rooms not in use, and so on

Cleanroom classifications are confirmed by measuring particle counts per cubic meter in the *dynamic* state. ISO 14644-1 details three occupancy states for clean room classification: "as built," "static," and "dynamic." Of the three states "dynamic" is more representative of in-use conditions and represents the "worst case." For these reasons the dynamic state is the condition of clean rooms selected for classification purposes.

Classification of critical cleanrooms is confirmed in the *dynamic* state by taking nonviable particulate readings at a defined number of locations for 0.5 μm size particles at the following frequencies (as stated in ISO 14644-2). It is good practice to reclassify (or recertify) cleanrooms annually, with aspartic processing areas assessed every 6 months.

With cleanrooms it is important to define the "critical" and "supporting areas." These terms generally relate to sterile manufacturing. The definitions are important in that the environmental monitoring program should be biased toward the most critical areas of the manufacturing process. This general philosophy should also apply to nonsterile manufacturing.

EUROPEAN REGULATIONS

In Europe, EU GMP Regulations (such as the Guide to good manufacturing practice for medicinal products) specify the limits for different grades of cleanroom (refer to Annex 1) (Eudralex, 2009). It should be noted that the European Pharmacopeia does not directly refer to environmental monitoring.

Central to European GMP is Annex 1. The purpose of the current Annex is to emphasize that the manufacture of sterile products is subject to special requirements. The scope, since 2018, has also been broadened to include nonsterile pharmaceutical products, in terms of those aspects which are applicable. These requirements are necessary in order to minimize risks of microbiological, particulate, and pyrogen contamination of sterile products and also to provide guidance as to how sterile products are best protected. This guidance embraces personnel training, equipment qualification, cleanroom design, and environmental monitoring.

Throughout Annex 1, reference is made here to quality risk management (QRM), especially in relation to microbial contamination control. That QRM needs to be a proactive exercise is emphasized and repeated several times throughout the document. Reference is also made to personnel, indicating early on that people are critical to processes. The point made is about the importance of employing personnel with the appropriate skills, training, and attitudes. Given the centrality of people as a major source of contamination (a point made several times in this book), this point is well made.

NORTH AMERICAN

The main regulatory issues arising from North America are centered on the USP and the FDA.

The United States Pharmacopeia (USP) guidance chapter <1116> "Microbiological control and monitoring of aseptic processing environments" (which applies to aseptic filling environments only) (USP, n.d.-b). Until its 2011 revision the chapter gave recommended values for environmental monitoring limits. In 2011 the scope of the chapter was narrowed to aseptic processing only and there was a change from quoting limits to a focus on the frequency of occurrence. This was a marked change in philosophy for environmental monitoring in that it mattered less what the count was and more on how often environmental monitoring excursions occurred. There is, therefore, a contrast in the approach taken by EU GMP guidelines and the USP.

Other USP chapters are also of relevance. For example, general chapter <797>, titled "Pharmaceutical compounding–sterile preparations." This chapter states that sterile compounding procedures require clean facilities, specific training for operators, air quality evaluations, and a sound knowledge of sterilization and stability principles.

In 2014 the Pharmacopeial Forum (which is part of the USP) issued a draft chapter aimed at nonsterile environments: USP <1115>—Bioburden control of nonsterile drug substances and products. The chapter contains reference to the environmental monitoring of nonsterile environments. The draft guidance chapter suggests using a risk-based approach to identify the microbial control risks during the development and manufacturing of nonsterile products. Specifically, the chapter covers a wide range of important information that should be reviewed when performing a risk assessment including US regulatory guidance outlined in the Food and Drug Administration's good manufacturing practices, considerations during development and manufacturing, microbial control, assessments of environments, and overall quality management (USP, n.d.-a).

In relation to FDA Inspections, the FDA guide to aseptic manufacturing (last issued in September 2004) is a very important document (FDA, n.d.). This document identifies how the manufacturing of sterile products should be undertaken and defines certain elements of critical environments. The document also published some guidance values, which indicate what an FDA inspector will expect to see in terms of cleanroom standards.

The FDA's view on biocontamination control and environmental monitoring is also captured in the Code of Federal Regulations, especially 21 part

211, which relates to aseptic manufacture (specifically FDA CFR 211.42). The 21 CFR 211.113 (a) Control of microbiological contamination establishes that appropriate written procedures, designed to prevent the objectionable microorganisms in drug products not required to be sterile, shall be established and followed. Other relevant sections include 21 CFR 211.42: Design manufacturing areas, which ensures suitable size, construction, and location for manufacturing activities; 21 CFR 211.46: HVAC ventilation, air filtration and air heating and cooling system, must control space pressurization, microorganisms, dust, humidity, and temperature for drug product manufacturing; 21 CFR 211.56(c): sanitation: pest control (i.e., rodenticides, insecticides, fungicides, and fumigating agents). This also includes cleaning and sanitizing agents to prevent contamination of equipment, product containers, and so on.

In addition, documents issued by the US Parenteral Drug Association (PDA), although not regulatory, are commonly held up to be examples of good practice. In relation to environmental monitoring, PDA Technical Report No. 13 details some aspects of the practical approach taken to constructing an environmental monitoring program.

SYNERGY OF US AND EUROPEAN REGULATIONS

Although the US and European regulations differ, there are some common factors that need to be considered when assessing and implementing biocontamination control. These are as follows:

1. Buildings, facilities, and utilities (e.g., water for injection and HVAC) systems that are used in for pharmaceutical and healthcare products production need to be designed, constructed, and maintained to control microbial and particulate contamination.
2. Product components, containers, and closures should be tested or certified (and results are compared to specifications), treated, and handled to detect, prevent, and eliminate microbial and other contamination.
3. A contamination control monitoring program needs to be in place. This is defined by procedure and implemented to assure that conditions are suitable for producing pharmaceutical products.
4. Personnel must be qualified through a combination of training and experience in effective microbial control and preventive measures. Personnel should wear clean (or sterilized) clothing while working in critical, controlled areas and engage in good sanitation practices and health habits.
5. The effectiveness of processing is demonstrated and documented through qualification and validation.

6. Controls should be implemented to reduce risks that could adversely affect the production of pharmaceutical products.
7. Quality inspection and laboratory testing of various types are used to demonstrate that processes are producing acceptable results.
8. Batch record reviews for release of products with microbiological concerns need to be carefully performed, taking those microbiological concerns into account in addition to those normally considered.

INTERNATIONAL

The International Standards Organisation (ISO), jointly with the Committee for European Normalisation (CEN), is the main provider of international guidance relating to environmental monitoring and cleanroom design. The ISO produces so-called voluntary standards (Schicht, 2003).

These include:

- ISO 13408, which relates to the Aseptic processing of healthcare products (ISO, 2008).
- ISO 14698 Cleanrooms and associated controlled environments—biocontamination control and microbiological monitoring methods. This set of standards refers to viable monitoring techniques and contamination control.
- ISO 14644, which relates to cleanroom construction and design. These standards were first issued in 1999, and various updates have been completed since, of which the most important were the December 2015 updates to Parts 1 and 2.

ISO 14644

The ISO 14644 standard uses different "classes" of cleanrooms and this is used internationally, with the exception of Europe where "Grade" (A, B, C, and D) remains in use. These standards assess: design, performance, and testing criteria. There are many parts to ISO 14644, and this covers a range of industries. For pharmaceuticals and healthcare, the most important are as follows:

- ISO 14644-1:2015—Part 1: Classification of air cleanliness by particle concentration (ISO, 2015a).
- ISO 14644-2:2015—Part 2: Monitoring to provide evidence of cleanroom performance related to air cleanliness by particle concentration (ISO, 2015b).

ISO 14644-1 describes different phases in relation to the testing and monitoring of cleanrooms. These are as follows:

- *Commissioning*: This is testing, proving, and documenting a facility system to demonstrate and satisfy the safe functionality in accordance with the design criteria.
- *Validation*: Qualification practices, fully documented, to provide the necessary assurance, through predefined test/s to prove that the critical systems operate in accordance with the facility design criteria. Validation and qualification are required in a regulatory regime.

Classification is the process of qualifying the cleanroom environment by the number of particles using a standard method. The end result of the activity is that cleanroom x is assigned ISO Class y. Importantly classification is distinct from routine environmental monitoring and distinct from process monitoring, such as the requirement in EU GMP Annex 1 for continuous monitoring of aseptic filling.

Cleanrooms are certified according to principles outlined in ISO 14644 Part 1 and monitored according to the methods described in ISO 14644 Part 2. To classify pharmaceutical grade cleanrooms either:

- The number of particles equal to and $>0.5\,\mu m$ per cubic meter of air is measured and this count is used to identify the cleanroom class. The concentration of $5\,\mu m$ particles may also be measured if required to meet regulatory grades.
- Or, the class is assigned, and this is either proven correct or not through an assessment of the number of particles equal to and $>0.5\,\mu m$ measured in one cubic meter of air.

Selecting the approach will be dependent upon a local policy. For aseptic filling, the clean zone must be ISO Class 5/EU GMP Grade A. Therefore the area is designed to this specification and testing is carried out to ensure if the device can meet this classification.

The tests listed in ISO 14644 are divided into mandatory and optional tests. Optional tests may be included where they are of relevance to the cleanroom (such as an assessment of temperature and humidity). The range of tests may also differ where the cleanroom is undergoing validation in contrast to commissioning.

The designation for cleanroom classification needs to include the following elements:

- The room classification number expressed as "ISO Class N."
- The occupancy state.

- The considered particle size. It is also possible to certify a cleanroom at multiple sizes; if this is the case then the sample volume requirement for the largest particle size is used.

With occupancy state, the certification state of the cleanroom must be defined in advance of testing, by selecting one of three possible occupancy states:

- *As Built*: condition where the cleanroom or clean zone is complete with all services connected and functioning but with no equipment, furniture, materials, or personnel present.
- *At Rest*: condition where the cleanroom or clean zone is complete with equipment installed and operating in a manner agreed upon, but with no personnel present.
- *In Operation*: agreed condition where the cleanroom or clean zone is functioning in the specified manner, with equipment operating and with the specified number of personnel present.

With the "at rest" and "in operation" states, for most areas, the operational state is preferred as this represents a greater challenge as the cleanroom has equipment running and people are present (Sharp, Bird, Brzozowski, & O'Hagan, 2010). Cleanrooms are classified according to the number and size of particles permitted per volume of air. ISO 14644-1 gives a method to classify cleanrooms by the concentration of airborne particles.

Some of the key steps involved with cleanroom classification are outlined as follows.

Particle Sizes to be Measured

For pharmaceuticals and healthcare, to meet FDA regulations, particles of a size $\geq 0.5\,\mu m$ are required to be measured. For those wishing to classify using $\geq 5.0\,\mu m$ size in addition, the standard requires that the outcome is expressed using a macroparticle size descriptor, namely:

$$ISO\,M\,(20;\ \geq 5.0\,\mu m);LSAPC$$

where M = macroparticles, 20 = class limit (value taken from EU GMP Annex 1), $\geq 5.0\,\mu m$ = the particle size under consideration, LSAPC = Light scattering airborne particle counter (reference to the test instrumentation).

So, with for EU GMP:

> Grade A
>> ISO 5; at rest, operational; $\geq 0.5\,\mu m$
>> ISO M $(20; \geq 5.0\,\mu m)$; at rest, operational; LSAPC

Grade B
>   ISO 5; at rest; $\geq 0.5\,\mu m$, and M (29; ≥ 5.0); at rest, LSAPC
>   ISO 7; operational; $\geq 0.5\,\mu m$, 5.0.

Number of Locations to be Measured Within the Cleanroom

A significant change with the standard is the method for selecting the number (and position) of particle counter locations within a cleanroom. The method is based on a look-up table. The table uses a range of cleanroom sizes and provides the number of locations required (if the exact room size is not listed, the user selects the next largest room size and picks the appropriate number of locations). These numbers are based on a statistical method called hypergeometric distribution. This is very different to the square root approach, which was based on binominal distribution. Without going into statistical detail, the former approach assumed that in each location a particle counter was placed, the particle in the cleanroom was normally distributed. In contrast, the revised approach is based on particles not being normally distributed. The new approach allows each location to be treated independently (Rice, 2007).

The hypergeometric distribution is used to calculate probabilities when sampling without replacement. This is perhaps best illustrated using a nonparticle counting example. Consider a pack of playing cards. If we randomly sample one card from a deck of 52 and next, without putting the card back in the deck, we sample a second card. Following this, suppose we sample a third card, again without replacing any cards, and so on. Considering this sampling procedure, what is the probability that exactly two of the sampled cards will be aces? (For noncard players, 4 of the 52 cards in the deck are aces). The probability is very low.

If the exercise was carried out again, but the cards were replaced, this would be an example of binomial distribution (which the 1999 version of the standard was based on). The realities of particle counting are such that once particles in a given volume of air have been sampled they are not replaced; hence, hypergeometric distribution is more realistic than binominal distribution.

For the user, the approach is simpler because no calculations are required. In addition, for rooms with <9 particle count locations, the requirement to perform a 95% upper confidence level check has been removed. With the assigned numbers there is an in-built confidence interval of 95%. This means when a cleanroom is monitored there is a 95% level of confidence that 90% of the cleanroom complies.

In general, the new approach leads to an increase in particle count locations compared with the previous standard.

Location of Particle Counters Within the Cleanroom

Once the number of locations has been selected, the room is divided up into sectors and a particle counter placed in each sector. With the previous standard, these sectors were equal in size and a counter placed in approximate center. With the revised standard, the position where the counter is placed within each sector is determined by the user. The standard allows counters always to be placed at the same point within the sector, randomly placed within the sector, or evenly distributed, or selected by risk. The risk-based approach would be the best one to adopt. A risk-based decision could be based on variables like room layout, equipment type, airflow patterns, position of air supply and return vents, air change rates, and room activities.

The reason for not selecting the center of the location relates back to the issue of particle distribution: particles counts no longer assumed to be homogenous within a sector. Furthermore, additional locations can be added at the discretion of the facility. This might arise from the room-by-room risk assessment.

Volume of Air to be Sampled

A further change is with the volume air that requires sampling in each location. The theory behind this is that the volume of air sampled needs to be sufficient to detect at least 20 particles of the largest particle size selected. The revised standard supplies a formula to be used. The outcome is the number of liters that need to be sampled in each location. The standard requires a minimum of 2 L per location; the application of the formula can result in this being higher. Generally, the lower the particle count limit, the greater the volume to be sampled (so a larger volume is taken from an EU GMP Grade B room compared with a Grade C room). It should be noted that the Pharmaceutical Inspection Convention and Pharmaceutical Inspection Co-operation Scheme (PIC/S), to which EU GMP inspectors and the FDA are members, states in guide PE 009 that for routine testing the total sample volume should not be less than $1\,\mathrm{m}^3$ for Grade A and B areas and preferably also in Grade C areas. It is up to each manufacturer how this guidance is interpreted (PIC/S, 2009).

When operating a particle counter in unidirectional airflow, for example, Grade A, the counter probe must be oriented into the airflow or pointed upwards for turbulent flow air.

Assessing Results

Assessment of results involves:

1. Recording the results for each location.
2. Convert the results to particles per cubic meter.
3. This is set out using the formula published in the standard.
4. It should be noted that the formula states "number of particles at each location or average." This is because an option exists to add more than one particle count location per sector. When this occurs the results are averaged and the average used as the number to proceed with the previous calculation. Individual results may fall outside of the class, provided that the mean is within.
5. Although assessment is based on an average, each individual result must be within limits. Those out of limits need to be investigated.

Should out-of-limits results be obtained an investigation should be performed into the origin of the particle counts. This should conclude consideration of room design, equipment, and operator activities. Once a root cause has been identified, and corrective measures put in place, the exercise should be repeated. A risk assessment will be required to assess activities performed in the cleanroom between classification exercises.

Once a cleanroom has been fully classified there are certain aspects that need to be maintained such that the cleanroom operator can continue to claim that the cleanroom continues to meet the classification and in which state that classification was made. This is where the second part of the ISO 14644 standard comes into play. Cleanroom classification needs to be repeated on a frequency defined by ISO 14644-2. Part 2 of ISO 14644 additionally outlines the requirements of a risk assessment to be performed in determining the details of a monitoring plan, these include:

- What level of monitoring is required?
- Which action and alert limits will be set?
- What should happen should an action or alert limit be exceeded?

It is also required that the system being used to demonstrate control over the environment be based upon a written design and that design should take into account the risks associated with the activities being performed and the best practice to both monitor the environment and establish suitable control limits.

- ISO 14644-3:2005—Part 3: Test methods (ISO, 2005).

  In Part 3, tests are specified for two types of cleanrooms: unidirectional flow and nonunidirectional flow (or turbulent flow). The test methods recommend what test apparatus and test procedures are required and where appropriate an alternative procedure is suggested. The most important objectives of this document are to provide an internationally common basis of measurement and evaluation of cleanrooms and, at the same time, not to prevent the introduction of new technologies.

The ranges of tests are as follows:

1. Airborne particle count for classification and test measurement of cleanrooms and clean air devices,
2. Airborne particle count for ultrafine particles,
3. Airborne particle count for macroparticles,
4. Airflow test,
5. Air pressure difference test,
6. Installed filter system leakage test,
7. Airflow direction test,
8. Airflow visualization,
9. Temperature test,
10. Humidity test,
11. Electrostatic and ion generator test,
12. Particle deposition test,
13. Recovery test,
14. Containment leak test.

The reader should note that not all of these tests are applicable for the pharmaceutical, medical device, or healthcare sectors.

- ISO 14644-4:2001—Part 4: Design, construction and start-up (ISO, 2009).

  ISO 14644 Part 4 specifies the requirements for the design and construction of cleanroom installations. It provides the details for all the important elements for the design and construction of a new cleanroom or clean facility. The standard includes sections on defining requirement; the planning and design of the cleanroom, construction, and start-up; the testing and approval of the delivered facility and the documentation required to hand over the facility to the end user.

- ISO 14644-5:2004—Part 5: Operations (ISO, 2004a).

  ISO 14644-5 provides a source for addressing the primary functions of how a cleanroom should be used and the operations that are essential to their use. These include operational systems, cleanroom clothing, personnel, stationary equipment, portable equipment and materials, and also the cleaning and disinfection of the cleanroom.

The standard includes these sections as being a requirement of cleanroom operations and as such must be followed or have a procedure against each one, it then expands on each section to give more information regarding how each can be implemented.

- ISO 14644-7:2004—Part 7: Separative devices (clean air hoods, gloveboxes, isolators, and mini-environments) (ISO, 2004b).

  This part of ISO 14644 specifies the minimum requirements for the design, construction, installation, testing, and approval of separative devices in those respects where they differ from cleanrooms as described in ISO 14644-4 and 14644-5. Separative devices range from open to closed systems and include isolators and Rapid Access Barrier Systems (RABS). Isolators are commonly used for aseptic processing.

The issuing of the ISO 14644 and ISO 14698 standards represented the first time that a group of standards had been created collectively for cleanrooms. However, the scope of these chapters covers a diverse range of industries including food, pharmaceutical, and cosmetics.

Reference to environmental monitoring is also made by the World Health Organisation (WHO). WHO Technical Report 823 covers similar ground to EU GMP (WHO, 1992).

ISO 14698 Biocontamination Control and Microbiological Monitoring Methods

The ISO 14698 twin standards deal specifically with the microbiological contaminants and how to manage an efficient control plan. The standards explain the general principles and global methodology to evaluate and monitor both the air and surface biocontamination control in such controlled environments. The standards also specify the required methods to guarantee a coherent monitoring of the critical areas and to apply the right preventive and corrective actions in case of contamination.

ISO 14698-1 describes the principles and basic methodology for a formal system to assess and control biocontamination, where cleanroom technology is applied, in order that biocontamination in zones at risk can be monitored in a reproducible way and appropriate control measures can be selected (ISO, 2003a). The approach is based around the Hazard Analysis and Critical Control Points (HACCP) risk assessment tool.

ISO 14698-2 gives guidance on basic principles and methodological requirements for all microbiological data evaluation, and the estimation of biocontamination data obtained from sampling for viable particles in zones at risk, as specified by the system selected. This is not intended for testing the performance of microbiological counting techniques of determining viable units (ISO, 2003b).

cGMP

Outside of published standards there is a raft of "best practices" that fall within the blanket phrase "current Good Manufacturing Practice" (cGMP). In many place, cGMP refers to generally agreed Goof Manufacturing Practices that have yet to be codified. However, all GMP is sometimes referred to as "cGMP." The "c" stands for "current," reminding manufacturers that they must employ technologies and systems which are up to date in order to comply with the regulation.

For "current" GMPs that have yet to be captured in a regulatory document, these are in part driven by regulatory inspections, where an inspector will wish to seek assurance that there is proper directional flow of air, controlled material transfer, and people movement. cGMPs also reflect changes to technology and what is available to the cleanroom manager or microbiologist at a given time (nevertheless, whether or not every technological change advances patient safety is a matter of contention). As it stands, not every cGMP initiative needs to be adopted. Each manufacturer needs to decide individually how to best implement the necessary controls by using scientifically sound design, processing methods, and testing procedures.

Some recent cGMP developments relate to the design of cleanrooms, where "quality by design" has been incorporated into the process flow and the types of equipment used. In relation to air handling systems, computational flow dynamics allow predictions to be made as to how the air might move. With monitoring, the most significant advances have been with rapid and alternative microbiological methods.

THE ISSUE OF LIMITS: COMPETING STANDARDS

The different regulations share a requirement for the user to establish alert and action levels against which the environmental monitoring data will be assessed. However, one of the problems in assessing the different standards is that they can be contradictory. Furthermore, often, when a company manufactures products for different product markets, some kind of rationale needs to be developed so that "one" environmental monitoring program can be used to conform with the different regulatory standards pertaining to one product market. This often means that the strictest limits from the different standards are to be taken as the maximal limits (although, as examined later, each facility must develop alert and action levels below these recommended values).

The following tables attempt to compare the different current (and recently superseded standards) in relation to cleanroom classification. The classification of cleanrooms is explored later in this module.

Comparisons have been divided into two cleanroom operational states. These are static and dynamic (or, "at rest" and "operational"), as presented in Tables 2 and 3. The withdrawn FDA 209E (Federal Standard, 1992) and USP <1116> standards have been included because these are still referred to in many references (particularly the 209E classes). However, the reader should avoid using these when discussing cleanroom grades or classes.

Until the 2015 revision of ISO 14644, ISO Class 5 was equivalent to ISO Class 4.8. This was because the particle limit for 5.0 µm size particles for in EU GMP was slightly tighter (at 20) than the equivalent limit for ISO Class 5 (which was, until it was dropped, 29).

For *static* conditions (or "at rest"), there is a difference between European/ISO and US standards. The EU GMP defines the static state as a room

Table 2 Cleanroom classification, static state

	For *static* conditions, these are:		
U GMP	US 209E (withdrawn)	USP <1116> (withdrawn)	ISO 14644-1
A	Class 100	M 3.5	5
B	Class 100	M 3.5	5
C	Class 10,000	M 5.5	7
D	Class 100,000	M6.5	8

Table 3 Cleanroom classification, dynamic state

	For *dynamic* (or "in operation") conditions, the equivalences are:		
EU GMP	US 209E (withdrawn)	USP <1116> (withdrawn)	ISO 14644-1
A	Class 100	M 3.5	5
B	Class 10,000	M 5.5	7
C	Class 100,000	M 6.5	8
D	Not stated	Not stated	9

without personnel present, following 15–20 min "clean up time," but with equipment operating normally. The US standards indicate that equipment is not running.

Dynamic conditions (or "operational") are typically defined as rooms being used for normal processing activities with personnel present and equipment operating. The following table is a summary of the tightest levels taken from the applicable standards. EU GMP grades have been used as reference categories.

With viable limits, the EU GMP requirements are presented in Table 4.

Prior to the 2018 EU GMP Annex 1 revision process, the Grade A values of "1" were expressed as "<1" and there was also an accompanying statement about these being "average values." From 2018, the limit simply became "1 cfu."

Table 4 EU GMP viable count limits

Parameters	EU GMP Grade A/ISO Class 5	EU GMP Grade B/ISO Class 7 (dynamic)	EU GMP Grade C/ISO Class 8 (dynamic)	EU GMP Grade D/ISO Class 9 (dynamic)
Air samples (active) Dynamic state	cfu/m^3 Action = 1	cfu/m^3 Action = 10	cfu/m^3 Action = 100	cfu/m^3 Action = 200
Air samples: Settle plates (passive) Dynamic state	cfu/event Action = 1	cfu/event Action = 5	cfu/event Action = 50	cfu/event Action = 100
Surface samples at working height Contact plates Dynamic state	$cfu/25cm^2$ Action = 1	$cfu/25cm^2$ Action = 5	$cfu/25cm^2$ Action = 25	$cfu/25cm^2$ Action = 50
Surface samples at working height Swabs Dynamic state	cfu/swab Action = 1	cfu/swab Action = 5	cfu/swab Action = 25	cfu/swab Action = 50
Surface samples Floor contact plates/swabs	cfu/device Action = 1	cfu/device Action = 10	Not defined	Not defined
Drain swabs	N/A	N/A	Not defined	Not defined
Finger plates Dynamic state	cfu/plate (hand) Action = 1	cfu/plate (hand) Action = 5	cfu/plate (hand) N/A	cfu/plate (hand) N/A
Gowning (suit contact plate) Dynamic state	$cfu/25cm^2$ Action = N/A	$cfu/25cm^2$ Action = N/A	$cfu/25cm^2$ N/A	$cfu/25cm^2$ N/A

Table 5 FDA aseptic processing microbial limits

ISO Class (in operation)	Active air samples (cfu/m³)	Settle plates (cfu/4-h exposure)	Surface samples (cfu)
5	1	1	Not stated
7	10	5	Not stated
8	100	50	Not stated
9	Not stated	Not stated	Not stated

With the FDA 2004 guidance, the limits described here are (as per Table 5).

With USP <1116>, issued in 2012, most references to "limits" have been removed. Instead, a contamination rate metric has been added. This is defined as: "The contamination recovery rate is the rate at which environmental samples are found to contain any level of contamination. For example, an incident rate of 1% would mean that only 1% of the samples taken have any contamination regardless of colony number."

The initial contamination rate metrics from the USP are presented in Table 6.

The published recommended limits are, however, normally applicable only to newly build facilities. The microbiologist should therefore set limits that are meaningful to the performance of the facility and its operations. This is performed by a historical review of the data. Local alert limits usually operate tighter than published limits and *must never* be allowed to be lower. Once set, limits should be periodically reexamined using further collected, historical data.

Table 6 Initial nonzero contamination rates

Room classification	Active air sample (%)	Settle plate (9 cm/4 h exposure) (%)	Contact plate or swab (%)	Glove or garment (%)
Isolator or closed RABS (ISO Class 5)	<0.1%	<0.1%	<0.1%	<0.1%
ISO Class 5	<1%	<1%	<1%	<1%
ISO Class 6	<3%	<3%	<3%	<3%
ISO Class 7	<5%	<5%	<5%	<5%
ISO Class 8	<10%	<10%	<10%	<10%

Where limits are exceeded, the standards indicate that these should be examined as individual excursions and as part of time-based trends. Before doing so, each result should be subject to an Out-of-Specification (or more accurately an Out-of-Limits) examination. This is a procedure employed by a laboratory to distinguish between results of genuine product failure from laboratory error. When dealing with microbiological results from environmental monitoring such assessments are not always clear-cut.

COMMON GMP DEFICIENCIES

Regulatory bodies do not only provide standards, for inspection and audit are key parts of the licensing process. The cycle of inspections requires the manufacturer to be aware of current practices and inspectorate trends. A good source for this is the Gold Sheet or the FDA website. When drawing up an approach to environmental monitoring and considering the different standards, the manufacturer must also be aware of *current* Good Manufacturing Practice (cGMP). A review of some FDA warning letters between 2012 and 2018, which were published on the internet, indicated some common deficiencies relating to environmental monitoring. Such cGMP deficiencies accounted for some 50% of FDA 483 warning letters.

Commonly cited warnings included:

- Failure to monitor in all aseptic filling areas;
- Not responding fast enough to out-of-specification events;
- Inadequate corrective actions;
- Failure to follow written procedures;
- Inadequate documentation;
- Failure to monitoring environmental conditions (such as temperature and humidity);
- Failure to adequately test, calibrate, and standardize equipment used for the generation, measurement, or assessment of data;
- An inadequate environmental; monitoring program;
- Failure to validate cleaning and sanitization techniques;
- Not having a defined environmental monitoring program;
- Failure to trend environmental monitoring data;
- Failure to find root causes;
- Not identifying microorganisms to species level;
- Not trending microflora;
- Poor laboratory procedures and techniques.

Pharmaceutical manufacturers should regularly review such inspectorate issues and modify their environmental programs as necessary.

DOCUMENTATION AND RECORD KEEPING

It is important to comply with cGMP regulations when recording the results of a monitoring session and when reading environmental monitoring data. A high degree of accuracy and standard of paperwork is essential. However, in terms of examination of the data the results of individual monitoring sessions are rarely of importance. The importance of environmental monitoring is in the trend or the "big picture." Documenting the "big picture" from environmental monitoring is not easy. There is often an immense amount of data and a range of potential variables which affect the data. Unit six explores possible approaches to the trending and reporting of environmental monitoring in greater detail.

The approach to environmental monitoring must be captured in a company policy or rationale. Such documents should detail and explain all of the themes explored in this module.

SUMMARY

There are an array of different regulations and guidances, under the umbrella of GMP, that impact on the way pharmaceuticals and healthcare products are manufactured, released, and distributed. A number of these provide direction and advice for microbial control and for the design of controlled environments within which products are manufactured. This chapter has presented these and, where appropriate, has outlined the key differences (areas such as monitoring limits) and where there are synergies in approach. While the scope of regulations is extensive, the reader will also note there are gaps and many important control elements are not covered or only given brief and underdeveloped reference. Hence, the need, in many ways, for this book.

REFERENCES

Eudralex. The rules governing medicinal products in the European Community, Annex 1, published by the European Commission: Brussels, Belgium, 2009 (draft issued in 2018).

FDA. (n.d.) Food and Drug Administration's guidance for industry sterile drug products produced by aseptic processing—current good manufacturing practice.

Federal Standard: Federal Standard 209E: Airborne particulate cleanliness classes in cleanrooms and clean zones. September 11, 1992.

ISO ISO 13408-1:2008, Aseptic processing of health care products—Part 1: General requirements, ISO, Geneva, Switzerland, 2008.

ISO ISO 14644-1, Cleanrooms and associated controlled environments–Part 1: Classification of air cleanliness by particle concentration, ISO, Geneva, Switzerland, 2015a.

ISO, ISO 14644-2, Monitoring to provide evidence of cleanroom performance related to air cleanliness by particle concentration, ISO, Geneva, Switzerland, 2015b.

ISO ISO 14644-3:2005, Cleanrooms and associated controlled environments—Part 3: Test methods, ISO, Geneva, Switzerland, 2005.

ISO ISO 14644-4:2001, Cleanrooms and associated controlled environments—Part 4: Design, construction and start-up, ISO, Geneva, Switzerland, 2009.

ISO ISO 14644-5:2004, Cleanrooms and associated controlled environments—Part 5: Operations, ISO, Geneva, Switzerland, 2004a.

ISO ISO 14644-7:2004, Cleanrooms and associated controlled environments—Part 7: Separative devices (clean air hoods, gloveboxes, isolators and mini-environments), ISO, Geneva, Switzerland, 2004b.

ISO, ISO 14698-1, Cleanrooms and associated controlled environments—biocontamination control, Part 1: General principles and methods, ISO, Geneva, Switzerland, 2003a.

ISO, ISO 14698-2, Cleanrooms and associated controlled environments—biocontamination control, Part 2: Evaluation and interpretation of biocontamination data, ISO, Geneva, Switzerland, 2003b.

PIC/S (2009). *PIC/S Pe 009-9, Guide to good manufacturing practice for medicinal products*. Geneva, Switzerland: Pharmaceutical Inspection Convention and Pharmaceutical Inspection Co-operation Scheme.

Rice, J. A. (2007). *Mathematical statistics and data analysis* (3rd ed., p. 42): New York: Duxbury Press.

Schicht, H. H. (2003). The ISO contamination control standards—a tool for implementing regulatory requirements. *European Journal of Parenteral and Pharmaceutical Sciences, 8*(2), 37–42.

Sharp, J., Bird, A., Brzozowski, S., & O'Hagan, K. (2010). Contamination of cleanrooms by people. *European Journal of Parenteral and Pharmaceutical Sciences, 15*(3), 73–81.

USP (n.d.-a) USP Chapter <1115>, Bioburden control of nonsterile drug substances and products. Pharm Forum 2013, 39(4) July/August; accessed on-line at: http://blog.microbiologynetwork.com/wp-content/uploads/2013/08/394-In-Process-Revision_-_1115_-BIOBURDEN-CONTROL-OF-NONSTERILE-DRUG-SUBSTANCES-AND-PRODUCTS.pdf (accessed 1st August 2013).

USP (n.d.-b) "USP Chapter <1116>, Microbiological control and monitoring of aseptic processing environments", USP #36, pp. 784–794.

WHO, Provisional guidelines on the inspection of pharmaceutical manufacturers. WHO Technical Report Series 823, Annex 2, 1992, WHO, Geneva, Switzerland.

Chapter 4

Biocontamination Control Strategy

CHAPTER OUTLINE

Introduction 47

Regulatory Expectations 49

Biocontamination Control Strategy 50

Understanding the Design of Both the Plant and Process 50

Detail of Equipment and Facilities 50

Training and Control of Personnel 51

Control of Utilities 51

Raw Materials Control 52

Product Development 53

In-Process Controls 53

Product Containers and Closures 54

Vendor Approval 54

Outsourced Services 54

Process Risk Assessment 55

Process Validation 57

Preventative Maintenance 58

Cleaning and Disinfection 58

Monitoring Systems 58

Prevention 60

Data Recording and Handling 61

Continuous Improvement 61

Summary 62

References 62

INTRODUCTION

Pharmaceutical and healthcare products can be at risk to biocontamination, and such contamination can present a health risk to the patient or consumer in receipt of these products. By "biocontaminant," this term refers to a contaminant that is a viable microorganism; a virus; or a contaminant of biological origin, such as bacterial endotoxin or other pyrogenic substance (viruses are not directly considered in this book, however some of the measures described will be useful in maintaining virus-free areas). These risks exist

Biocontamination Control for Pharmaceuticals and Healthcare. https://doi.org/10.1016/B978-0-12-814911-9.00004-3

with both sterile and nonsterile pharmaceuticals. Microbial contamination can arise from a number of sources, ranging from water, to raw materials, to the processing environment and personnel. Addressing such issues is fundamental to biocontamination control. Moreover, biocontamination control can provide guidance on best practice in microbiological measuring methods to be used including investigating, trending, and tracking of potentially disinfectant-resistant microorganisms (Sandle, 2015a).

While each element is important, too often contamination sources and their associated risks have been looked at independently, an approach which can lead to a failure to see all of the interconnections. In addition, the lessons from a contamination event, following the identification of the most probable root cause and the setting of corrective or preventative actions, are not reviewed historically (to assess if other batches might have been subject to the same risks); or reviewed across other areas, to see what other aspects of the process might be subject to similar risks; or always effectively forwards, in terms of avoiding future reoccurrences. In other words, assessment of contamination is not always "holistic."

The way to capture the holistic nature is to design an effective and robust biocontamination control strategy: one that looks at good process design; appropriate equipment selection; understands bioburden reduction throughout the process; has appropriate, science-based monitoring in place, and so on.

A further requirement is with understanding the nature of the product and its application. While all sterile products suspected of being microbially contaminated present a potential risk to patients (especially given that many patients dependent upon the products are very ill, and likely immunocompromised), with nonsterile products some are at greater risk than others. According to Clontz, products with moderate to high water activity and availability, products containing sugars, and products in multidose containers will fall into the greatest risk categories (Clontz, 2008). Coupled with this, the types of microorganisms isolated from the product, of from the manufacturing environment, will present different risk factors.

Hence the objective of a biocontamination control strategy is to minimize microbial contamination in the environment and in the product (these two concepts are intimately connected), and for aseptically filled products, to achieve sterility assurance. These outcomes are intrinsically dependent upon a process specifically purposed to impart this desired state, consistently. This should take the form of a formal, holistic contamination control strategy; a document which reflects a facility-wide strategy for minimizing contamination control (Sandle, 2015b).

REGULATORY EXPECTATIONS

A biocontamination control strategy is a fundamental requirement in order to meet the expectations of EU GMP Annex 1 (Eudralex, 2009), and aspects of the control strategy set out in this chapter will enable an organization to best meet the expectations of the Annex.

There are two major, global guidance documents for sterile products manufacture: the FDA guidance (FDA, 2004) and Annex 1 of EU GMP. Both documents signal the approach from regulators around the safeguards needed for sterile products manufacture, in terms of understanding microbial risk (EMA, n.d.). Many aspects can also be applied to nonsterile manufacturing.

There are three broad requirements of the Annex 1 and these are reflected at various intervals in the document (often through repeated occurrences). These areas are as follows:

1. The global acceptance and implementation of ICH Q9 (Quality risk management) and Q10 (Pharmaceutical quality system) is not reflected in the current Annex. The new draft contains many references to quality risk management (QRM) in particular, emphasizing that QRM should be used as a proactive tool. There are now 92 instances of the word "risk" in the new draft, an increase from 20 in the previous version.
2. There have been advances in sterile manufacturing technology, especially with RABS and isolators. There have also been advances with rapid microbiological methods, which the draft Annex acknowledges.
3. Annex 1 is often beyond sterile manufacturing, including aspects of nonsterile manufacturing. The scope of the Annex reflects this.

The adoption of risk management for pharmaceutical manufacturing and healthcare is also part of "Quality risk management." Quality risk management is a systematic process for the assessment, control, communication, and review of risks to the quality of the medicinal product. Quality risk management has been promoted by European medicines inspectors and by the FDA as fundamental to 21st century GMPs. The most widely used GMP approach to quality systems is outlined in International Conference on Harmonization (ICH) Q10 "Pharmaceutical quality system" (ICH, 2008). This document requires that quality risk management becomes embedded into an organization's quality management system (QMS) (ICH, 2008).

The two primary principles of quality risk management as per ICH Q9 are as follows:

- The evaluation of the risk to quality should be based on scientific knowledge and ultimately linked to the protection of the patient; and

- The level of effort, formality, and documentation of the quality risk management process should be commensurate with the level of risk.

Hence the development of a biocontamination strategy is a regulatory expectation. Regulatory expectations are detailed in Chapter 3.

BIOCONTAMINATION CONTROL STRATEGY

Each facility should have a detailed, facility-specific contamination control strategy. To be effective there needs to be an approach that can assess seemingly isolated contamination events holistically and which is capable of putting appropriate corrective and preventive actions (CAPA) in place (Lowry, 2001).

The main elements of such a control strategy, together with a short interpretation of what needs to be considered, are set out as follows.

Understanding the Design of Both the Plant and Process

Pharmaceutical and healthcare facilities use cleanrooms (or controlled environments) as the surrounding space for manufacturing. Good design of these, and the equipment within them, is of importance. Importantly, these are designated spaces in which the concentration of biocontaminants in air and on surfaces is controlled and specified. To achieve this these spaces need to be constructed and used in a manner to minimize the introduction and impact of contamination (Utescher, Franzolin, Trabulsi, & Gambale, 2007).

Hence the quality of the design is important for controlling contamination. This includes reducing the number of process steps; using closed systems, where possible; and reducing the numbers of personnel permitted to be in a cleanroom. Process maps should be available for each step. Understanding of the effectiveness of process design can also be achieved, in the context of sterile products, through conducting aseptic processing trials (media filling trials). Here the media fills need to be representative of conditions during processing and that they reflect the greatest challenges (Farquharson & Whyte, 1999).

Detail of Equipment and Facilities

The manufacturer should have a thorough understanding of the equipment used and the types of repairs required and justification of the calibration frequency. The best available technologies should also be used, or plans should be in place to adopt them, such as the use of equipment such as, in the case of sterile products manufacturing, RABS, isolators, or closed systems for aseptic processing. Such barrier technology reduces the need for interventions into the Grade A (ISO 14644 Class 5) environment and hence minimizes the risk of contamination. An underlying principle with sterile products manufacturing should be with the removal of personnel from Grade A environments, given that people are the primary cause of any contamination detected in such environments.

Training and Control of Personnel

How well personnel behave, especially in cleanrooms, is critical toward achieving contamination control. The minimum basis for a training program for a sterile facility would include hygiene, cleanroom practices, contamination control, aseptic techniques, and potential safety implications to the patient of a loss of product through contamination with an objectionable microorganism or loss of sterility, as well as with the basic elements of microbiology.

Control of Utilities

Utilities need to be controlled and operated within their design parameters. This includes compressed gases, HVAC systems, and water systems. Controls also need to be assessed in conjunction with monitoring. The microbiological plan for assessing a water system, for example, needs to justify the sampling frequencies and times. In addition, appropriate alert and action levels need to be set.

Assessment of water needs to include tests of bioburden and for bacterial endotoxin. Bacteria are present in feed (or raw water), in higher numbers and as a myriad of species, of both Gram-positive and Gram-negative morphological types. The exact types will be reflective of the nutrients available and water sources. The pharmaceutical plant will contain steps to reduce these numbers, and here the low nutrient conditions tend to result in only Gram-negative bacteria being present. Whereas some organisms will be present in purified water; the recovery of bacteria from Water for Injections should represent a rare event, one which is normally linked to poor outlet or tubing management.

Bacterial endotoxin derives from dying Gram-negative bacteria, where the lipopolysaccharide component of the cell wall functions as a pyrogenic toxin when it comes into contact with the mammalian blood stream. The term "endotoxin" refers to the stable lipopolysaccharide being endogenous to the bacterial cell structure.

The key to minimizing microbial contamination is with good utility design, such as with the materials of construction, water flow velocities, absence of dead legs, and so on (Collentro, 2011). In addition, controls need to be in place wherever maintenance occurs, especially when a system is broken into (such as to repair a valve or pipework). Each period of maintenance must be followed by system sanitization and microbial monitoring, in order to assess system suitability prior to the water being returned for production use. Chapter 13 considers microbial risks from water systems in more detail.

Raw Materials Control

Control of raw materials is not only a factor of testing (such as use of the microbial limits test), but it also relates to controls in place when containers are opened: are sterile sampling tools used?; is the environment within which materials are sampled the same as the environment within which materials are dispensed or used in production?; what safeguards are in place to ensure containers are stored in dry environments?, are among the types of questions that need to be considered in a strategy document.

For example, microbial contamination of raw materials used to manufacture dry formulations (like tablets) is often reduced as a consequence of the pharmaceutical manufacturing process, where bioburden reduction is a factor of process temperatures and the chemical nature of the intermediate product. The metabolic properties of any contaminating organisms are also factor in terms of how likely they are to survive when subject to process temperatures and pressures. Other products, based on aqueous formulations or containing sugars (such as syrups) are at greater risk due to the products containing growth factors or environmental conditions commensurate to microbial survival.

A typical product risk hierarchy (from high to low) is:

1. Metered-dose and dry powder inhalants
2. Nasal sprays
3. Otics
4. Vaginal suppositories
5. Topicals
6. Rectal suppositories
7. Oral liquids (aqueous)
8. Liquid-filled capsules
9. Compressed tablets and powder-filled capsule.

Based on the type of product, the process should be reviewed in terms of the contamination control steps in place to reduce microbial survival. These steps can include:

- Physical, such as dry heat, moist heat, cold temperatures, freezing, ultraviolet radiation, ionizing radiation, filtration.
- Chemical, such as ethylene oxide, use of acids or esters, alcohols, aldehydes, other disinfectants.
- Combination process like heat and chemical combinations or thermoradiation.

Product Development

The application of biocontamination principles is an important feature with new product development, such as assessing where samples are to be taken in the process and for assisting with evaluating the risks associated with phase-appropriate GMP. Points to be considered when assessing the potential microbial risk associated with nonsterile drug products include (Sandle, 2018):

- Synthesis, isolation, and final purification of the drug substance;
- Microbiological attributes of the drug substance;
- Formulation and physicochemical attributes of the drug product;
- Water activity of the drug product;
- Manufacturing process;
- Packaging and delivery system;
- Storage conditions of the drug substance and product;
- Route of administration;
- Expected treatment procedure and dosage regimen;
- Age and health condition of the intended recipients of the drug.

By addressing these factors early, biocontamination risks can be assessed prior to the production of a commercial product and ideally "designed out," or risk minimized, to avoid many opportunities for contamination to develop.

In-Process Controls

Understanding process controls has been a long-established part of biochemical testing, such as assessing product potency. Bioburden and endotoxin control need to be part of the same control mechanism. Appropriate points in the production process need to be selected for monitoring and appropriate limits set. A risk tool like Hazard Analysis Critical Control Points (HACCP) can be effective for achieving this.

Product Containers and Closures

Damaged containers, with nonsterile products, can lead to product adulteration, ranging from loss of activity, through odors and off-flavors, to patient risk where microbial ingress has occurred and where the products are applied to areas like open skin, or via the eyes or lungs. With sterile products, loss of sterility will occur since "sterile" is a temporary and transient state. A sterile product can quickly become nonsterile if a nonintegral (i.e., uncapped) container is exposed to non-Grade A air or if the sealed container is breached. This requires a review of Grade A containment of vials, setting maximum exposure time of sterilized containers and closures prior to closure and in ensuring crimping is conducted expediently, and a robust container closure integrity qualification. Assessment of container closure integrity should extend through the shelf life of the product, being part of formal stability studies.

Vendor Approval

Understanding where materials come from, whether they have been prepared and processed properly, and whether they remain the same as those components used in previous validation are important parts of the quality assurance system. With vendor approval, this obviously extends to key component suppliers. Also of consideration, however, is the sterilization of components and the suitability of single-use systems and services.

Single-use systems and technologies are becoming more widely used and their use is generally encouraged. There are some key aspects with the use of single-use technology that need to be addressed. These are the interaction between the product and product contact surface (notably adsorption, leachable, and extractables).

Outsourced Services

It is not simply sufficient for a manufacturer to outsource services and accept certification when items are delivered, especially with items that have undergone a sterilization step. Sufficient evidence must be provided to the contract giver to ensure the process is operating correctly. This includes audit.

Assessment also needs to extents, where applicable, to expert review of the sterilization process to ensure that it is suitable for the processed items. This is particularly so for items that interact with a Grade A environment, such as gloves.

Process Risk Assessment

An effective microbial control program will begin with an understanding of the hazards presented to manufacturing processes, including an identification of potential contaminants and the points in the process where these contaminants may occur. The hazards should be expressed as risks and a risk assessment conducted.

A formal risk assessment should be in place for each process step, beginning with the start of the manufacturing process, capturing processing, through to packaging. The results obtained from the risk assessment should be assessed in terms of risk reduction. Furthermore, risk assessments should be used during facility and equipment designs; and for establishing equipment and personnel flows, which will provide the basis of the environmental monitoring program (a tool such as Hazard Analysis Critical Control Points (HACCP) is especially useful here) (Jahnke, 1997).

As an example, HACCP could assess (Sandle, 2013):

1. Raw materials
2. Excipients
3. Utilities, for example, water, compressed gases
4. Cleanroom design and HVAC
5. Temperature and humidity control
6. Facility construction design
7. Cleaning validation
8. Cleaning and disinfection requirements
9. Equipment design
10. Equipment flow
11. Personnel flow
12. Open and closed processing.

Risk assessments can also consider (Sandle, 2006):

1. Points in the process where contamination could occur. This includes good facility design, such has having nonporous walls, ceilings and floors that are readily cleanable. In addition, there should only be floor drains that can be closed during processing or fitted with an air break if opened during area and equipment cleaning.
2. Cleanroom air is also an important consideration. Ventilation and air filtration should be adequate to maintain the specified cleanliness, space pressurization, temperature, and humidity.
3. The process flow is also important. Here material, equipment, and personnel flows should avoid contamination.

4. For bioburden control equipment should have the following attributes:
   a. Sanitary design.
   b. Readily cleaned preferably using a CIP system.
   c. Self-draining to eliminate stagnate water.
   d. Preventative maintenance program to periodically replace valves, seals, filters, and hosing.
   e. Inclusion of microbial monitoring in cleaning validation protocols.
5. Points in the process where organisms could survive.
6. Points in the process where organisms could proliferate.
7. Process hold times.
8. Suitable points in the process for monitoring.
9. Equipment cleaning and disinfection (or sterilization) procedures.
10. Equipment hold times, both clean and dirty.
11. Degree of personnel involvement in the process, and measures to control or reduce this involvement. For sterile manufacturing, this would include removing personnel from Grade A/ISO 14644 Class 5 areas. It is important to restrict access only to essential personnel.

Sound risk assessments also develop the microbial testing program, considering (Jahnke & Kuhn, 2003):

1. How often to test each type of raw material and the appropriate test methods.
2. Testing of ingredient water.
3. Intermediate bioburden testing.
4. Environmental monitoring.
5. Developing a list of objectionable organisms of concern, in terms of posing a particular process or product risk.
6. End product testing.

With environmental monitoring, consideration needs to be given to the appropriateness of the test method. Factors to consider here include (Ljungqvist & Reinmuller, 1996):

- The time and duration of the controlled environment activities
- Accessibility into the controlled environment for the sampling device
- The effect of the sampling device on the process or environment to be monitored.
- The efficiency and precision of the sampling method.

Across these lists, process hold times represent a key area of concern and an area that needs to be tightly controlled and one which must reflect process validation (where bioburden testing is performed at the start of the hold time and at the end of the hold time). Time limits for each process stage must be established and adhered to. Extended hold times are commonly associated with microbial risks.

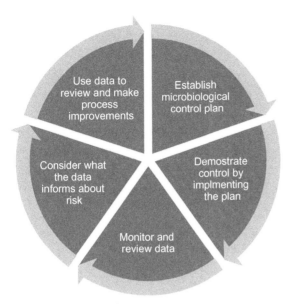

■ **FIG. 1** Contamination control review cycle.

Risk assessments also assist with the review of contamination events, allowing good control and preventive measures to be implemented. With contamination events, there needs to be an investigation system in place to consider out-of-limits, out-of-specification, and out-of-trend incidents. The process for these also needs to account for the possibility of laboratory error, and, as part of data integrity requirements, assess the accuracy of the data. A protocol or procedure needs to be in place that describes the investigation process (Allen Jr., 2016).

The information from monitoring and control should be regularly reviewed and this information should be used to inform about improvements to the monitoring program. This can be summarized as per Fig. 1.

Given the commitments of Good Distribution Practice, risk assessments should extend to the point where the recipient receives the product. Of particular concern is packaging and container closure integrity.

Process Validation

Process validation refers to the analysis of data gathered throughout the design and manufacturing of a product. This is reviewed in order to confirm that the process can reliably output products of a determined standard. Importantly, process validation is an ongoing process and it should be frequently reviewed and adapted as manufacturing feedback is gathered.

An essential part of this is knowledge of contamination rates, particularly in relation to in-process bioburden and to the supporting manufacturing environment.

Preventative Maintenance

The regular maintenance of equipment and premises, as either planned and unplanned maintenance, is of importance to ensure product quality and for a consistent process. It is important that these are conducted to a standard that will not add significant risk of contamination. To achieve this means having engineering staff who are knowledgeable about contamination; undertaking risk assessment or process impact assessments prior to any works being undertaken; and then assessing the impact of postworks, which can include the monitoring of the engineers (such as finger plates) and the monitoring of the cleanroom environment at the end of the activity.

Cleaning and Disinfection

Cleaning and disinfection practices are an essential part of contamination control in healthcare and in the pharmaceutical industry. These practices can be divided into two key parts:

- Cleaning and disinfection of cleanrooms, and
- Cleaning of equipment (which requires cleaning validation to verify the effectiveness of the cleaning).

Cleaning and disinfection are important steps for maintaining control. Cleanrooms are invariably well designed; the concern that often arises is when people begin to work within them. Having a sound cleaning (use of a detergent) and disinfection (rotation of two biocides with different modes of activity) regime in place helps to address the risks of microorganisms introduced into cleanrooms. There should be a rationale in place justifying the use of each disinfectant agent, together with supporting data to show efficacy in terms of microcidal kill, on surfaces of a similar type used within the manufacturing area.

Monitoring Systems

The environmental monitoring program used to assess biocontamination should be reviewed and assessed. A strong program will include:

- Methods appropriate for the monitoring of water, air, compressed gases, surfaces, personnel, and clean steam as appropriate.
- Appropriate culture media and incubation conditions.

- Verification that all operators and technicians are trained and qualified to operate the program.
- Defined locations for monitoring.
- Defined frequencies for monitoring.
- Procedures for data collection, analysis, and trending.
- Procedures in place for the investigation of microbial data deviations and resolution of issues.
- Identification of microbial contaminants using qualified methods.

Chapter 10 provides greater details on the requirements of a robust environmental monitoring program.

To assess whether cleanrooms and utilities are functioning as designed regular checks are required, such as of airflows or pressure differentials. To be effective the monitoring methods need to be continuous, so that data can be trended, and equipped with audible alarms. The use of monitoring systems should extend to microbiological assessments, such as continuous particle counters and consideration of rapid microbiological methods, like spectrophotometric counters which incorporate fluorescence-based optical spectroscopy. This method detects microbiological particles, with no discrimination as to whether they are viable, culturable, or nonculturable, in real time (Sandle, 2012).

Rapid and alternative microbiological methods endeavor to reduce time to results, increase sensitivity, accuracy, precision, and reproducibility compared to the established culture-based method. Some of these methods utilize established culture-based sample collection methods but use technologies that decrease the time at which actively growing microorganisms can be detected; others do not rely on growth and proliferation of microorganisms to facilitate detection.

The use of alternative monitoring systems deploys alternative metrics to measure microbiological contamination, in terms of units applicable for the technology used and these may not be directly comparable to conventional growth culture-based measurements, reported as colony-forming units (cfus). A complexity for the user is how to establish and understand the relationship of the results with those reported by the established culture-based methods. It thus follows that alert and action levels based on established culture-based methods may not be applicable when using an alternative method. For example, if the new method has improved sensitivity, results that exceed the alert or action level may occur and may not be indicative of a change in the state of control. Additionally, as AMM produce results reported in some other unit than cfu, new levels applicable to the method used must be set and a new risk assessment completed.

There is also, at least potentially, for a different philosophy to be applied when using alternative microbiological methods for the assessment of biocontamination control. Conventional culture-based methods provide time-delayed results which generally only permit reactive actions to be taken to attempt to return any adverse microbiological contamination to a state of control. The use of an alternative method, that provides results in real time, gives the opportunity for the microbiologist to take proactive actions to return to an area of process to a state of control. This could include, for instance, taking immediate steps to remove or segregate any potentially implicated product, while, at the same time, ensuring that the remainder of the product is appropriately secured (Sandle, Leavy, Jindal, & Rhodes, 2014).

The expansion of technologies under the title "process analytical technology" (PAT) can assist with biocontamination control, even where this is not directly microbial (and here progress with microbial monitoring has been slower than compared with chemical or physical measures). PAT can be used to assess environmental parameters, for example; and chemical testing, under the philosophy of taking laboratory tests out of the laboratory environment and into the process area, can signal failures with pH, for instance, which may inform about an enhanced risk of microbial proliferation.

The key principles of PAT are (Koch & Chrisman, 2012) as follows:

1. Targeting the product profile.
2. Determining Critical Quality Attributes (CQA).
3. Linking raw material attributes and process parameters to CQAs.
4. Developing the design space for operating the process.
5. Designing and implanting a process control strategy.
6. Managing the product life cycle.
7. A data-driven approach to process improvements.

With biocontamination an established and relatively mature technology, like a continuous particle monitoring system, fits within the PAT paradigm.

Prevention

A biocontamination control strategy should have in place a good system for addressing corrective and preventive actions. To arrive at effective CAPA there needs to be a system in place for trending, conducting investigations, arriving at root causes, and then for suggesting and implementing appropriate corrective and preventive actions. These activities hinge on effective investigational tools. A sound contamination control strategy will have already identified the main contamination risks and areas where contamination may occur, together with the impact and severity should such an event occur.

Data Recording and Handling

To ensure that all information is readily available, clear procedures for data recording and handling should be developed and implemented, designed to meet records and data integrity requirements. This applies to both paper-based and electronic systems.

Data recording should consider the following aspects:

- Raw data;
- Meta-data ("data about data," such as time of sampling);
- The list of types of information held in the records;
- The identification and location of laboratory documents, or computerized records;
- Control of the use of workbooks, worksheets or computers or other appropriate means to record the various types of observations, calculations, and other relevant information;
- List of the procedures to be followed for recording, checking, correcting, signing and countersigning of observations, calculations, and reports;
- Recommendations for consistent results interpretation;
- Any specific, legal, or regulatory requirements.

Continuous Improvement

No biocontamination control strategy should stand still and it should be regularly reviewed and updated. As part of any review, continuous improvement should drive necessary changes, based on information gathered from the above areas. This can range from addressing circumstances where the same event leads to more than one contamination event occurring within the same review period to having knowledge of new technologies and having plans in place to implement improvements to reduce contamination likelihoods throughout the manufacturing process.

With each of these different elements it is notable that the draft Annex does not see these as simply confined to biocontamination, since reference is also made to subvisible particles (the classic appearance tests) and the overall appearance of the pharmaceutical product.

ISO and other standards which should be reviewed when putting a control strategy together (this would infer attention is paid to ISO 14698 Parts 1 and 2) (ISO 14698-1:2003, n.d.). Also, to be considered in the strategy should be rapid microbiological methods. Manufacturers need to continually survey industry trends for the best available technologies to ensure contamination control.

SUMMARY

A biocontamination control strategy is a documented approach, outlining a facilities approach to assessing, controlling, and monitoring microbial concerns. For this work, such a strategy needs to be supported by risk assessment. With risk assessment, the focus should be on the proactive and, when contamination events occur, there must be a sound system for risk escalation in place. Such a document will also include the rationale for addressing contamination events. When contamination events are reviewed, the holistic nature of the strategy is important—with each contamination event it is important to pose the question "what else may have been affected?" The purpose of the document is with protecting the patient, product, and process.

The aim of this chapter was to set out the key requirements for a biocontamination control strategy and to serve as the first substantive launch point for this book. For those with a strategy in place, the information contained in this article may act as a helpful benchmark; for those yet to write a document, the content here will act as a starting framework. In both cases, the strategy should be subject to regular review; in other words, it should be living document reflecting current best practices.

Importantly, a biocontamination control strategy, to be effective, must be regularly reviewed in terms of its appropriateness and also in terms of how well CAPA are being applied. This includes not only considering the effectiveness of investigation outcomes but also regular reviews of trend data.

REFERENCES

Allen, L. V., Jr. (2016). *The art, science and technology of pharmaceutical compounding* (5th ed., pp. 147–148). Washington, DC: American Pharmacists Association.

Clontz, L. (2008). *Microbial limit and bioburden test: Validation approaches and global requirements* (2nd ed., pp. 35–38). Boca Raton, FL: CRC Press.

Collentro, W. V. (2011). *Pharmaceutical water: System design, operation and validation* (2nd ed., pp. 388–390). New York: Informa Healthcare.

EMA. (n.d.) Concept paper on the revision of annex 1 of the guidelines on good manufacturing practice—manufacture of sterile medicinal products, EMA/INS/GMP/735037/2014, issued jointly by the European Medicines Agency and the

Pharmaceutical Inspection Convention: http://www.ema.europa.eu/docs/en_GB/document_library/Scientific_guideline/2015/02/WC500181863.pdf.

Eudralex The rules governing medicinal products in the European Union. Volume 4: EU guidelines to good manufacturing practice medicinal products for human and veterinary use. Annex 1: Manufacture of sterile medicinal products, European Commission, Brussels, Belgium, 2009: https://ec.europa.eu/health/sites/health/files/files/eudralex/vol-4/2008_11_25_gmp-an1_en.pdf.

Farquharson, G., & Whyte, W. (1999). The design of cleanrooms for the pharmaceutical industry. In W. Whyte (Ed.), *Cleanroom design* (2nd ed., pp. 79–114). London: Wiley.

FDA. Guidance for industry sterile drug products produced by aseptic processing—current good manufacturing practice, US Department of Health and Human Services, Food and Drug Administration, Bethesda, MD, 2004.

ICH (2008). "ICH Q10: Pharmaceutical quality system", International conference on harmonization of technical requirements for registration of pharmaceuticals for human use, ICH harmonized tripartite guideline, ICH, Geneva, Switzerland.

ISO 14698-1:2003 (n.d.) Preview Cleanrooms and associated controlled environments—Biocontamination control. Part 1: General principles and methods; Part 2: Evaluation and interpretation of biocontamination data, ISO, Geneva.

Jahnke, M. (1997). Use of the HACCP concept for the risk analysis of pharmaceutical manufacturing process. *European Journal of Parenteral Sciences*, *2*(4), 113–117.

Jahnke, M., & Kuhn, K.-D. (2003). Use of the hazard analysis and critical control points (HACCP) risk assessment on a medical device for parenteral application. *PDA Journal of Pharmaceutical Science and Technology*, *57*(1), 32–42.

Koch, M., & Chrisman, R. (2012). Introduction to process analytical technology in biopharmaceuticals. In C. Undey, D. Low, J. C. Menezes, & M. Koch (Eds.), *PAT applied in biopharmaceutical process development and manufacturing: An enabling tool for quality-by-design* (p. xxii). Boca Raton, FL: CRC Press.

Ljungqvist, B., & Reinmuller, B. (1996). Some observations on environmental monitoring of cleanrooms. *European Journal of Parenteral Science*, *11*, 9–13.

Lowry, S. (2001). Designing a contamination control program. In R. Prince (Ed.), *Microbiology in pharmaceutical manufacturing* (pp. 203–266). DHI/PDA Publishing.

Sandle, T. (2006). Environmental monitoring risk assessment. *Journal of GXP Compliance*, *10*(2), 54–73.

Sandle, T. (2012). Real-time counting of airborne particles and microorganisms: A new technological wave? *Clean Air and Containment Review*, *9*, 4–6.

Sandle, T. (2013). Contamination control risk assessment. In: R. E. Masden, & J. Moldenhauer (Eds.), *Vol. 1. Contamination control in healthcare product manufacturing* (pp. 423–474). River Grove, IL: DHI Publishing.

Sandle, T. (2015a). Contamination control risk assessment. In K. Z. McCullough, & J. Moldenhauer (Eds.), *Microbial risks and investigations* (pp. 783–836). River Grove, IL: DHI/PDA.

Sandle, T. (2015b). Development of a biocontamination control strategy. *Cleanroom Technology*, *23*(11), 25–30.

Sandle, T. (2018). Microbiological control and testing for phase appropriate GMP. In T. Deeks (Ed.), *Phase appropriate GMP for biological processes: Pre-clinical to commercial production*. Arlington Heights, IL: PDA/DHI Book.

Sandle, T., Leavy, C., Jindal, H., & Rhodes, R. (2014). Application of rapid microbiological methods for the risk assessment of controlled biopharmaceutical environments. *Journal of Applied Microbiology, 116*(6), 1495–1505.

Utescher, C. L. A., Franzolin, M. R., Trabulsi, L. R., & Gambale, V. (2007). Microbiological monitoring of clean rooms in development of vaccines. *Brazilian Journal of Microbiology, 38*, 710–716.

Cleanrooms and Environmental Monitoring

CHAPTER OUTLINE
Introduction   65
Cleanrooms and Clean Air Devices   66
Isolators, Gloveboxes, and Hatches   67
Contamination Control   68
Particles   73
Cleanroom Classification   74
    Assessing Results   77
Ongoing Environmental Monitoring   79
Summary   81
References   81

INTRODUCTION

This chapter introduces cleanrooms and cleanroom technology and considers the types of microorganisms that inhabit the cleanroom ecological niche. Cleanrooms are common to much of the pharmaceutical industry, providing a controlled environment for the preparation of medicinal products (Beaney, 2006). Cleanrooms are also used within healthcare (such as surgical units or with small-scale medicine dispensing), and for the manufacturing of consumables, test kits, and medical devices. The objective of the controlled environment is to minimize the levels of contamination and to protect the product.

A cleanroom can be considered as a room which the concentration of airborne particles is controlled, and which is constructed and used in a manner to minimize the introduction, generation, and retention of particles inside the room and in which other relevant parameters, such as temperature, humidity, and pressure, are controlled as necessary.

Biocontamination Control for Pharmaceuticals and Healthcare. https://doi.org/10.1016/B978-0-12-814911-9.00005-5

The most important control issue within the cleanroom design is air, given that air can distribute contamination around the cleanroom. While a risk arises from the influx of contaminated air this is less likely to occur within a correctly functioning cleanroom with effective air filtration; the greater risk is with what happens to particles shed from people working within the cleanroom when such particles enter the airstream. The contamination risk is from microbial carrying particles (primarily skin detritus, where microorganisms can be carried on skin flakes). This is minimized through staff working within cleanrooms wearing appropriate garments particles that are shed by operators are controlled through effective air movement and air changes within the cleanroom. A third contamination source is from surfaces, and these are controlled through effective cleaning and disinfection procedures (Sandle, 2016).

This chapter examines the most important criteria in relation to the design, construction, specification, testing, and continual use of cleanrooms. The focus, in keeping with the theme of this book, is with biocontamination control.

CLEANROOMS AND CLEAN AIR DEVICES

Cleanrooms and clean air devices are typically classified according to their use (the main activity within each room or zone) and confirmed by the cleanliness of the air by the measurement of particles. For pharmaceutical cleanrooms, air cleanliness is either based on EU GMP guidance for aseptically filled products and the EU GMP alphabetic notations are adopted (Euradlex, 2009); or by using the International Standard ISO 14644, where numerical classes are adopted. The World Health Organization uses the same cleanliness grades as EU GMP. The cleanliness of the air is controlled by an HVAC system (heating, ventilation and air-conditioning). The key aspect is that the level of cleanliness is controlled.

By prescribing a grade or a class to a cleanroom, the areas are then regarded as controlled environments. A controlled environment can be considered as any area in an aseptic process system for which airborne particulate and microorganism levels are controlled to specific levels, appropriate to the activities conducted within that environment.

Within some cleanrooms are various clean air devices are used. The terminology of ISO 14644-7, Cleanrooms and associate controlled environments—Part 7, uses the term "Separative Devices" to collectively describe clean air hoods, gloveboxes, isolators, and mini-environments. These devices include unidirectional airflow (UDAF) devices, biosafety cabinets (microbiological safety cabinets), and isolators. Such devices normally operate at EU GMP Grade A/ISO Class 5. The term "cabinet" is used more widely within Europe and the term "hood" used more widely in the United States.

Whereas most cleanrooms operate with a turbulent airflow, clean air devices are designed to minimize turbulence; for turbulence can lead to dust and dirt collection air pockets. To overcome this, the devices operate with the air blowing in one direction (hence "unidirectional"), where the design feature is to move air away from the critical activity to ensure that any contamination is blown away to a less critical area. With UDAF devices these are either constructed with horizontal flow or vertical flow. Specially designed UDAFs are biosafety cabinets. These are "self-contained" enclosures which provide protection for personnel, environment, and/or products in work with hazardous microorganisms. The cabinets provide protection by creating an air barrier at the work opening and by filtration of exhaust air. Class I cabinets protect the operation or the product from personnel contamination, whereas Class II cabinets protect personnel, environment, and products.

With some UDAF devices, gloves are fitted in order to restrict the number of personnel interventions. Such devices are described as restrict access barrier systems (RABS). These stand partway between a conventional UDAF and an isolator. Another special type of cabinet is the powder containment cabinet. These are compact containment cabinets with inward airflow and filtration that provides protection for operators and the environment from powders generated by processes such as compounding of pharmaceuticals.

ISOLATORS, GLOVEBOXES, AND HATCHES

The most intrinsically safe clean air device is an isolator. Isolators are superior to cleanrooms in that the contamination risk is reduced through the construction of a barrier between the critical area (sometimes called the "microenvironment") and the outside environment. Isolators are used for sterility testing, aseptic filing, and other applications where a clean environment is required. It is important that any possibility of contamination is avoided so that a "false positive" does not occur (Akers & Agalloco, 2000).

Isolators enable the isolation between the operator and the process. An isolator is an arrangement of physical barriers that are integrated so that the workspace (an enclosed environment) within the isolator is sealed from the outside environment. The barrier to the outside is measured in terms of a routine leak test and the maintenance of pressure differential, both of which are assessed within specified limits. The isolator allows manipulations to be performed within the workspace in a way which does not compromise the integrity of the isolator.

An isolator consists of either a flexible film, for the outer wall, or it has a solid wall envelope. These barriers serve to separate the inside of the isolator from the surrounding environment. Except for handling certain medicinal products, such as cytotoxic drugs, isolators used for sterility testing, when operative, are at positive pressure relative to the room and have a HEPA (high efficiency particulate air) filtered airflow. The pressure level of the isolators is normally demonstrated by pressure alarms and readings. Isolators are most commonly sanitized using surface contact disinfectants: hydrogen peroxide vapor (an alternative is ionized hydrogen peroxide) or peracetic acid (Sandle, 2013).

A variation of an isolator is a glovebox. A glovebox is an enclosure, fitted with sealed gloves, that allows external manual manipulations in controlled or hazardous environments (Farquharson, 1996). In addition to the clean air devices mentioned before, many cleanrooms contain pass-through hatches. These are hatches with double doors that protect critical environments while allowing transfer or materials to or from adjoining rooms. They are typically installed within the walls of cleanrooms. The hatches allow materials to be transferred with minimal loss of room pressure and without the need for personnel movement between rooms. Some pass-through hatches have localized HEPA filters.

CONTAMINATION CONTROL

The primary objective of cleanrooms in pharmaceutical processing is to minimize and control microbial and particulate contamination. There are many sources of contamination. The atmosphere contains dust, microorganisms, condensates, and gasses. Manufacturing processes will also produce a range of contaminants. Wherever there is a process which grinds, corrodes, fumes, heats, sprays, turns, and so on, particles and fumes are emitted and will contaminate the surroundings.

People, in clean environments, are the greatest contributors to contamination emitting body vapors, dead skin, microorganisms, skin oils, and so on. The typical person sheds 1,000,000,000 skin cells per day, of which 10% have microorganisms on them (hence some particles are referred to as microbial carrying particles). This phenomenon of "shedding" demonstrates the importance of wearing cleanroom suitable clothing and wearing this clothing correctly. The risk of personnel depositing particles into the airstream of a cleanroom can be increased through physical behavior like fast motion and horseplay or from physiological concerns like room temperature, humidity or from psychological concerns like claustrophobia, odors, and workplace attitude (Reinmüller, 2001).

In general, people produce contamination via:

- *Body regenerative processes*: skin flakes, oils, perspiration, and hair.
- *Behavior*: rate of movement, sneezing and coughing.
- *Attitude*: work habits and communication between personnel.

A degree of protection is provided through cleanroom clothing. Cleanroom gowns are manufactured from special materials which are designed to minimize the amount of contamination which can be shed from the skin, provided that the gown is not worn for an excessive time and that the temperature is not too high. Special apparel includes nonshedding gowns or coveralls, head covers, face masks, gloves, footwear, or shoe covers. The requirements for cleanroom garments will vary from sector to sector. Gloves, face masks, and head covers are standard in nearly every cleanroom environment. Second to people, another important contamination source is water. Outside of aseptic filling areas the use of water is unavoidable for water is the main ingredient in many products, and it is used widely throughout the processing areas for equipment cleaning, preparation of cleaning solutions, and so on. Water is a concern because it is both a vector and a growth source for microorganisms.

Most cleanroom microorganisms are found in the air. If they settle on a dry surface they are unlikely to survive and ideally any contamination is removed from the room through the air control system. However, if any microorganisms within the air could be potentially directed toward a critical location, then this could present a major risk. Therefore the primary risk within cleanrooms arises from the air and this is how contamination can be moved around the cleanroom. However, air is also a solution within cleanroom design to this contamination risk (Ljungqvist & Berit, 1997). Hence, air is both a means to ensure that cleanrooms are clean, and it can be a source of contamination.

In order to ensure that cleanrooms are operating correctly, air is monitored through:

- Formal classification of cleanrooms (as defined by air cleanliness, which relates to the number of airborne particles),
- Through physical measurements of HVAC operations,
- Through nonviable particle monitoring,
- Through viable particle monitoring.

To understand the potential contamination risk from air, consider this: even in clean rural areas air is contaminated with about 10^8 particles of 0.5 μm and greater per m^3, many of these will be microorganisms depending on the nature of the area and the season of the year. Thus air is a contamination problem. However, in the pharmaceutical industry airflow is the answer to many contamination problems.

There are four principles applying to control of airborne microorganisms in cleanrooms. These are (Sandle, 2015):

- Filtration (through the use of HEPA filters): The air entering a cleanroom from outside is filtered to exclude dust, and the air inside is constantly recirculated through HEPA (high efficiency particulate air) filters (alternative filters are ultra-low penetration air (ULPA) filters, although these mainstays of the electronics world are uncommon in the pharmaceutical sector). Filtration is controlled through an HVAC (heating, ventilation, and air conditioning) system.
  - HEPA filters function through a combination of three important aspects. First, there are one or more outer filters that work like sieves to stop the larger particles of dirt, dust, and hair. Inside those filters, there is a concertina—a mat of very dense fibers—which traps smaller particles. The inner part of the HEPA filter uses three different mechanisms to catch particles as they pass through in the moving airstream:
    1. Impaction, where larger particles are unable to avoid fibers by following the curving contours of the airstream and are forced to embed in one of them directly; this effect increases with diminishing fiber separation and higher airflow velocity. Thus at high air speeds, some particles are caught and trapped as they smash directly into the fibers.
    2. Interception, where particles following a line of flow in the airstream come within one radius of a fiber and adhere to it.
    3. Diffusion, an enhancing mechanism that is a result of the collision with gas molecules by the smallest particles, especially those below $0.1\,\mu m$ in diameter, which are thereby impeded and delayed in their path through the filter (via Brownian motion). This occurs at lower air speeds.
  - Together, these three mechanisms allow HEPA filters to catch particles that are both larger and smaller than a certain target size. HEPA filters are protected from blockage by prefilters which remove up to about 90% of particles from air.
  - There are different grades of HEPA filters based on their "efficiency ratings." One of the most commonly used HEPA filter is the H14 filter (defined by European Norm EN 1822:2009 or United States Department of Energy), which is designed to remove 99.997% of particles from the air. The 99.997% efficiency is based on particle sizes $0.3\,\mu m$ and larger (i.e., theoretically only 3 out of 10,000 particles at 0.3 m size can penetrate the filter).

- In addition to assessing the efficiency of HEPA filters, they are also subject to leak testing. Because potential leakage is not confined to the filter media there is a requirement to perform an in-situ filter integrity test. This is commonly called the DOP test after dioctyl phthalate one of the first substances used as an aerosol challenge for this test.

- Dilution (to ensure that particles generated in cleanrooms, in addition to those which pass the filters, are carried away by diluting the area with new "clean" air).

  - Each cleanroom grade should have a set number of required air changes per hour. Air changes are provided in order to dilute any particles present to an acceptable concentration. Any contamination produced in the cleanroom is theoretically removed within the required time appropriate to the room grade. This is important because particles would otherwise build up in enclosed spaces if there is no ventilation.

  - Ventilation is the process by which any particles generated in cleanrooms (in addition to those which pass the filters) are carried away for any remaining in the room to be diluted with new "clean" air. The minimum ventilation rate expected in pharmaceutical cleanrooms is 20 air changes per hour (the modern requirement up to twice as many as this, and up to 75 for a changing room), the air in a cleanroom is replaced at least every 3 min. In contrast, an office might have 2–3 air changes per hour.

  - Connected to air changes is the time taken for a clean area to return to the static condition, appropriate to its grade, in terms of particulates. Cleanup times are sometimes referred to as "recovery tests." This is assessed by the room being subject to a level of particles above the room class and then measuring, through the use of an optical particle counter, how long the room takes to return to the level of particles required for the room class. The typical target is for a room to "clean up" within 15–20 min.

  - The conducting of cleanup times is an optional test to be considered at the time of room classification; following substantial changes to room design; for newly built cleanrooms or as part of an investigation.

  - Monitoring air changes is necessary because the recirculation of filtered air is important for maintaining control of the clean area. Air change rates stated are the minimum and should be calculated from supply air volume and room volume measurements.

- Directional airflow (to ensure that air blows away from critical zones, as particles and microorganisms cannot "swim upstream" against a directional airflow). This is achieved through pressure differentials.
  - Airflows are monitored using an anemometer. The air velocity is designed to be sufficient to remove any relatively large particles before they settle onto surfaces. This monitoring should be performed routinely and during requalification exercises.
- Air movement (rapid air movement is important for as long as particles and microorganisms stay suspended in the air they are not really a problem, for it is only when they settle out that they become an actual cause of contamination).
  - Connected to the measurement of airflow is the maintenance of positive pressure. In order to maintain air quality in a cleanroom the pressure of a given room must be greater relative to a room of a lower grade. This is to ensure that air does not pass from "dirtier" adjacent areas into the higher-grade cleanroom. Generally, this is set at 15–20 Pa, although some areas of the same grade will also have differential pressure requirements due to specific activities, such as where dust is generated through the weighting of powders.
  - Pressure differentials are the relative pressures from a higher-grade area into a lower one. Pressurization is defined as a method by which air pressure differences are created mechanically between rooms to introduce intentional air movement paths through room leakage openings. With this the relative quantities of air that are delivered and removed from each space by the ducted air system, air transfer system and losses. These openings could be either designated, such as doorways, or undesignated, such as air gaps around doorframes or other cracks.
  - To help achieve the required pressure differential between cleanrooms of different grades airlocks are used. An airlock is an airtight room which adjoins two cleanrooms. The airlock acts as a buffer zone between two independent areas of unequal pressure. A pressure differential of ≥ 15 Pa is typically maintained between the inner room and the air lock; and between the air lock and the external.

Other contamination control measures, that form part of good cleanroom practices, include (Sandle, 2017a):

- Staff enter and leave through airlocks and wear protective clothing such as hats, face masks, gloves, boots, and coveralls.
- Equipment inside the cleanroom is designed to generate minimal air contamination. There are specialized mops and buckets. Cleanroom furniture is also designed to produce a low number of particles and to be easy to clean.

- Common materials such as paper, pencils, and fabrics made from natural fibers are excluded from the most critical areas, like an aseptic filling suite.
- Cleanroom HVAC systems also control the humidity to low levels. This, along with temperature is designed to reduce the likelihood of personnel perspiring and to protect the integrity of the cleanroom suits. Sometimes extra precautions are necessary to prevent electrostatic discharges. The other functions of HVAC are as follows:
  o To heat the air.
  o To supply ventilation (the process of replacing air in a room in order to remove heat, dust, and airborne bacteria).
  o To condition air. This involves the control of humidity (dehumidification) or the removal of heat to cool the air to required level.
  o Maintain room pressure: areas that must remain "cleaner" than surrounding areas must be kept under a "positive" pressurization (a concept examined later).
- In conjunction with HEPA filters, to control airborne particulates and microorganisms.
- Contamination control also requires personnel to practice aseptic techniques, wear specially designed clothing, to clean the areas to the correct standard, and to behave in ways which will minimize contamination.

In summary, contamination control is critical to all aspects of pharmaceutical manufacturing. Practices are put in place to ensure that the air is of the correct standard, that opportunities for contamination are not present (like water puddles on the floor), and that the opportunities for contamination carried on people being deposited into the airstream are minimized.

PARTICLES

"Particle" in the context of a cleanroom is a general term for all subvisible matter. From this definition, airborne particles simply refer to particles suspended in air. Air contains a variety of different particles of a range of different sizes. These are particles of dust, dirt, skin, microorganisms, and so on. The unit of measurement for subvisible particles is the micrometer (often abbreviated to the "micron"). This is symbolized as μm. The micron is a unit of length equal to one millionth () of a meter. As discussed before, the function of cleanrooms is to reduce the number of airborne particles. To illustrate this: air in an office building air contains from 500,000 to 1,000,000 particles of a size 0.5 μm or larger per cubic foot of air. In contrast, an ISO Class 5/EU GMP Grade A cleanroom is designed not to allow >100 particles of a size 0.5 μm or larger per cubic foot of air.

With cleanrooms the regulatory standards, which are discussed later, focus on two cutoff sizes of particles which are selected due to the potential risk that they pose. These are:

- $\geq 0.5\,\mu m$ size particles, which are close in size to many microorganisms;
- $\geq 5.0\,\mu m$ size particles, which are close in size to skin flakes, on which many microorganisms are bound to (and arguably are more likely to be detected within pharmaceutical cleanrooms than are "free floating" microorganisms).

With European GMP, there is concern with both types of particle size. With the FDA, the primary focus is upon the $0.5\,\mu m$ size.

Particles are generated from a variety of sources. These can include (Sandle, 2017b):

- Facilities, such as walls, floors, and ceilings; paint and coatings; construction material; air-conditioning debris; room air and vapors; spills and leaks.
- People, including skin flakes and oil; cosmetics and perfume; spittle; clothing debris (such as lint, fibers, and so on); hair.
- Equipment generated, including friction and wear particles, lubricants and emissions, vibrations.
- Cleaning equipment, like brooms, mops and dusters; cleaning chemicals.
- Fluids, arising from spillages.
- Particulates floating in air, primarily bacteria, fungi, organic material, and moisture.
- Compressed gasses.
- Product generated.

Methods of assessing particle counts are discussed in Chapter 8.

CLEANROOM CLASSIFICATION

Cleanrooms used within the pharmaceutical industry are classified according to international standards: ISO 14644. Outside of classification requirements, for the production of sterile products, both FDA and EU GMPs require continuous monitoring. In addition, there is a separate ISO standard for biocontamination control which is divided into two parts:

- ISO 14698-1: Cleanrooms and associated controlled environments—Biocontamination control—Part 1: General principles and methods.
- ISO 14698-2: Cleanrooms and associated controlled environments—Biocontamination control—Part 2: Evaluation and interpretation of biocontamination data.

ISO 14644 is the internationally recognized cleanroom standard and it is the only standard to which the US Food and Drug Administration (FDA) and the United States Pharmacopeia refer. It is important to understand that ISO 14644 is not a pharmaceutical standard; as a cleanroom standard it applies to all industries (such as healthcare and electronics). This means that not all parts are applicable to the pharmaceutical sector. The ISO 14644 standard classifies cleanrooms according to the concentration of particles in a given volume of air ($1\,m^3$) and based on this a class is defined and the cleanroom is assigned a class number.

ISO 14644 describes different phases in relation to the testing and monitoring of cleanrooms. These are:

- *Commissioning*: This is testing, proving, and documenting a facility system to demonstrate and satisfy the safe functionality in accordance with the design criteria.
- *Validation*: Qualification practices, fully documented, to provide the necessary assurance, through predefined test/s to prove that the critical systems operate in accordance with the facility design criteria. Validation and qualification are required in a regulatory regime.

Classification is the process of qualifying the cleanroom environment by the number of particles using a standard method. The end result of the activity is that cleanroom x is assigned ISO class y. Importantly classification is distinct from routine environmental monitoring and distinct from process monitoring, such as the requirement in EU GMP Annex 1 for continuous monitoring of aseptic filling.

Cleanrooms are certified according to principles outlined in ISO 14644—Part 1 (ISO, 2015a) and monitored according to the methods described in ISO 14644—Part 2 (ISO, 2015b). To classify pharmaceutical grade cleanrooms either:

- The number of particles equal to and $>0.5\,\mu m/m^3$ of air is measured and this count is used to identify the cleanroom class. The concentration of $5\,\mu m$ particles may also be measured if required to meet regulatory grades.
- Or, the class is assigned, and this is either proven correct or not through an assessment of the number of particles equal to and $>0.5\,\mu m$ measured in $1\,m^3$ of air.
- Selecting the approach will be dependent upon a local policy. For aseptic filling, the clean zone must be ISO Class 5/EU GMP Grade A. Therefore the area is designed to this specification and testing is carried out to ensure if the device can meet this classification.

The tests listed in ISO 14644 are divided into mandatory and optional tests. Optional tests may be included where they are of relevance to the cleanroom (such as an assessment of temperature and humidity). The range of tests may also differ where the cleanroom is undergoing validation in contrast to commissioning.

For pharmaceuticals and healthcare, to meet FDA regulations, particles of a size $\geq 0.5\,\mu m$ are required to be measured. For those wishing to classify using $\geq 5.0\,\mu m$ size in addition, the standard requires that the outcome is expressed using a macroparticle size descriptor, namely:

$$ISO\,M\,(20;\ \geq 5.0\mu m);LSAPC$$

where M = macroparticles, 20 = class limit (value taken from EU GMP Annex 1), $\geq 5.0\,\mu m$ = the particle size under consideration, LSAPC = Light scattering airborne particle counter (reference to the test instrumentation).

So, with for EU GMP:

> Grade A
>> ISO 5; at rest, operational; $\geq 0.5\,\mu m$
>> ISO M (20; $\geq 5.0\,\mu m$); at rest, operational; LSAPC
> Grade B
>> ISO 5; at rest; $\geq 0.5\,\mu m$, and M (29; ≥ 5.0); at rest, LSAPC
>> ISO 7; operational; $\geq 0.5\,\mu m$, 5.0.

As part of the assessment, the method for selecting the number (and position) of particle counter locations within a cleanroom should be noted. This method is based on a look-up table. The table uses a range of cleanroom sizes and provides the number of locations required (if the exact room size is not listed, the user selects the next largest room size and picks the appropriate number of locations). These numbers are based on a statistical method called hypergeometric distribution. This is very different to the square root approach, which was based on binominal distribution. Without going into statistical detail, this is based on particles not being normally distributed. The new approach allows each location to be treated independently.

The hypergeometric distribution is used to calculate probabilities when sampling without replacement (Rice, 2007). This is perhaps best illustrated using a nonparticle counting example. Consider a pack of playing cards. If we randomly sample one card from a deck of 52 and next, without putting the card back in the deck, we sample a second card. Following this, suppose we sample a third card, again without replacing any cards, and so on. Considering this sampling procedure, what is the probability that exactly two of the sampled cards will be aces? (for noncard players, 4 of the 52 cards in the deck are aces). The probability is very low. If the exercise was carried out again, but the cards were replaced, this would be an example of binomial distribution. The realities of particle counting are such that once particles in a given volume of air have been sampled they are not replaced; hence, hypergeometric distribution is more realistic than binominal distribution.

For the user, the approach is simpler because no calculations are required. In addition, for rooms with <9 particle count locations, the requirement to perform a 95% upper confidence level check has been removed. With the assigned numbers there is an in-built confidence interval of 95%. This means when a cleanroom is monitored there is a 95% level of confidence that 90% of the cleanroom complies.

Once the number of locations has been selected, the room is divided up into sectors and a particle counter placed in each sector. With the previous standard, these sectors were equal in size and a counter placed in approximate center. With the revised standard, the position where the counter is placed within each sector is determined by the user. The standard allows counters always to be placed at the same point within the sector, randomly placed within the sector, or evenly distributed, or selected by risk. The risk-based approach would be the best one to adopt. A risk-based decision could be based on variables like room layout, equipment type, airflow patterns, position of air supply and return vents, air change rates, and room activities.

The reason for not selecting the center of the location relates back to the issue of particle distribution: particles counts no longer assumed to be homogenous within a sector. Furthermore, additional locations can be added at the discretion of the facility. This might arise from the room-by-room risk assessment.

With assessing the volume of air to be sampled, the standard supplies a formula to be used. The outcome is the number of liters that need to be sampled in each location. The standard requires a minimum of 2 L per location; the application of the formula can result in this being higher. Generally, the lower the particle count limit, the greater the volume to be sampled (so a larger volume is taken from an EU GMP Grade B room compared with a Grade C room). When operating a particle counter in unidirectional airflow, for example, Grade A, the counter probe must be orientated into the airflow or pointed upwards for turbulent flow air.

Assessing Results

When assessing the results from the cleanroom classification exercise, each individual result must comply. Assessment of results involves:

1. Recording the results for each location.
2. Convert the results to particles per cubic meter.

3. This is set out using the formula published in the standard.
4. It should be noted that the formula states "number of particles at each location or average." This is because an option exists to add more than one particle count location per sector. When this occurs, the results are averaged, and the average used as the number to proceed with the previous calculation. Individual results may fall outside of the class, provided that the mean is within.
5. Although assessment is based on an average, each individual result must be within limits. Those out of limits need to be investigated.

Should out-of-limits results be obtained an investigation should be performed into the origin of the particle counts. This should conclude consideration of room design, equipment, and operator activities. Once a root cause has been identified, and corrective measures put in place, the exercise should be repeated. A risk assessment will be required to assess activities performed in the cleanroom between classification exercises.

Once the exercise is complete, test certificates in relation to cleanroom classification must be issued. It is good practice for certificates to indicate:

- Name and address of the testing organization.
- Date of testing.
- No. and year of the publication of the relevant part of ISO 14644, for example, ISO 14644-1:2015.
- Location of cleanroom (or clean zone).
- Specific representation of locations, for example, diagram.
- Designation of cleanroom.
- ISO class (plus EU GMP).
- Occupancy.
- Particle count sizes considered.
- Test method used (and any departures or deviations).
- Identification of test instrument and calibration certificate.
- Test results.

Additional guidance for testing is provided in ISO 14644-3:2005—Part 3: Test methods. In Part 3, tests are specified for two types of cleanrooms: unidirectional flow and nonunidirectional flow (or turbulent flow). The test methods recommend what test apparatus and test procedures are required and where appropriate an alternative procedure is suggested. The most important objectives of this document are to provide an internationally common basis of measurement and evaluation of cleanrooms and, at the same time, not to prevent the introduction of new technologies.

The ranges of tests are as follows:

- Airborne particle count for classification and test measurement of cleanrooms and clean air devices,
- Airborne particle count for ultrafine particles,
- Airborne particle count for macroparticles,
- Airflow test,
- Air pressure difference test,
- Installed filter system leakage test,
- Airflow direction test,
- Airflow visualization,
- Temperature test,
- Humidity test,
- Electrostatic and ion generator test,
- Particle deposition test,
- Recovery test,
- Containment leak test.

The reader should note that not all of these tests are applicable for the pharmaceutical, medical device, or healthcare sectors.

ONGOING ENVIRONMENTAL MONITORING

In drawing in risk assessment criteria, environmental monitoring assesses whether the necessary controls are being maintained through providing a detection mechanism. Environmental monitoring is a program which evaluates the cleanliness of the manufacturing environment, the effectiveness of cleaning and disinfection program, and the operational performance of environmental controls. As such, pharmaceutical manufacturers of both sterile and nonsterile products, and medical devices, are required to demonstrate that manufacturing processes and procedures minimize any potential contamination to the product from the manufacturing environment. Contamination can arise from several sources: water, air, surfaces, and personnel, each of which poses a potential risk to product (Sandle, 2012).

These risks of contamination are avoided by putting environmental controls in place (through correct grade of air supply, satisfactory cleaning and disinfection practices, and so on). Where controls cannot offset every contamination risk, and also as a means to demonstrate the level of control, environmental monitoring programs are devised and put into action (this is an important point repeated throughout the module—environmental control and environmental monitoring are related but different). In the context of this book, environmental control is biocontamination control, and the monitoring as part of the overall biocontamination control strategy.

With environmental monitoring, data review is of great importance. The interpretation of environmental monitoring data is itself a complex activity. This is because the surrounding environment (people, equipment, and rooms) are potential, and variable, sources of significant contamination. Furthermore, it is impossible to monitor and measure this potential contamination at all times. Therefore a manufacturer is reliant upon a well-designed program and the retrospective review and trending of data. Such data includes microbial counts and microbial flora, both which are indicators of the degree of control and of what has changed. The key thing here is time. Results of environmental monitoring allow changes over time to be examined and particularly good environmental monitoring programs allow predictions to be made as to the future direction of the data.

The data gathered allows the manufacturer to propose changes to the way that products are manufactured, such as, in developing effective cleaning and disinfection programs. Such information also impacts upon facility design, process flow, and working practices. The data can also provide a degree of assurance, particularly to those tasked with batch release.

Despite the importance of the data, what environmental monitoring can achieve in practice, is however, fairly limited. This relates to (Sandle, 2017c):

- The results from monitoring are not available for several days after the event due to the need to incubate samples;
- Only limited periods of manufacturing can be monitored, because few monitoring techniques lend themselves to continuous monitoring (and even then, this needs to be offset against cost and the high volume of data generated);
- The results of monitoring are rarely reproducible on reexamination;
- The data generated is generally only a crude measure of environmental stability. The most important consideration is invariably the long-term trend.

Despite these quite considerable limitations, environmental monitoring is very important. It allows the microbiologist to know when environmental control breaks down, what the possible origin or source of the contamination was, such as, in relating back to the categories of air, water and personnel contamination, and material transfer.

To do so requires the use of viable monitoring methods and particle counting. These approaches are discussed in Chapters 6 and 8, respectively, while the overall monitoring program is outlined in Chapter 10.

SUMMARY

Cleanrooms are the basis for most manufacturing activities within the pharmaceutical sector, providing the required space and environment for an appropriate level of air and surface cleanliness. This chapter has outlined the important aspects of cleanroom design, construction, and operation. This has included the importance of particle counting and the operation of optical particle counters.

The chapter has also discussed cleanroom classification, in line with ISO 14644 requirements. Importantly, ISO 14644 and the emphasis upon particle control represent only one part of contamination control. Moreover, ISO 14644, while it addresses ongoing compliance, remains focused on the classification of cleanrooms and this can be an unrepresentative activity. Other aspects of environmental control and environmental monitoring need to be considered alongside the ISO 14644 requirements.

The objective of the chapter has been to provide the reader with an understanding of how cleanrooms and clean air devices work and how they function to protect the product and to minimize contamination. The chapter, in outlining the theme of contamination, thus provides the context for other chapters which follow.

REFERENCES

Akers, J., & Agalloco, J. (2000). Isolators: validation and sound scientific judgment. *Journal of Pharmaceutical Science and Technology*, *54*(2), 110–111.

Beaney, A. M. (2006). *Quality assurance of aseptic preparation services* (4th ed.). London: Pharmaceutical Press.

Euradlex. The rules governing medicinal products in the European Community, Annex 1, published by the European Commission, Brussels, Belgium, 2009 (draft issued in 2018).

Farquharson, G. J. (1996). Technical and cost optimisation of industrial scale aseptic processing isolators. *European Journal of Parenteral Sciences*, *1*(1), 3–7.

ISO ISO 14644-1, Cleanrooms and associated controlled environments–Part 1: Classification of air cleanliness by particle concentration, ISO, Geneva, Switzerland, 2015a.

ISO, ISO 14644-2, Monitoring to provide evidence of cleanroom performance related to air cleanliness by particle concentration, ISO, Geneva, Switzerland, 2015b.

Ljungqvist, B., & Berit, R. (1997). *Cleanroom design—Minimizing contamination through proper design.* Buffalo Grove, IL: Interpharm Press.

Reinmüller, B. (2001). People as a contamination source-clothing systems. In *Dispersion and risk assessment of airborne contaminants in pharmaceutical cleanrooms* (pp. 54–77). Stockholm: Royal Institute of Technology, Building Services Engineering Bulletin No. 56.

Rice, J. A. (2007). *Mathematical statistics and data analysis* (3rd ed., p. 42). New York: Duxbury Press.

Sandle, T. (2012). Environmental monitoring: a practical approach. In: J. Moldenhauer (Ed.), *Vol. 6. Environmental monitoring: A comprehensive handbook* (pp. 29–54). River Grove, IL: PDA/DHI.

Sandle, T. (2013). Controlled environments for sterility testing. In T. Sandle (Ed.), *Sterility testing of pharmaceutical products* (pp. 129–160). Bethesda, MD: DHI/PDA.

Sandle, T. (2015). Cleanroom design. In: J. Moldenhauer (Ed.), *Vol. 7. Environmental monitoring: A comprehensive handbook* (pp. 3–28).

Sandle, T. (2016). Application of disinfectants and detergents in the pharmaceutical sector. In T. Sandle (Ed.), *The CDC handbook: A guide to cleaning and disinfecting cleanrooms* (pp. 168–197). Surrey: Grosvenor House Publishing.

Sandle, T. (2017a). Clean room design principles: focus on particulates and microbials. In S. C. Esteves, A. C. Varghese, & K. C. Worrilow (Eds.), *Clean room technology in ART clinics: A practical guide* (pp. 75–91). Boca Raton, FL: CRC Press.

Sandle, T. (2017b). Distribution of particles within the cleanroom: a review of contamination control considerations. *Journal of GXP Compliance*, *21*(6), 1–10.

Sandle, T. (2017c). Environmental control and environmental monitoring in support of aseptic processing. In T. Sandle, & E. C. Tidswell (Eds.), *Aseptic and sterile processing: Control compliance and future trends* (pp. 447–540). Bethesda, MD: DHI/PDA. ISBN 9781942911128.

Chapter 6

Viable Environmental Monitoring Methods

CHAPTER OUTLINE
Introduction   83
Application of Environmental Monitoring Methods   84
Settle Plates   85
   Assessing Suitability of Settle Plates   87
Active (Volumetric) Air Samplers   88
   Air Sampler Efficiency   92
   Practical Use of Air Samplers   94
   Compressed Gas Sampling   94
Surface Sampling   95
   Swabs   96
   Qualification Criteria for Swabs   97
   Contact Plates   98
   Selection of Contact Plates and Sampling Methods   99
Personnel Monitoring   99
Summary   99
References   100

INTRODUCTION

Environmental monitoring, as Chapter 5 has explained, involves the collection of data relating to the numbers or incidents of microorganisms present on surfaces, in the air, and from people. In addition, particle counting, a physical test, is undertaken in conjunction with viable monitoring because of the relationship between high numbers of airborne particles and microorganisms. Particle counting is assessed as part of Chapter 8.

Viable microbiological environmental monitoring is a key aspect of any sterility assurance program and is necessary to assess the number of viable

Biocontamination Control for Pharmaceuticals and Healthcare. https://doi.org/10.1016/B978-0-12-814911-9.00006-7

microorganisms present in the cleanroom environment. An environmental monitoring program requires the use of a range of different techniques. These can be divided into air samples, surface samples, and personnel samples. Air samples include both passive (settle plates) and active (using a sampling device) techniques.

This chapter examines the four standard techniques for the examination of viable microorganisms in the sterile or nonsterile production environment. Through the discussion, the reader will appreciate that each technique has considerable limitations and that a combination of all four is required for any comprehensive monitoring program. The chapter does not address rapid microbiological methods; these are discussed in Chapter 9.

APPLICATION OF ENVIRONMENTAL MONITORING METHODS

There are different sources of microbiological contamination within clean environments—water, air, surfaces (both within the room and from equipment), and personnel. These hazards, as Chapter 4 has outlined, should be evaluated by the microbiologist in terms of the relative risks to the product, and the environmental monitoring program should be oriented toward the points of greatest risk. In order to evaluate these sources, each of the different environmental monitoring methods plays an important part.

The objective of viable environmental monitoring is to enumerate the numbers of microorganisms present at a location within a cleanroom or

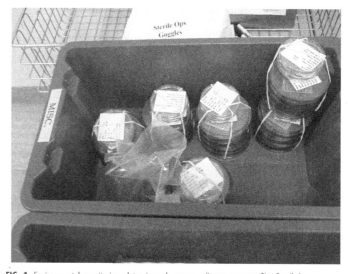

■ **FIG. 1** Environmental monitoring plates in a cleanroom. *(Image courtesy Tim Sandle.)*

controlled environment (Fig. 1). This is undertaken using a range of different air and surface counting methods (Sandle, 2012):

- *Active air sampling*: volumetric air sampler,
- *Passive air sampling*: settle plates,
- *Surface samples*: contact (replicate organism detecting and counting—RODAC) plates and swabs,
- *Personnel samples*: finger plates and gown plates.

Although these methods are well established there are several practical aspects to consider when using each of these methods. These are considered later.

SETTLE PLATES

Settle plates are Petri dishes, typically of either 9 or 14 cm diameter, containing different fill volumes of agar (normally between 20 and 30 mL). Settle plates are designed to detect any viable microorganisms that may directly settle on or in the product (i.e., microorganisms that are carried in the airstream, although a person who leans over a plate can also potentially deposit microorganisms). At determined monitoring locations (ideally positioned and exposed either side of the testing environment) the lids of the dishes are removed and the plates are exposed to the air for a defined period of time. In theory, microorganisms and units containing microorganisms settle out of the air under gravity and are deposited onto horizontally positioned agar plates. This theoretically works better in turbulent or laminar airflows. The efficiency can be described as the "settling rate" (Whyte, 1986).

The settling rate depends partly on the characteristics of the particles and on the airflows. Larger units will tend to settle faster (due to gravitational effects) and settling is facilitated by still airflows (which should not occur within a correctly designed unidirectional airflow zone). Smaller particles have a lower tendency to settle due to air resistance and air currents. The principle behind settle plates is that most microorganisms in air are in association with particles. Generally the "complete particle" (microorganism in association with the "carrier") is 12 µm diameter or larger.

Outside of unidirectional air, such as the main cleanroom itself, then the greater the degree of turbulence there is. The amount of air turbulence is proportional to the amount of time that particles remain suspended in the air. Thereby, the greater the amount of air turbulence then the longer the particles will remain suspended in the air (this is not always a bad thing, as particles can be blown away from a critical zone, depending upon the design of the room). This can, however, influence the reliability of the settle plate and here the additional use of active air samplers can provide additional assurance for the microbiologist assessing the cleanroom cleanliness.

The phenomenon of gravitational settling is, however, a debatable issue. The prevailing view, as discussed before, is that as most microorganisms are associated with physical particles they will be large enough to settle out of the air due to gravity. The dissenting view is that microorganism carrying particles or any microorganisms not associated with units as being light enough to remain in the airstream for several minutes and possibly be carried out of the airstream and not settle. Much of this debate thereby centers on the size of the particles in the air and the airflow (Sykes, 1970).

The results from settle plates can either be simply assessed as the number of microorganisms per plate or in a semiquantitative way by calculating the number of microorganisms settling per 4 h. For example, guidelines such as EU GMP express alert and action levels as cfu (colony-forming unit) per 4 h.

Where settle plates provide semiquantitative data this is not fully quantitative data because the information from the plate does not quantitatively relate to the level of contamination per unit volume of air (unlike the information obtained from an active air sampler). However, as the surface area of the Petri dish and the exposure time are known, the number of contaminants likely to settle in the airstream can be calculated. This concept is examined in the risk assessment unit in this module.

A further issue for the interpretation of settle plate data is with the actual "value" of 1 cfu on a settle plate. The single colony-forming unit could be the representation of one microorganism or several hundred microorganisms that were carried on a skin unit. Such uncertainty restricts the interpretative value of the settle plate (Fig. 2).

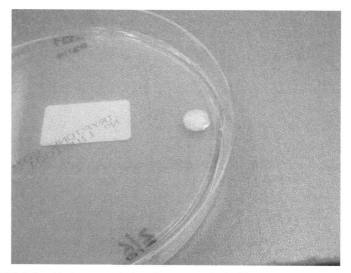

■ **FIG. 2** Bacterial colony on a settle plate. *(Image courtesy Tim Sandle.)*

The exposure time of the settle plate can be varied, although there is probably little value in exposing plates for <1 h. For consistency of sampling, for aseptic filling, the EU GMP Guide recommends a four-hour exposure time. This time should not be exceeded without strong justification, and even then there will probably be a challenge from the regulatory authority. For exposure times under 4 h, such as when a shorter activity is being monitored, the result obtained should be extrapolated using the simple equation:

$$\text{Count} \times 240 = \frac{\text{cfu}/4\,\text{h}}{\text{Time exposed (min)}}$$

The risk from any exposure is desiccation. The depth and condition of the agar are the key variables, as is the cleanroom environment. The agar in the plate will dry out faster if the airflow is excessively high or if the air humidity is low. Therefore, the exposure time of settle plates under the conditions of use (a particular cleanroom or unidirectional airflow cabinet) must be validated.

Settle plates are not universally accepted by all regulators. Generally, they are considered to be of less value by inspectors from the United States compared with Europe. When using settle plates, it should be noted that the use is required and accepted within Europe as a "quantitative measurement"; the FDA considers them semiquantitative at best and inferior to active air samples (Food and Drug Administration, 2004), a point expressed in the USP aseptic processing chapter (USP <1116>) (USP, 2017). This is unfortunate as the data generated from settle plates can be meaningful, especially if located correctly as this provides an indication of what could have been directly deposited into a critical area or product. The safest approach for a global manufacturer is to combine the use of settle plates with active air samplers (although the inherently higher cost of active air samplers will always be an issue of consideration).

Settle plates can be filled with any agar. Commonly this is either tryptone soya agar (for general microbial recovery) or, in two media situations, a specific fungal medium is used (refer to Chapter 7). Agar in settle plates does not ordinarily contain neutralizers. This is because neutralizers may affect the ability of the plate to withstand the harsher airflow under unidirectional conditions, leading to the agar cracking.

Assessing Suitability of Settle Plates

As settle plates are exposed over time they undergo a loss of weight due to desiccation. The degree of weight loss varies depending upon the environment in which the plate is exposed. The weight loss is greater when plates are exposed under Grade A/ISO Class 5 UDAFs. The desiccation of the agar may be detrimental to the viability of any microorganisms which may have settled onto the surface of an exposed agar plate. The process of desiccation can be considered of in terms of total water loss or by reduced access to moisture due to the formation of a "skin layer" onto the agar surface.

In order to demonstrate that settle plates can be exposed without undue moisture loss leading to concerns with growth promotion, a validation assessment should be performed. This is to show if settle plates retain the ability to support microbial growth after the maximum exposure time (which, as indicated before, is a four-hour exposure).

When designing a validation test protocol to examine the impact of weight loss there are a number of factors to consider. These include:

- The type of culture medium;
- The use of neutralizers in the culture medium (this may or may not be a factor depending on the application of the plates);
- The placement of plates (locations and schedule);
- The hydration state of the medium and the impact of this upon the rate of desiccation;
- The metabolic and physical state of any microorganism that may be deposited onto the plate surface;
- The length of the exposure time;
- The environment used (e.g., exposure under a unidirectional airflow unit).

There are different approaches to take when designing when and how settle plates will be assessed. The optimal approach is to expose plates for 4 h under a representative UDAF, then incubate them for the maximum incubation time, and then to perform growth promotion testing using a suitable range of microorganisms (Sandle, 2011a).

ACTIVE (VOLUMETRIC) AIR SAMPLERS

One of the more difficult choices facing an organization is which type of active air sampler to select. The use of active air samplers is highlighted by all the regulators and in the international cleanroom standard ISO 14698-1 (ISO, n.d.-a), as being of fundamental importance to any environmental monitoring regimen. Active air samplers allow the number of microorganisms in a given volume of air or measured over a set period of time to be captured onto a microbiological culture medium and then to be enumerated.

Microorganisms are not evenly distributed in air and several factors like moisture, temperature, electrostatic charge, light, air movement, and so on, influence their distribution. There are many variations in the type of active air sampler and in the efficiency of different models. No single model or type has universal acceptance and each model has strengths and weaknesses. This unit details some of the variations associated with active air sampling, with an aim in guiding the reader into making an informed choice.

Active (or volumetric or bioaerosol) air samplers are a slightly different measure of microorganisms in air than settle plates. As indicated earlier, the settle plate indicates the number of microorganisms that may deposit onto a surface; whereas, the active air sampler indicates the number of microorganisms present in a given volume of air within the range of the air sampler. Both of these approaches have merits and any comprehensive program will use both active air samples and settle plates.

Active air samplers sample a defined quantity of air. The volume of air sampled is normally one cubic meter of air. This allows the data to be quantified as cfu/m^3. Within a Grade A (ISO 5) cleanroom environment the number of microorganisms present would be expected as $<1\,cfu/m^3$, therefore the efficiency and accuracy of the sampler is of great importance in being able to capture and culture low levels of airborne microorganisms (Fig. 3).

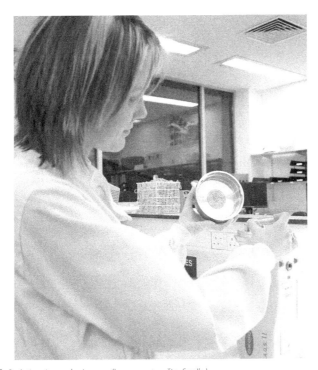

■ **FIG. 3** Active air sampler in use. *(Image courtesy Tim Sandle.)*

There are some variations with all types of active air sampling. These include:

- The nonrandom distribution of microorganisms in the environment;
- Imprecision in the various sampling techniques;
- The rate of sampling. At lower velocities there is a danger that microorganisms will not be deposited onto the agar medium, whereas at higher velocities there is a danger of desiccation of the culture medium.

These variations must be considered when choosing between different sampler types and models. The type of air sampler used has an important bearing on the data. There are limitations with accuracy and recovery when selecting between air samplers and there is no one model on the market that overcomes all of the difficulties. In examining different models, the first problem is that the results from different types of model (especially those using different sampling techniques) are not comparable. There are also competing ways to validate the samplers, which are discussed in a separate unit in this module.

There are three main types of active air sampler: impaction, centrifugal, or filtration. However, other types of sampler are available. In assessing the three main types, an impaction air sampler functions by accelerating air, at an angle of 90 degrees, through holes in the head of an air sampler (often a "sieve like" design) and impacting any microorganisms onto an agar strip or plate. A centrifugal air sampler draws air into the sampler head through a rotating vane mechanism. The vane causes microorganisms to be thrown out of the air and onto the agar through the effect of the centrifugal force. For filtration air samplers air is sucked through a filter and any microorganisms are captured onto a membrane filter which is then transferred to the surface of a culture medium and this is then incubated.

Effective air samplers must be able to precipitate particle sizes of at least 2 μm. In relation to most cleanrooms particles sized 5 μm or larger are more meaningful. This is because most airborne microorganisms are typically of a size between 5 and 15 μm and this increases to 15–18 μm for naturally occurring airborne particles, like skin flakes, many of which contain bacteria (Kaye, 1986; Meir & Zingre, 2000). There are also differences in the sampling volumes of different model samplers, with most models capable of sampling at least 1000 L.

A summary of the most common types of air sampler and the methods of operation is (Sandle, 2010):

a. Slit-to-Agar Air Sampler (STA)—The air is drawn by a self-contained vacuum pump through a standardized slit below which is placed on a slowly revolving Petri dish containing agar. Units in the air that have sufficient mass impact on the agar surface. The agar plates are incubated and viable organisms are allowed to grow out.

This type of air sampler is especially suited for compressed air-line monitoring. A general sampling method involves reducing the pressure of the compressed air line (which usually is 160 pounds per square inch or greater), using a built-in or external regulator; attach a flow meter, and adjust the flow to a suitable rate, for example, 1 cubic foot per minute; and attach the air impaction sampler which has been prepared with a Petri plate.

b. Sieve Impactor—The apparatus consists of a container designed to accommodate a Petri dish containing agar. The cover of the unit is perforated, with the perforations of a predetermined size. A vacuum pump draws a known volume of air through the cover and the particles in the air containing microorganisms impact on the agar medium in the Petri dish. Some samplers are available with a cascaded series of containers containing perforations of decreasing size.

There are variations in terms of the air sampler heads with such models:

- Single-Stage (contact plates or Petri dishes)
- Multi-Stage Cascade (Stacked perforated plates)
- Sterilizable Atrium (Stainless Steel head collection device)
- Single-Use Sterile Atrium (Disposable)

The previous two methods allow the determination of the distribution of the size ranges of particulates containing viable microorganisms based on which size perforations admit the units onto the agar plates. Other air sampler types include:

c. Centrifugal Sampler—The unit consists of a propeller or turbine that pulls a calculated volume of air into the unit and then propels the air outward to impact on a tangentially placed nutrient agar strip set on a flexible plastic base.

d. Sterilizable Microbiological Atrium—The unit is a variant of the single-stage sieve impactor. The unit's cover contains uniformly spaced orifices. The base of the unit accommodates one Petri dish containing a nutrient agar. Air is drawn through the unit by vacuum and allowed to impact on the agar surface.

e. Surface Air System Sampler—This integrated unit consists of an entry section that accommodates an agar contact plate. Immediately behind the contact plate is a motor and turbine that pulls air through the unit's perforated cover over the agar contact plate and beyond the motor, where it is exhausted.

f. Filter Samplers—The unit consists of a vacuum pump with an extension hose terminating in a filter holder that can be remotely located in the critical space. The filter consists of random fibers of gelatine capable of retaining airborne microorganisms. After a specified exposure time, the filter is aseptically removed and dissolved in an appropriate diluent and then plated on an appropriate agar medium to estimate its microbial content. The filter may also be plated directly on an agar surface.

The types of filters used include polycarbonate, cellulose acetate, or gelatine filters.

g. Impinger (use of liquid medium for particle collection)

Low shear-force liquid impingers are used for the recovery of stressed organisms and therefore they are claimed to show the best recovery over a wide range of airborne microorganisms. Yet, using an impinger sampler is less portable, more time consuming, and requires a greater degree of laboratory sophistication, and therefore is not the first choice for use in routine sampling.

Air Sampler Efficiency

In addition to the wide choice of various sampler types, different models of air sampler vary in their efficiency. Some devices themselves can generate nonviable particle counts, and this should be considered in the design qualification of such devices. The key concern if these are at a level that could be detected by discrete unit counters and therefore generates "false" count data when processes are being monitored. Other design considerations include the suitability of the sampler to any sanitization procedure for equipment to enter the cleanroom and the sampler's operation as an isokinetic sampler (that is to match the airflow speed within the UDAF).

There are two primary measures for air samplers: physical collection efficiency and biological collection efficiency. The physical collection efficiency measures the collection efficiency of inert particles. This is assessed in relation to air of the d50 value concept. Because of differences in physical characteristics, samplers differ in collection efficiency, often referred to as "cutoff" size (d50) (e.g., the particle size above which 50% or more of the particles are collected). As most air samplers have very sharp cutoff characteristics, most particles larger than the d_{50} are collected (Nevalainen, Pastuszka, Liebhaber, & Willeke, 1992). The d50 size is often used to describe the impact efficiency of a sampler, it being the particle size at which 50% of the particles are collected, and 50% pass through the sampler because that are too small to impact.

A further important measure is the flow rate (Ljungqvist & Reinmüller, 1998). The flow rate accuracy for the different models of air samplers varies by manufacturer; the specifications can range from $\pm2.5\%$ to $\pm10\%$ of the volume collected, depending upon the model. In critical environments such as cleanrooms, the sampling times are typically a full cubic meter of air and the counts are very low. In this environment, accurate sample collection is important. Assuming a sampling volume of 1000 L (m^3) the difference in collection accuracy is as follows:

- At $\pm2.5\%$ accuracy the variance in the volume collection is ±25 L of air.
- At $\pm10\%$ accuracy the variance in volume collection is ±100 L of air.

This is a difference of ±75 L of air in overall volume collection accuracy between different models. It is possible for the target organism to be missed by the instrument with lower accuracy. Flow rate accuracy should be considered based on the manufacturing environment when choosing a system.

There is also a consideration to be made about the relationship between sampling time and sampling volume. When comparing two different air samplers with different flow rates, the results can vary depending on whether the same air volume or the same total sampling time is used for both devices; the total sampling time rather than sampling volumes should be identical. To ensure equivalent representative samples, both units must be set to start and stop at the same time. Once the plates are read the results can then be multiplied to obtain cfu/m^3. When running systems with the same flow rates, identical sampling volumes may be used.

Air samplers are also assessed in terms of their biological collection efficiency. This is assessed in a bioaerosol chamber. This assessment requires specialized equipment in order to generate bioaerosols (such as a Collinson spray) and testing requires the use of a Class III microbiological safety cabinet (or, alternatively a scaled ventilation chamber). For this, there are a number of variables relating to the airborne particles and to the air samplers which depend on the inertial properties of the particles, such as size, density, and velocity, and on the physical parameters of the impactor, such as inlet nozzle dimensions, jet-to-plate distances, and airflow velocities and paths (Henningson & Ahlberg, 1994).

Practical Use of Air Samplers

There are a number of important issues to consider when using active air samplers, especially in critical zones. There are arguments against and in favor of active air samples in the Grade A/ISO Class 5 environment. This debate centers on the extent of the disruption of the airflow caused by the operation of the air sampler (all air samplers disrupt the airflow to some degree). The number of active air samples taken during a session should also be considered. The location is also important because air samplers must not counteract the protective airflow patterns in critical areas of the cleanroom. The effect of the air sampler location and number of samplers can be examined through airflow visualizations (or "smoke") studies where the disruption of the airflow can be visualized by smoke studies (at a time when the cleanroom is decommissioned).

A further area of consideration is the effect of dehydration on the culture media used in the active air sampler. This is an area that organizations will need to examine for themselves, rather than drawing upon validation data provided by the air sampler manufacturers, because the rate of moisture loss will relate to the type of culture media used (and the fill volume). Weight loss will also depend upon the incubation conditions, times, and temperatures. Such studies should be performed postincubation and use a range of microorganisms with which the growth-promoting properties of the culture medium should be assessed (Whyte & Niven, 1987). It is common to include isolates from the manufacturing facility in such studies.

Compressed Gas Sampling

Compressed gasses are used at different stages of the pharmaceutical manufacturing process. Applications include weighing of vials on process line or the removal of fallen vials. Furthermore, compressed gasses such as air, nitrogen, and carbon dioxide are deployed in operations involving purging or overlaying. Compressed gas sampling for microorganisms is an important part of contamination control assessment (Sandle, 2013). While sampling is important, the method of sampling can be hindered by the design of the gas system, where sampling is not easily conducted in an aseptic manner, or by the design of the air sampling instrument. Specialized samplers are available for this purpose or add-on devices are available to adapt standard model air samplers.

Compressed gas requires assessment against a number of parameters, including particles and viable microorganisms. The part of the standard used for making assessments is ISO 8573 Compressed air—Part 7: "Test method for viable microbiological contaminant content" (ISO, n.d.-b). When sampling compressed air for microorganisms, it is important that the air is depressurized and that the flow rate is controlled. Control of the flow rate is important to ensure that a cubic meter of air is sampled within the required sampling time (this time will be instrument dependent). With this, compressed gas is typically at 160 pounds per square inch or greater. An external regulator will be needed to bring this down to the sampling rate of instrument. If the air sampler takes 36 min to capture a cubic meter of air, then it will be sampling at one cubic foot per minute. The regulator will need to reduce the air down to allow for this. This is assessed using a flow meter. Pressure reduction to atmospheric conditions is of great importance and knowing the flow allows the agar exposure time to be assessed, so that one cubic meter of air is sampled.

It is also important that isokinetic sampling of the air occurs and that air velocity is reduced until it is within the range of the sampler as identified by the manufacturer. This is not only necessary for obtaining the correct sample size but it also impacts on the possibility of microbial survival. The level of impact stress has been shown to affect microbial recovery on agar and be dependent upon the impaction velocity of the cells into the agar as well as the design and operating parameters. Due to the fact that any microorganisms present are transported under pressure and then suddenly released into atmospheric conditions, they may be damaged by the immediate expansion of the gas and the resulting shearing forces (Stewart et al., 1995).

SURFACE SAMPLING

Surface sampling can reveal important information concerning the state of the manufacturing environment and risk of contamination transference (through proximity to the critical zones); surface sampling is arguably of greatest value when commissioning a new cleanroom, restarting an existing cleanroom after a shutdown period, or with determining the effectiveness of cleaning and disinfection.

Surfaces are assessed by taking contact (or RODAC) plates and swabs. There is contradictory evidence as to whether a contact plate is superior to a swab (particularly with the wider use of flocked swab) (Angelotti, Wilson, Litsky, & Walter, 1964; Dalmaso, Bini, Paroni, & Ferrari, 2008); however, as a general point, contact plates tend to be preferred where there is a flat surface. This is because the contact plate can be standardized, taken for a defined time using a set pressure (achieved using commercially available activator devices). After use, the residue should always be wiped clean with a suitable sanitizer. Swabs are typically used for sampling from nonflat surfaces such as tubes, seals, and valves.

Swabs

Swabs are typically made up of sterile cotton tips, although swabs vary in the materials used for the applicator stick (either wood or plastic) and the tip (where materials like cotton, viscose, alginate, etc. are used). A more recent innovation are flocked swabs, which appear to provide higher recoveries of microorganisms from surfaces in comparison to standard cotton or Rayon swabs (or "plain" swabs) (Halls, 2004).

Flocked swabs comprise of a solid molded plastic applicator shaft with a tip that can vary in size and shape. The tip of the applicator is coated with short Nylon fibers that are arranged in a perpendicular fashion. This perpendicular arrangement results from a process called flocking, where the fibers are sprayed onto the tip of the swab, while it is held in an electrostatic field. This process creates a highly absorbent thin layer with an open structure. Unlike traditional fiber wound swabs, which resemble a mattress or cushion, flocked swabs have no internal absorbent core to disperse and entrap the specimen—the entire sample stays close to the surface for fast and complete elution. The perpendicular Nylon fibers act like a soft brush and allow improved collection of cell samples. Capillary action between the fiber strands facilitates strong hydraulic uptake of liquid sample, and the sample stays close to the surface allowing easy elution.

Some types of swabs require prewetting using a diluent (such as Ringer's Solution, phosphate buffered saline, sodium hexametaphosphate, sterile water, etc.) before use. Other types of swabs are contained with a transport medium. They are either contained within a transport medium or require prewetting with a suitable recovery medium. Swabbing is performed by rubbing a surface while rotating the swab—so that all parts of the tip are exposed—through a number of strokes (typically between 10 and 25). Dry swabbing is not recommended as this will result in a low recovery from surfaces.

Following the sampling, the swab can either be streaked out onto an agar plate (which is the least efficient method) or, where the appropriate tip has been used, dissolved in a diluent and either tested by pour plate or by membrane filtration (of which the latter is the most efficient method). The membrane filter will be either 0.45 or 0.22 μm, and this technique carries a further advantage in that disinfectant residues can be overcome through rinsing the filter. A development of the concept of rinsing involves immersing a surface or device into a sterile fluid and subjecting it to agitation (using manual or ultrasonic energy techniques). The fluid can then be membrane filtered. This development has the advantage that an entire surface can be tested, although validation can be problematic and it is often impracticable to remove surfaces. An alternative is where the swab tip is incubated in broth, for the detection of growth (Sandle, 2011b). These types of swabs are best suited to Grade A environments where presence or absence of contamination is the matter at hand.

Some degree of quantization can be introduced for swabbing by using a sterile template. The use of a template can be used to give the same approximate surface area as the contact plate. However, given that swabs tend to be used when there are uneven or irregular surfaces, the use of such templates is often not practicable.

The advantages of the swab method are that they are more applicable to surfaces that are flexible, uneven, or where the area is too small for a contact plate to make a "complete contact." The swabbing technique is also superior where a high level of contamination is suspected. The contact plate, by virtue of "replicating" a surface, can create a distortion through overcrowded and overlapping colonial growth. In contrast, the swabbing method breaks down microcolonies and aggregates and can more often reflect where a higher count is present.

Qualification Criteria for Swabs

With swabs some factors to consider are as follows:

A. The pack density of the swab (a source of variation);

B. Operator practice. This is highly variable because of the following factors:
   a. How is the swab rotated?;
   b. What level of pressure is applied to the swab?;
   c. What is the effect of different surfaces?;
   d. What is the surface area that is swabbed?);
   e. Transfer efficiency from surface to swab;
   f. Transfer efficiency from swab to culture media. Factors include:
      i. The hydration state of the culture media;
      ii. How the swab is rotated;
      iii. The degree of pressure that is applied;
      iv. Whether the swab diluent is vortex mixed beforehand;
   g. Whether different types of microorganisms are extracted from the swab with the same efficiency.
   h. The effect of different media and cultural conditions (incubation time and temperature).

Some of these are points to be standardized and others need to be assessed through surface recovery studies. There are two approaches here: either representative surfaces in pharmaceutical cleanrooms can be artificially inoculated using different environmental strains (an *in vitro* study) or naturally inoculated floors can be swabbed with swabs types (an in situ study).

Contact Plates

Surface contact plates are a common test for surface contamination. Contact plates are Petri dishes filled with microbiological agar. The plate is filled to a level above the rim of the plate so that the agar surface extends upwards when dry (that is it is convex). The plate has a typical diameter of 50–55 mm and a surface area of $25\,cm^2$. The bottom of the plate has a $1\,cm^2$ square grid, which facilitates the counting of grown microbes. The raised surface allows the agar to be pressed onto a surface. The design of the contact plate is therefore different to the standard Petri dish, where the agar is contained within the Petri dish.

The contact plate is a quantifiable method, because the contact between the plate and the surface provides a "mirror image" of the surface. Following incubation, this image transfer provides information relating to the number of microbial colonies and their relative position. The quantification is derived from recording the number of colony-forming units (cfu) per square centimeter. This act of replication gives the contact plate its alternative name: RODAC. This is an acronym for "replicate organism detection and counting," and the term is more commonly applied in North America and it is a trade mark of a certain brand of plates.

In terms of microbial recovery from surfaces, there are many considerations of efficiency which affect this (Tidswell, 2017). These include the nature of the surface, physicochemical forces holding microorganisms to the surface, the type of agar, pressure and time applied, incubation conditions, and so on. Generally, the "smoother" or "flatter" the surface, the better the recovery. For monitoring of surfaces, which might contain residues of antibiotics or disinfectants it is recommended to use agar media supplied with inactivating agents like lecithin, Tween 80, histidine, sodium thiosulfate, or enzymes like beta-lactamases.

One issue with the use of contact plates that needs to be observed is that the plate leaves traces of nutrients, so the postsampled surface should be wiped with a suitable disinfectant.

Selection of Contact Plates and Sampling Methods

With contact plates some factors to consider are (Niskane & Pohja, 1997):

- The selection of the culture media and whether the culture media should contain a disinfectant neutralizer;
- The pressure and time requirements;
- The hydration state of the culture media;
- The recovery rates from different surfaces.

As with swabs before, some of these are points to be standardized and others need to be assessed through surface recovery studies.

PERSONNEL MONITORING

With sterile processing activities, personnel monitoring is undertaken. This consists of swabs or contact plates taken from garment surfaces, isolator sleeves, and finger plates of gloved hands. Such samples are normally only taken for sterile manufacturing in Grade A/ISO Class 5 and Grade B/ISO Class 7 cleanrooms. However, there may be other applications, especially in relation to investigations of particular microorganisms that maybe personnel related, where such samples will be of use.

Sleeves and gowns are sampled by using contact plates, whereas finger plates are taken of impressions of the fingers of each hand onto a 9 cm agar plate. Therefore, both sample types can be quantified as cfu, either as cfu per five fingers per hand or as cfu per 25 cm^2. Due to the regular spraying of gloves with disinfectant hand rubs, it is important that the culture medium used contains appropriate neutralizers. The areas that have come into direct contact with the agar should be disinfected after use or the gown changed.

Finger plates are known by several terms: glove print, finger print, finger dab, and so on. This all refers to the same thing: the placement of the tips of four fingers and the thumb, of each gloved hand, onto an agar plate. The gloves worn by personnel, immediately after performing critical activities or as part of an ongoing check, are sampled. It is good practice to replace the gloves after each finger plate has been taken. However, some firms justify the spraying of disinfectant onto the glove to remove agar residues.

SUMMARY

This chapter has presented the conventional methods for environmental monitoring. Even with the advent of some rapid microbiological methods, these approaches make up the majority of the types of environmental monitoring performed. While these methods are well described in literature, this chapter has looked at these methods from the prism of reliability and variability, focusing on some of the factors that need to be considered for method selection and qualification. Paying attention to this provides the basis for a sound environmental monitoring program and increases assurance as to the validity of that program.

REFERENCES

Angelotti, R., Wilson, J. L., Litsky, W., & Walter, W. G. (1964). Comparative evaluation of the cotton swab and Rodac methods for the recovery of *Bacillus subtilis* spore contamination from stainless steel surfaces. *Health Laboratory Science*, *1*(4), 289–296.

Dalmaso, G., Bini, M., Paroni, R., & Ferrari, M. (2008). Validation of the new irradiated nylon™ Flockedn QUANTISWAB™ for the quantitative recovery of microorganisms in critical clean room environments. *PDA Journal of Pharmaceutical Science and Technology*, *62*(3), 191–199.

Food and Drug Administration. (2004). *Guideline on sterile drug products produced by aseptic processing*. Rockville, MD: FDA.

Halls, N. (2004). Microbiological environmental monitoring. In N. Halls (Ed.), *Microbiological contamination control in pharmaceutical clean rooms* (pp. 23–52). Boca Raton, FL: CRC Press.

Henningson, E. W., & Ahlberg, M. S. (1994). Evaluation of microbial aerosol samplers: a review. *Journal of Aerosol Science*, *25*, 1459.

ISO ISO 14698-1 & 2 (Part 1: Cleanrooms and associated controlled environments—biocontamination control—General principles and methods and Part 2: Evaluation and interpretation of biocontamination data. ISO, Geneva, Switzerland.

ISO ISO 8573-7:2003, Test method for viable microbiological contaminant content, ISO, Geneva, Switzerland.

Kaye, S. (1986). Efficiency of biotest RCS as a sampler of airborne bacteria. *Journal of Parenteral Science and Technology*, *42*(5), 147–152.

Ljungqvist, B., & Reinmüller, B. (1998). Active sampling of airborne viable particles in controlled environments: a comparative study of common instruments. *European Journal of Parenteral Science*, *3*(3), 59.

Meir, R., & Zingre, H. (2000). Qualification of air-sampler systems: MAS-100. *Swiss Pharma*, *22*, 15–21.

Nevalainen, A., Pastuszka, J., Liebhaber, F., & Willeke, K. (1992). Performance of bioaerosol samplers: collection characteristics and sampler design considerations. *Atmospheric Environment*, *26A*, 531–540.

Niskane, A., & Pohja, M. (1997). Comparitive studies on the sampling and investigation of microbial contamination of surfaces by contact plate and swab method. *Journal of Applied Bacteriology*, *42*, 53–63.

Sandle, T. (2010). Selection of active air samplers. *European Journal of Parenteral and Pharmaceutical Sciences*, *15*(4), 119–124.

Sandle, T. (2011a). Microbial recovery on settle plates in unidirectional airflow cabinets. *Clean Air and Containment Review*, (6), 8–10.

Sandle, T. (2011b). A study of a new type of swab for the environmental monitoring of isolators and cleanrooms (the Heipha ICR-swab). *European Journal of Parenteral and Pharmaceutical Sciences*, *16*(92), 42–48.

Sandle, T. (2012). Environmental monitoring: a practical approach. In J. Moldenhauer (Ed.), *Vol. 6. Environmental monitoring: A comprehensive handbook* (pp. 29–54). River Grove, IL: PDA/DHI.

Sandle, T. (2013). Contamination control risk assessment. In R. E. Masden, & J. Moldenhauer (Eds.), *Vol. 1. Contamination control in healthcare product manufacturing* (pp. 423–474). River Grove, IL: DHI Publishing.

Stewart, S. L., Grinshpun, S. A., Willeke, K., Terzieva, S., Ulevicius, V., & Donnelly, J. (1995). Effect of impact stress on microbial recovery on an agar surface. *Applied and Environmental Microbiology*, *61*, 1232–1239.

Sykes, G. (1970): The control of airborne contamination in sterile areas. Aerobiology: Proceedings of the 3rd international symposium, in Silver, I. H. (ed.), Academic Press, London.

Tidswell, E. C. (2017). Bioburden control. In T. Sandle, & E. C. Tidswell (Eds.), *Aseptic processing: Control, compliance and future trends* (pp. 163–192). River Grove, IL: DHI Publishing.

USP General chapter <1116> Microbiological control and monitoring of aseptic processing environments, USP 40. US Pharmacopeial Convention, Rockville, MD, 2017, 1430–1443.

Whyte, W. (1986). Sterility assurance and models for assessing airborne bacterial contamination. *Journal of Parenteral Science and Technology*, *40*, 188–197.

Whyte, W., & Niven, L. (1987). Airborne bacteria sampling: the effect of dehydration and sampling time. *Journal of Parenteral Science and Technology*, *40*, 182–188.

Chapter 7

Selection and Application of Culture Media

CHAPTER OUTLINE

Introduction   104
Defining Culture Media   104
Supply of Culture Media   105
Types of Culture Media Used for Biocontamination Control   105
   Tryptone Soy Agar   106
   Nutrient Agar   107
   Sabouraud Dextrose Agar   108
   Blood Agar   109
Quality Control Testing   109
Incubation Strategies for Environmental Monitoring   110
Temperatures of Incubation and Microbial Recovery   111
General-Purpose Culture Media   112
Incubation Strategies   112
   Studies to Evaluate Two-Tiered Incubation   114
   Marshall's Study   114
   Sandle's Study   115
   Gordon' Study   117
   Sage's Study   117
   Symonds' Study   118
   Guinet's Study   119
   Summary of Studies   119
Incubation Time   120
Summary   121
References   122

Biocontamination Control for Pharmaceuticals and Healthcare. https://doi.org/10.1016/B978-0-12-814911-9.00007-9

INTRODUCTION

This chapter examines what has arguably, even in the context of many emerging types of rapid methods at least, the foundation of all microbiological testing: culture media; here, the focus is on different types of media used for biocontamination control assessments.

Microbiological culture media is essential for the cultivation and growth of microorganisms. Microbiological culture medium is a substance which encourages the growth, support, and survival of microorganisms. Culture media contains nutrients, growth-promoting factors, energy sources, buffer salts, minerals, metals, and gelling agents (for solid media). The ISO 11133 definition is:

> *"Formulations of substances in liquid, semi-solid or in sold form, which contain natural and/or synthetic constituents intended to support the multiplication, or to preserve the viability, of microorganisms".*

(ISO, 2014)

DEFINING CULTURE MEDIA

Culture media contains the nutrients needed to sustain a culturable microorganism; beyond this, culture media vary in the many ingredients added, allowing the media to select for or against microbes. Culture media can be subdivided into:

a. Liquid culture media. This is commonly called "broth."
b. Solid and semisolid culture media. This media contains a solidifying material which may be agar–agar or gelatine or some other analogous substance. This media is commonly called "agar," irrespective of the type of solidifying agent used.

With agar, when "agar" is used, this is a gelatinous substance derived from seaweed. The gelling agent is an unbranched polysaccharide obtained from the cell walls of some species of red algae, primarily from the genera *Gelidium* and *Gracilaria*, or other algae like *Sphaerococcus euchema*.

Further subdivisions that can be considered are as follows:

a. Growth media,
b. Transport media,
c. Preservation media,
d. Resuscitation media,
e. Enrichment media,
f. Selective growth media,
g. Differential media.

It is important to note that such subdivisions, while commonplace, are to an extent arbitrary and then are different ways that can be considered by which media can be grouped. It is also worth mentioning that some of the previously listed may have multiple uses.

SUPPLY OF CULTURE MEDIA

In terms of how culture media reaches the point of being used, media can be obtained as:

a. Ready to use (from a supplier);

This is culture media supplied in containers in a ready-to-use form (e.g., Petri dish or tubes or a similar carrier).

b. Partially completed;

This is culture media which requires one or more additional working steps before its intended use (e.g., melting or pouring).

c. As a dehydrated formulation (which requires manufacturer within the facility).

The preparation of culture media requires consistent practices and a dedicated area for preparation; this is commonly described as the "media kitchen."

In addition to culture media, diluents and rinsing solutions are widely used to support microbiological tests. Diluents are sterile solutions, often isotonically balanced, designed to either promote the recovery of microorganisms or to remove microorganisms from a surface. Diluents are considered in a later chapter.

With the above means of receiving culture media, culture media is normally derived from two sources: either it is prepared on site, or, more increasingly, it is prepared by a commercial supplier. Whichever the source, the microbiologist must have confidence in the supplier's ability to make consistent and high-quality media. Much of the chemical tests which underpin the quality control of culture media, like pH, gel strength, clarity, and color, will be performed by the supplier. Here the microbiologist is reliant upon internal or external quality audits and from performance of the media, in practice, between batches and over time (Mossel et al., 1980).

TYPES OF CULTURE MEDIA USED FOR BIOCONTAMINATION CONTROL

The pharmaceutical and healthcare sciences microbiology laboratory will use a range of culture media depending upon the application required. The two common general medium types are nutrient agar or broth; and tryptone soya agar or broth (as described by early writers like Pflug, Smith, and Christensen (1981)). Tryptone soya agar, in particular, is widely used for environmental monitoring. Both tryptone soya and nutrient media are undefined culture media because the amino acid source contains a variety of compounds with the exact composition being unknown. These media contain the essential ingredients that most bacteria need for growth and are nonselective, so they are used for the general isolation, cultivation, and maintenance of bacteria kept in culture collections.

The approach taken with culture media for environmental monitoring is to use a general-purpose medium: tryptone soya agar, blood agar, or nutrient agar together with a mycological agar (to assess bacteria and fungi separate) or to use a general-purpose culture medium to detect both.

Expanding upon this, the more common types of media found within a pharmaceutical microbiology laboratory are given below.

Tryptone Soy Agar

Tryptone soya agar (TSA) is equivalent to soybean casein digest medium (as described in the compendial texts)—a medium for the isolation and cultivation of nonfastidious and fastidious microorganisms. This medium is used for environmental monitoring and in-process bioburden testing. This medium may contain a neutralizer when used for environmental monitoring so that disinfectant residues can be neutralized. Some samples of this medium will also be irradiated where it is used in the manufacturing facility.

The general formula is presented in Table 1.

The medium contains enzymatic digests of casein and soybean meal, which provide amino acids and other nitrogenous substances, making it a nutritious medium for a variety of organisms. Glucose provides the energy source. Sodium chloride maintains the osmotic equilibrium, while dipotassium

Table 1 Formula for tryptone soy agar	
Formula	**gm/L**
Pancreatic digest of casein (a peptone)	15.0
Enzymatic digest of soybean (sometimes called soytone)	5.0
Sodium chloride	5.0
Agar	15.0
pH 7.3 ± 0.2 @ 25°C	

phosphate acts as buffer to maintain pH (Abbott & Graham, 1961). Agar is added to form a gel.

With growth promotion testing, the common test organisms are as follows:

- Bacillus subtilis (ATCC 6633)
- *Candida albicans* (ATCC 10231)
- Aspergillus brasiliensis (ATCC 16404)
- *Staphylococcus aureus* (ATCC 6538)
- Pseudomonas aeruginosa (ATCC 9027)

The use of these organisms ensures that testing meets the different pharmacopeia chapters which describe the use of the medium. Chapter 16 looks at some general applications of this medium.

Nutrient Agar

Nutrient agar is a general-purpose medium for the cultivation of nonfastidious microorganisms. This is a general growth medium and is primarily used for preserving microbial cultures. There have been various formulations developed since *circa* 1910.

A typical formula is given in Table 2.

With the formulation, peptic digest of animal tissue, beef extract and yeast extract provide the necessary nitrogen compounds, carbon, vitamins, and also some trace ingredients necessary for the growth of bacteria. Sodium chloride maintains the osmotic equilibrium of the medium.

Table 2 Formula for nutrient agar	
Formula	**gm/L**
Yeast extract	4.0
Tryptone	5.0
Glucose	50.0
Potassium dihydrogen phosphate	0.55
Potassium chloride	0.425
Calcium chloride	0.125
Magnesium sulfate	0.125
Ferric chloride	0.0025
Manganese sulfate	0.0025
Bromocresol green	0.022
Agar	15.0
pH 5.5 ± 0.2	

Nutrient agar is ideal for demonstration purposes where a more prolonged survival of cultures at ambient temperature is often required without risk of overgrowth that can occur with more nutritious substrate. Unmodified the medium used for the cultivation and enumeration of bacteria which are not particularly fastidious. The addition of different biological fluids such as horse or sheep blood, serum, egg yolk, and so on, makes the medium suitable for the cultivation of related fastidious organisms (Lapage, Shelton, & Mitchell, 1970).

Suitable organisms for testing the medium include:

- *Escherichia coli* (ATCC 25922)
- *Pseudomonas aeruginosa* (ATCC 27853)
- Salmonella Typhi (ATCC 6539)
- *Staphylococcus aureus* (ATCC 25923)
- Streptococcus pyogenes (ATCC 19615)

Sabouraud Dextrose Agar

Sabouraud dextrose agar (SDA) (equivalent to Sabouraud glucose agar) is used for the isolation and cultivation of fungi, especially dermatophytes. While the medium has been adapted, it remains based on the formulation of its creator. The formulation was later adjusted by Chester W. Emmons when the pH level was brought closer to the neutral range and the dextrose concentration lowered to support the growth of other microorganisms (Sandven & Lassen, 1999).

An example formulation is given in Table 3.

With the formulation, mycological peptone provides nitrogenous compounds. Dextrose provides an energy source. High dextrose concentration and low pH favor fungal growth and inhibits contaminating bacteria from test samples.

Microorganisms used for testing the medium include:

- *Candida albicans* (ATCC 1023)
- *Aspergillus brasiliensis* (ATCC 16404)

Table 3 Formula for Sabouraud dextrose agar

Formula	gm/L
Mycological peptone	10.0
Glucose (dextrose)	40.0
Agar	15.0
pH 5.6 ± 0.2 @ 25°C	

In terms of appearance, when in Petri dishes, the medium appears a light amber color, clear to slightly opalescent as a gel.

An alternative agar is malt extract agar, which contains malt extract and dextrose and mycological peptone; moreover, other agar that can be selected for the cultivation of fungi such as Rose Bengal Chloramphenicol Agar Base or Potato Dextrose Agar. Despite these other types of mycological media being available, SDA is more common.

Blood Agar

Blood agar, such as Columbia blood agar, is a highly nutritious general-purpose agar. Blood Agar is a general-purpose enriched medium often used to grow fastidious organisms and to differentiate bacteria based on their hemolytic properties. This medium is used for some microbiological identification tests.

Of the agars described it is most common for TSA to be used, either solely or in conjunction with SDA. Nutrient agar is a nutrient medium most effectively used for the cultivation of microorganisms supporting growth of a wide range of nonfastidious organisms, and blood agar is most appropriate for human-related organisms, in clinical practice.

QUALITY CONTROL TESTING

It is important that each batch of such media undergoes some form of quality control before it is released for general use. This can either be by the manufacturer (assuming the culture medium is not manufactured in house) or by the recipient laboratory (a debate which is perennial, and which is discussed in this chapter). This provides some measure of confidence for the results issued from microbiology laboratories and forms an essential part of internal quality assurance (Martin, 1991). Without knowing if the culture media are any good, how can the microbiologist have any confidence in the results that are produced? Many of the approaches to media quality control used within the pharmaceutical and healthcare sectors have been adopted from the food industry (as will be apparent in some of the references cited for this chapter), and to a lesser degree from clinical microbiology practices.

Quality control testing of culture media typically consists of (Martin, 1991):

- physical appearance
- pH
- contamination check
- gel strength (for plate media)
- growth promotion.

An assessment of the growth promotion properties of culture media is the "bedrock" underpinning microbiology laboratory activities. The growth promotion test is an assessment of the growth-promoting properties of microbiological culture media and an assessment of the ability of any diluents to support the survival of microorganisms (that is, not causing inhibition). This "nutritive properties" test involves challenging media with a pure culture of a selected microorganism and assessing the recovery of that known microorganism (Bridson, 1998). This is often a known population to be recovered within 50%–200%, within a specified time frame.

INCUBATION STRATEGIES FOR ENVIRONMENTAL MONITORING

While the selection of media is of importance, which medium (or media) is selected and the incubation strategies applied represent important choices. For many laboratory tests, such as sterility testing or the microbial limits test, these are well described in the pharmacopeia. One area, essential to the assessment of environmental control, is with the environmental monitoring program and its associated methods. With the growth in rapid microbiological methods acknowledged (Jimenez, 2011), it remains that the main component of an environmental monitoring regime involves the application of microbiological culture media in association with established monitoring methods. These methods consist of air samples (including settle plates and active air sampling using a volumetric air sampler); surface samples (contact plates and swabs); and, where necessary, samples of personnel working within cleanrooms (finger dabs and gown plates) (Sandle, 2012). Data is assessed for individual excursions against defined alert and action levels and for trends over representative periods of time.

While the requirement for environmental monitoring is well established, there is no regulatory guidance on appropriate culture media or incubation parameters (time and temperature). With US and European GMP, there is, however, an expectation that monitoring methods are capable to assessing areas for bacteria and for fungi (Marshall, Poulson-Cook, & Moldenhauer, 1998). Hence the culture medium used for the detection and enumeration of airborne and surface microorganisms should be suitable for the growth of these target microorganisms: aerobic bacteria and fungi (yeasts and molds). The medium should be tested, prior to use, for the absence of cell growth inhibitory substances (that is a test for "growth promotion"). One objective of testing for inhibitory substances is to confirm that the collection and growth of microorganisms will not be affected by the presence of alcohol, antibiotics, and so forth and to ensure that monitoring results are not altered by the quality of medium used.

In the author's experience the wider practice is to use a general-purpose agar. This is often because the alternative approach of using a medium for the detection of bacteria and a medium for the detection of fungi involves running double the number of samples. This is not only costly but the activity can also arguably enhance the risk to the process when monitoring the highest grades of cleanrooms, particularly in relation to aseptic manufacture. This is because such monitoring is invasive and the use of two media leads to a higher number of interventions being made. However, it is recognized that some users elect to use two culture media and the selection of an appropriate fungal medium is also considered in this chapter.

Where a general-purpose agar is used it is common for the agar to be incubated at two different temperatures, by incubating at one temperature first, for a defined period; and then transferring the media to a second temperature, for a second defined period of time, prior to the final read at which time the numbers of colony forming units are enumerated. The reason for a dual temperature incubation regime is to recover both bacteria and fungi.

The important question that stems from this is "at which temperatures?"; "Will a single temperature suffice?" Of if dual incubation is needed, "what is the required order of incubation?" (Guinet, Berthoumieu, Dutit, et al., 2017) These are questions that each facility must be prepared to consider and have an answer for (Moldenhauer, 2014).

TEMPERATURES OF INCUBATION AND MICROBIAL RECOVERY

The types of bacteria most likely to be recovered within cleanrooms are those transient or residential to human skin. Such bacteria will have adapted to growing in ecological habitats that represent the temperature variation found across the body. A large proportion of the skin microbiota generally consists of to the genera Staphylococci and Micrococci with *Corynebacterium* spp. recovered at slightly lower numbers (Sandle, 2011). The temperate habits for the human skin microbiome across which such microorganisms are found are between 29°C and 37°C (such distinct habitats are determined by skin thickness, folds, and the density of hair follicles and glands). It is on this basis that the most common temperature range for the recovery of cleanroom bacteria falls between 30°C and 35°C.

With fungi, literature suggests that the majority of fungi found in cleanrooms, including *Alternaria*, *Cladosporium* and Trichophyton, have an optimum growth of between 20°C and 25°C (Vijayakumar, Sandle, & Manoharan, 2012). This temperature range also applies to the most commonly isolated fungi from human skin: *Malassezia* spp. (Gao, Perez-Perez, Chen,

& Blaser, 2010). Moreover, most indoor molds, such as those that could be found within a cleanroom environment, do not efficiently grow at temperatures above 25°C (Fabian, Miller, Reponen, & Hernandez, 2005). However, there is some debate over this convention for other studies indicate that fungi like *Aspergillus* grow better at temperatures above 30°C (Abe, Ogawa, Tanuma, & Kume, 2009). Nonetheless, it is on this basis that most fungi appear to prefer temperatures below 25°C that a temperature range designed to select for the recovery of any fungi that might be present is incorporated.

GENERAL-PURPOSE CULTURE MEDIA

Where two media are used or with a two-tiered incubation scheme the typical culture medium selected for the recovery of bacteria (as with a two different media incubation scheme) or for bacteria and fungi (as with a dual incubation scheme), this is invariably tryptone soya agar (TSA). TSA is equivalent to the soybean casein digest medium described in the three main pharmacopeia (European, United States, and Japanese). The medium is a general microbiological growth medium, suitable for environmental monitoring. The medium supports the growth of a wide range of bacteria and fungi. Sometimes a fungal medium is desired, as set out in the previous chapter.

INCUBATION STRATEGIES

This substantive section of the chapter addresses incubation strategies. The primary concern is with the use of a single culture medium, although discussion inevitably spreads to the use of two different agars.

With incubation there are three approaches:

- To use two agars incubated at two different temperatures;
- To use one agar at one temperature;
- To use a dual incubation regime.

There is less preference for two agars, based on sample numbers, expense, and the risks involved with "double sampling" (especially for activities like aseptic processing). Thus many practitioners prefer one agar. As to one temperature or two, the literature for both is assessed here. With this, Marshall, Poulson-Cook, and Moldenhauer (1998) and Symonds, Martin, and Davies (2016) prefer one media at one temperature, whereas Sandle (2014), Gordon, Berchtold, Staerk, and Roesti (2014), and Guinet (2012) favor dual incubation. Where single incubation is recommended this is at 30–35°C, whereas the dual incubation advocates favor a different approach.

Before stepping into the discussion, it is worth noting that the only compendial text that addresses this issue in detail, the Japanese Pharmacopoeia (2011), states that 30–35°C is superior for recovering bacteria; 20–25°C is superior for recovering fungi and that an intermediate range (be that a mid-set point or dual incubation) is superior for recovering both types of microbes, albeit with recoveries slightly lower. This tallies, to an extent, with the USP, which describes a typical incubation regime of 20–35°C for 72 h or greater.

Regarding a two-tiered incubation regime there are two general approaches: to incubate at a higher temperature first followed by incubation at a lower temperature; or, alternatively, to incubate at a lower temperature first followed by a higher temperature. Based on the temperature ranges discussed before this translates as:

- *Option 1*: Incubating at 30–35°C followed by incubating at 20–25°C,
- *Option 2*: Incubating at 20–25°C followed by incubating at 30–35°C.

An additional consideration is required to determine the appropriate time the media is held for at each temperature; considering the time taken for the incubated plates to reach the required temperature and noting the time that plates are placed into an incubator and the day and time when they are removed (either for transfer to the second temperature range or for reading).

With the two different orders of incubation presented before there are different philosophical underpinnings. With the former, where the higher temperature is incubated first, the rationale behind this is that the overwhelming majority of microorganisms recovered from a properly functioning cleanroom will be bacteria with only a few fungi isolated. Therefore it is preferable to orientate the monitoring toward this temperature. Furthermore, there could also be the concern that should fungi be detected and where these fungi exhibit filamentous growth patterns (Sandle, Skinner, & Yeandle, 2013), then should the plates be incubated at the lower temperature first then there is a risk that fungal growth would obscure the plate rendering any bacteria present uncountable. Where plates are incubated at 30–35°C first, fungal growth is inhibited, allowing bacteria to be counted prior to transfer to the 20–25°C incubator and thereby avoiding obscuration by any fungi that might later grow across the agar surface.

The counter argument is that the recovery of fungi should be attempted first because higher temperatures may inhibit fungal growth, or even damage fungal lytic cellular enzymes preventing growth, leading to some fungi not being recovered and therefore resulting in an underestimation of the total count. With the lower temperature step being undertaken first, the argument runs that many bacteria will also be recovered or, where they do not grow at 20–25°C, they are recoverable at 30–35°C after a delayed incubation. It is also possible for some bacteria to be affected by being placed at a higher temperature first. According to Schumann (2000) a heat shock response in replicating microorganisms arising from a sudden increase in incubation temperature may lead to the unfolding of proteins, and hydrophobic amino acid residues normally buried within the interior of the proteins becoming exposed on their surface. This can cause retardation of growth or be life threatening to the cell.

Studies to Evaluate Two-Tiered Incubation

This debate with regards to the single growth medium has been discussed for several decades through various forums without any supporting data being presented in a published paper. Sandle (2014) devised a study which attempts to redress this (other studies have since followed, as presented later).

In approaching such a study, there are two possible approaches that can be taken: an in situ study, which involves assessing the microorganisms recovered in the cleanroom environment or an in vitro study, which involves the plating of cultured test microorganisms and observing the recovery under different incubation conditions. With in vitro studies the spectrum of microorganisms applied should be representative of those found in the manufacturing environment (it would be an error, e.g., to draw upon isolates that would be classed as clinical specimens). Even when this is addressed such studies can be prone to bias. On balance in situ methods are more representative of actual manufacturing conditions and thus this approach is preferred.

Marshall's Study

Prior to Sandle's (2014) study there had been few considerations of the incubation of environmental monitoring plates. One exception was Marshall et al. (1998). Here the authors adopt a direct plate challenge approach using laboratory cultures (an in vivo study). The authors concluded that the general-purpose medium TSA at 30–35°C was superior to the fungal medium SDA at 20–25°C for eight of the nine test organisms. The researchers also found that with the examination of SDA alone, SDA solely incubated at 30–35°C gave better recoveries than SDA solely incubated at 20–25°C.

With this study there is a possibility of an element of strain selection bias. This is because laboratory conditioning of the cultures used may have changed their recovery characteristics compared with naturally occurring strains of the same species isolated directly from the environment, leading to self-selecting pressure. It could also be that the fungi used (species of *Aspergillus* and *Candida* are atypical in preferring higher temperatures compared with those ordinarily recovered from cleanrooms). Moreover, there was no discussion as to why SDA was the appropriate fungal agar to select (fungal agars are discussed in the previous chapter).

Sandle's Study

With Sandle's (2014) study, the incubation times had been set through a previous study and represented a sufficiently long period of time in order to recover any microorganisms present (in addition, literature suggests that most bacteria grow within 2 days and most fungi grow within 5–7 days, although this depends upon the level to environmental stress to which the microorganisms have been subjected and level of sublethal damage). Thus while such length-of-incubation studies are important (Sandle et al., 2013), they were not addressed in detail here (this chapter briefly discusses assessing incubation time in the final section).

The basis of Sandle's study was to consider the use of a general-purpose culture medium incubated at two temperature regimes. Embedded in this was the consideration as to whether a delay in the optimal temperature simply delays growth so all is recovered in the end? Or does the wrong temp lead to loss of viability or countability? The study looked at two incubation regimes:

- Regime A was designed to recover bacteria first, and then to recover fungi, namely:
  - Incubation for a minimum of 2 days at 30–35°C, followed by a minimum of 5 days at 20–25°C.
- Regime B was designed to recover fungi (and some bacteria first), before recovering any other mesophilic bacteria present, namely:
  - Incubation for a minimum of 5 days at 20–25°C, followed by a minimum of 2 days at 30–35°C.

For the study, duplicate contact plates were taken side by side. This provided the closest estimate of "duplicate" that could be achieved. Air samples were not taken due to the considerable variability with sampling an equivalent volume of air given the nonnormal distribution of microorganisms in cleanroom air.

By running such a study there was one of two possible outcomes:

- That there is a significant difference between the two incubation regimes.
- That there is not a significant difference between the two incubation regimes.

When running the study, consideration was taken of Study took note of the time taken for the incubated plates to reach the required temperature, the time that the plates are placed into the incubator, and the day and the time that the plates are removed from the incubator (either for temperature transfer or final read).

The study looked at 39 different cleanrooms, each subjected to a wide variety of environmental conditions, and collected 136 samples. The collected data was examined for the total count (bacterial and fungal colonies). These data were then analyzed using an unpaired Student's t-test (0.05 significance level, 95% confidence interval). This was to determine if there was significant difference between the total numbers of colonies isolated by the two data sets. A summary of the data is presented in Table 4.

As Table 4 shows, the total colony count results for the incubation regime B gave a higher mean count than those from incubation regime A. Here:

- Regime A gave a mean count of 8 cfu/plate
- Regime B gave a mean count of 11 cfu/plate.

While the recoveries were different, significance testing revealed no significant difference between the two incubation regimes. This suggested that there was no optimum incubation regime for total count. However, putting the total count to one side and looking at fungal recoveries only from the 136 data sets, 15 sample results showed fungal colony growth. When these samples were considered it was found that a greater number of fungal colonies were isolated by incubation regime B incubation regime. Here:

Table 4 Collected results from Sandle's dual incubation study

Regime	Number and percentage of samples recording higher counts ($n = 136$)	Mean total (bacterial and fungal) colony count (cfu)
A	39 (28.7%)	8
B	54 (39.7%)	11
Data where results were equivalent	43 (31.6%)	<1

- Regime A recovered ∼ <1 fungal colony
- Regime B recovered ∼11 fungal colonies.

Unsurprisingly, when these findings were subjected to a significance test this time there was found to be a statistically significant difference. On this basis, Sandle's study concluded that incubation regime B produces a higher fungal count. This means an optimal approach for dual incubation would be:

- Regime B: 20–25°C for 5 days, followed by 30–35°C for 2 days

The commencement of the lower incubation temperature first supports the previously discussed literature that higher temperatures of incubation can inhibit fungal growth.

Gordon' Study

Shortly after Sandle's study was published, Gordon et al. (2014) published an incubation study analysis. The researchers showed that the highest recoveries for bacteria occur using TSA at 30–35°C. Whereas at 20–25°C there is a far better recovery of fungi. It was also found that a "two-tiered" incubation gave a statistically significant count when initiated at 20–25°C. When the dual incubation regime began at 30–35°C, significantly lower recoveries were recorded. This finding matched that of Sandle (2014), for the researchers found that recovery of fungi significantly falls with the increase to temperature. They conclude that many fungi found in cleanrooms only have a weak selective pressure to grow within the 30–35°C range. This provides support for a dual incubation regime in order to obtain the most representative count, following the pattern 20–25°C followed by 30–35°C.

Sage's Study

In 2014 Sage and colleagues published a study, where the focus was with a growth-based rapid microbiological monitoring method. This took the form, like Marshall et al. (1998) of an in vivo study where isolates were streaked onto plates and the time-to-result assessed. Three regimes were studied:

- 20–25°C for 5 days
- 30–35°C for 5 days,
- Serial incubation for 48 h at 20–25°C followed by 30–35°C for 72 h.

A reverse dual incubation scheme was not attempted based on previous research which showed that some filamentous fungi are temperature sensitive and hence their growth would be suppressed by being placed in at 30–35°C first (such as *Penicillium brevicompactum* and *Cladosporium halotolerans*). Indeed, the experimental findings found 30–35°C for 5 days to be comparatively weak at recovering fungi.

The outcome was that the "serial incubation" regime produced the highest recoveries. Further work, looking at ways to reduce the time to result found that a single temperature regime of 28°C produced counts that were statistically equivalent to the dual incubation regime.

Symonds' Study

In 2016 Symonds and colleagues published a paper outlining an incubation assessment study. This took a similar approach to Sandle where two samples were taken in the same location. One sample was subjected to a temperature of 20–25°C and the other at a temperature of 30–35°C. A second part of the study looked at dual incubation (20–25°C for 3 days followed by 2 days at 30–35°C). Across the board incubation was for 5 days. Two different culture media were considered: TSA and Sabouraud dextrose agar (SDA). Both contact plates and settle plates were used.

The researchers found that TSA was the most effective medium for the primary isolation of both bacterial and fungal/yeast microorganisms (which matches Sandle's study that TSA gives good recovery). However, there were differences at the two temperatures: bacteria were recovered best at 30–35°C with human commensals providing the largest numbers, while fungi and yeasts showed best recovery at 20–25°C. The use of dual temperature incubation at 20–25°C for 3 days followed by 2 days at 30–35°C gave reduced recovery for both types of microorganisms. The authors conclude that because fungi are relatively rare compared with human commensurable bacteria that a single incubation temperature of 30–35°C is the best approach to take. This can be supported, if necessary, with occasional monitoring at 20–25°C (e.g., following shutdowns).

However, the incubation times adopted in the study are relatively short (especially for a dual incubation strategy) and it could well be that the implementation of a longer initial incubation period at 20–25°C followed by a longer secondary incubation period at 30–35°C for dual temperature incubation could facilitate better fungal/yeast and bacterial recoveries, respectively, and overcome the need to have two sets of plates incubated at different temperatures. Symonds and colleagues to discuss this but they fear that this could extend the time between the occurrence of a contamination event and its detection and thereby delay any response. The Symonds study does not seek to evacuate the incubation time.

Guinet's Study

Another study looking into the order of incubation was undertaken by Guinet et al. (2017). The researchers looked at the following incubation regimes, using TSA:

- 20–25°C for 5 days;
- 30–35°C for 5 days;
- 20–25°C for 3 days followed by 30–35°C for 2 days;
- 30–35°C for 2 days followed by 20–25°C for 3 days.

To examine these regimes the researchers examined four different manufacturing sites. At each site they divided a test cleanroom into 10 squares and took quadruplicate replicates in each square, using settle plates and contact plates. While contact plates can sample approximately similar areas, it is less certain how settle plates can do so.

The analysis of the results showed that optimal growth occurred at 30–35°C, with the most common isolates being Gram-positive cocci, with some non-spore-forming Gram-positive rods. However, for fungi the optimal recovery occurred at 20–25°C (either as a single temperature or as the first incubation step). These patterns were replicated across the four manufacturing sites, with no differences found between them.

Based on the results the researchers drew two conclusions, either:

a. Run environmental monitoring at a single incubation temperature of 30–35°C (routinely) with additional monitoring at 20–25°C to periodically check for fungi, or;

b. Use an incubation regime of 20–25°C for 3 days followed by 30–35°C for 2 days.

Therefore Guinet and colleagues' study (2017) was similar in its conclusions to Sandle's (2014).

The researchers also looked at the optimal recovery conditions for media simulation trials, using tryptone soya broth (TSB), and reached the same recommendations.

Summary of Studies

Putting the findings of the main studies together is shown in Table 5.

The extent to which a consensus can be drawn indicates that while single temperatures of incubation may recover either bacteria or fungi individually each is weak at detecting the other class of organism. While it has been argued by some of the authors that reoccurrences of fungi should not occur

Table 5 Summary of incubation study outcomes (TSA medium only)

Study	Single temperature (20–25°C)	Single temperature 30–35°C	Dual incubation (30–35°C followed by 20–25°C)	Dual incubation (20–25°C followed by 30–35°C)
Marshall	Poor	Optimal	Not considered	Not considered
Sandle	Not considered	Not considered	Weak	Optimal
Gordon	Good fungi, poor bacteria	Good bacteria, poor fungi	Weak	Optimal
Sage	Good fungi, less good for bacteria	Good bacteria, very poor fungi	Not attempted, theoretically weak	Optimal (in addition to single temperature of 28°C).
Symonds	Good fungi, poor bacteria	Good bacteria, poor fungi	Not considered	Weak for bacteria and fungi individually.
Guinet	Good fungi, poor bacteria	Good bacteria, poor fungi	Weak	Optimal

in cleanrooms this does not necessary tally with reviews of cleanroom microbiota (Sandle, 2011) or pharmaceutical product recalls due to fugal contamination (Vijayakumar et al., 2012). Hence a strategy that stands a better chance of detecting bacteria and fungi might be better. With this, the studies suggest that incubating at 30–35°C followed by 20–25°C generates suppressed data and with it the risk of underestimating counts, whereas incubating at 20–25°C followed by 30–35°C leads to higher recoveries and thus more realistic counts.

INCUBATION TIME

Incubation time is as important as the incubation temperature. The question that initially arises is which to assess first? It is this author's view that incubation time needs to be decided once the dual media aspects and incubation temperature questions have been decided.

Once this has been settled, then the maximum incubation time should be assessed for the point at which do colony-forming units stop appearing. Here the research question is: "Is there a point when the media ceases to be able to support slow-growing microorganisms?"

As an example of how to conduct a study, Sandle et al. (2013) provide an experimental approach. The study involves holding plates in an incubator, removing them, counting them, putting them back, and so forth, until now more colonies are visible. Of course, the purist approach does not fit in with the demands of modern manufacturing and there will come a point when simply holding plates in an incubator serves no practical purpose in terms of product risk. What is key to such studies is, therefore, applying statistics to determine the point at which microbial recovery is no longer significant. The "art" behind Sandle's study is, therefore, no so much with conducting the study but interpreting the collected data. This chapter offers no recommendations since each cleanroom and its microbiota will differ. Thus each user will need to conduct their own analysis.

SUMMARY

This chapter has presented some of the common types of culture media used in the pharmaceutical and healthcare microbiology laboratory for environmental monitoring (there are, of course others as required for specialist tests or for use with different microbial identification methods). The chapter has presented some of the general formulations and looked at the applications. To this, some of the requirements for media quality control have been included; of these, the most important is growth promotion testing.

The main part of the chapter has looked at incubation strategies, since getting this right for a given facility is of importance to underpin the robustness of the collected environmental monitoring data.

The most important element is consistency of practice: to use the same incubation parameters so that results can be meaningfully compared over time. The second important consideration is whether to use one or two culture media. This consideration very much depends upon the typical microflora recovered from a facility and it is perhaps sensible to begin with two culture media and, if fungi are not present in high numbers or demonstrably grow equally well on selective and general-purpose agar, then move to adopting a general-purpose agar. A third consideration is the order of incubation (the focus of this chapter).

With the order of incubation, Sandle's investigation of a dual incubation regime where two alternate regimes were considered (to put crudely: higher temperature followed by lower temperature compared with lower temperature followed by higher temperature) showed that, based on total count (bacteria and fungi), the difference between the two incubation regimes was not satisfactorily significant when total count was considered. However, when only considering the fungal count as opposed to the total count, the alternative incubation regime beginning with the 20–25°C step produced statistically higher counts. It is possible to infer from this that an initial incubation at 30–35°C impairs fungal growth.

While this finding is of interest, it should be noted that the overall recovery of fungi was low and that when fungi were recovered, the numbers detected were also low. This supports the general assumption that a well-controlled environment, fungi only represent a small fraction of microorganisms recovered from environmental monitoring samples. Nonetheless, the data did provide sufficient grounds for considering the nature and purpose of incubation regimes for environmental monitoring. It could be, for instance, that rather than establishing a one-size-fits-all monitoring regime, some cleanrooms perhaps lend themselves to monitoring using a selective fungal agar or possibly that different incubation regimes be adopted for different types of cleanrooms.

REFERENCES

Abbott, J. D., & Graham, J. M. (1961). Colicine typing of *Shigella sonnei*. *Monthly bulletin of the Ministry of Health and the Public Health Laboratory Service*, *20*, 51–58.

Abe, M., Ogawa, Z., Tanuma, H., & Kume, H. (2009). Study of mycological examination methods in clinical laboratories—specimen pretreatment and isolation. *Nihon Ishinkin Gakkai Zasshi*, *50*(4), 235–242.

Bridson, E. Y. (1998). *Culture media. The oxoid manual* (8th ed., pp. 2–8). Hampshire, England: Oxoid Ltd. (8th ed., pp. 2–8).

Fabian, M. P., Miller, S. L., Reponen, T., & Hernandez, M. T. (2005). Ambient bioaerosol indices for indoor air quality assessments of flood reclamation. *Journal of Aerosol Science*, *36*, 763–783.

Gao, Z., Perez-Perez, G. I., Chen, Y., & Blaser, M. J. (2010). Quantitation of major human cutaneous bacterial and fungal populations. *Journal of Clinical Microbiology*, *48*, 3575–3581.

Gordon, O., Berchtold, M., Staerk, A., & Roesti, D. (2014). Comparison of different incubation conditions for microbiological environmental monitoring. *PDA Journal of Pharmaceutical Science and Technology*, *68*, 394–406.

Guinet, R. (2012). Les Contrôles Environneuataux site aux rencontres de microbiologie. *La Vague*, *35*, 17–19.

Guinet, R., Berthoumieu, N., Dutit, P., et al. (2017). Multicenter study on incubation conditions for environmental monitoring and aseptic process simulation. *PDA Journal of Pharmaceutical Science and Technology*, *71*(1), 43–49.

ISO (2014) ISO 11133-1:2014 Microbiology of food, animal feed and water—preparation, production, storage and performance testing of culture media, ISO, Geneva, Switzerland.

Japanese Pharmacopoeia Japanese Pharmacopoeia 16 (English Edition) Section G4: Microbiological evaluation of processing areas for sterile pharmaceutical products, 2011, pp. 1312–1316.

Jimenez, L. (2011). Molecular applications to pharmaceutical processes and cleanroom environments. *PDA Journal of Pharmaceutical Science and Technology*, *65*(3), 242–253.

Lapage, S. P., Shelton, J. E., & Mitchell, T. G. (1970). In J. R. Norris, & D. W. Ribbons (Eds.), *Vol. 3A. Methods in microbiology* (p. 116). London: Academic Press.

Marshall, V., Poulson-Cook, S., & Moldenhauer, J. (1998). Comparative mold and yeast recovery analysis (the effect of differing incubation temperature ranges and growth media). *PDA Journal of Pharmaceutical Science and Technology*, *52*(4), 165–169.

Martin, R. (1991). *"Culture media" in quality control: Principles and Practice in the Microbiology Laboratory* (p. 653). UK: Public Health Laboratory Service.

Moldenhauer, J. (2014). Justification of incubation conditions used for environmental monitoring. *American Pharmaceutical Review, 17*, 44–51.

Mossel, D. A. A., et al. (1980). Quality control of solid culture media: a comparison of the classic and the so-called ecometric technique. *Journal of Applied Bacteriology, 49*, 439–454.

Pflug, I. J., Smith, G. M., & Christensen, R. (1981). Effect of soybean casein digest agar lot on number of *Bacillus stearothermophilus* spores recovered. *Applied and Environmental Microbiology, 42*(2), 226–230.

Sandle, T. (2011). A review of cleanroom microflora: types, trends and patterns. *PDA Journal of Pharmaceutical Science and Technology, 65*(4), 392–403.

Sandle, T. (2012). Environmental monitoring: a practical approach. In J. Moldenhauer (Ed.), *Vol. 6. Environmental monitoring: A comprehensive handbook*: Davis Healthcare International Publishing.

Sandle, T. (2014). Examination of the order of incubation for the recovery of bacteria and fungi from pharmaceutical cleanrooms. *International Journal of Pharmaceutical Compounding, 18*(3), 242–247.

Sandle, T., Skinner, K., & Yeandle, E. (2013). Optimal conditions for the recovery of bioburden from pharmaceutical processes: a case study. *European Journal of Parenteral and Pharmaceutical Sciences, 18*(3), 84–90.

Sandven, P., & Lassen, J. (1999). Importance of selective media for recovery of yeasts from clinical specimens. *Journal of Clinical Microbiology, 37*(11), 3731–3732.

Schumann, W. (2000). Function and regulation of temperature-inducible bacterial proteins of the cellular metabolism. *Advances in Biochemical Engineering/Biotechnology, 67*, 1–33.

Symonds, I., Martin, D., & Davies, M. (2016). Facility-based case study: a comparison of naturally occurring species of bacteria and fungi on semi-solid media when incubated under standard and dual temperature conditions and its impact on environmental monitoring approach. *European Journal of Pharmaceutical Sciences, 21*(1), 7–15.

Vijayakumar, R., Sandle, T., & Manoharan, C. (2012). A review of fungal contamination in pharmaceutical products and phenotypic identification of contaminants by conventional methods. *European Journal of Parenteral and Pharmaceutical Sciences, 17*(1), 4–19.

Chapter 8

Particle Counting

CHAPTER OUTLINE

Introduction   125
Particle Counts and Contamination Risk   126
Particle Counters: Operation Basics   128
Limitations of Particle Counters   130
Operational Issues With Particle Counters   131
Limits Setting   133
Frequency of Particle Counting   134
Cleanroom Classification   135
    Particle Sizes   135
    Number of Locations   135
    Location of Particle Counters   136
    Air Volumes to be Sampled   136
    Results Assessment   137
Summary   137
References   138

INTRODUCTION

In addition to the monitoring of viable microorganisms in facilities, the other important consideration for environmental monitoring is an assessment of airborne particles. This is generally considered, erroneously, as *nonviable particle counting*. The act of particle measuring detects all particles of a given size, many of which will include bacteria or fungi attached to carriers in the airstream (so-termed "microbial carrying particles") (Whyte & Hejab, 2007) as well as other types of particles, ranging from liquid droplets, metal, or glass fragments, to clothing fibers (Whyte & Bailey, 1989). The ratio of inert particles to those which are "biologic" (microorganisms or microorganisms bound to matter) is unknown and experiments designed to produce a ratio have been shown to be inconsistent. Nevertheless, the continuous monitoring of particles for activities like aseptic processing can provide a useful measure of the maintenance of environmental controls (Raval, Koch, & Donnenberg, 2012).

Biocontamination Control for Pharmaceuticals and Healthcare. https://doi.org/10.1016/B978-0-12-814911-9.00008-0

Particle counting is performed using optical particle counters. The basis of these instruments dates to first cleanroom spaces developed for gyroscope manufacture during the Second World War (Whitby & Vomela, 1967). These devices detect aerosol particles as they flow through a narrow sensing zone where they are illuminated by an intense beam of white light. Light is then scattered at an angle and individual particles are detected via a photo-multiplier tube. The resultant electrical pulse of given amplitude is reflective of the particle size (Sandle, 2012).

The size of particles is measured in micrometers (commonly abbreviated to "microns"), which is a millionth part of a meter (or a thousandth part of a millimeter). To put size into perspective, visible particles are around 50 μm (e.g., a human hair would be say 50–150 μm), nonvisible particles such as bacteria are somewhere between sub 1 and 15 μm, with plant spores and pollens falling between the visible and nonvisible at around 10–100 μm.

The regulatory guidance is for two sizes of particles to be measured. The key particle sizes for pharmaceutical manufacturing and testing are 0.5 μm (and greater) and 5.0 μm (and greater). It has been speculated that the origins of these cutoff sizes lies in ≥ 0.5 μm particles being intended to represent the typical size of a microorganism and the ≥ 5.0 μm particles the typical size of a skin cell. This is most probably anecdotal since the probable origin of particle sizes relates to superseded NASA standards, which were the first standard written for particle monitoring in cleanrooms and these are provided in imperial measurements. These sizes are selected today because they conform to regulatory standards. There is a greater proportion of 0.5 μm size particles to 5.0 μm size particles in a typical cleanroom (Ensor, Donovan, & Locke, 1987).

In relation to biocontamination control, particle counting, in some senses, is the most important test as it can *dynamically* (and in real time) indicate the quality of the air continuously over time and hence the effectiveness of other clean room parameters, such as pressure differentials, HEPA filtration, and so on (Halls, 2004).

This chapter examines the approach taken for particle counting in cleanrooms and controlled environments, with a focus on the operation of particle counters. There are different types of particle counters found in the pharmaceutical environment: surface counters, liquid counters, and air counters. Given the subject matter of this book, the focus is with airborne monitoring via optical particle counters.

PARTICLE COUNTS AND CONTAMINATION RISK

As discussed in the introduction, a high level of particles may imply corresponding levels of microorganisms (although this relationship has never been determined, Ljungqvist and Reinmuller (1996), consider the relationship to be 10^5 particles: 1 microorganism). Others, however, argue that there is little correlation between viable and nonviable counts, or a fixed ration for comparing values. This becomes more so the cleaner the area, and any correlation relationship slips away (De Abreu, Pinto, & Oliveira, 2004). The best approach when considering the implications of particle counts is to look for changes to trend which may signal deterioration in standards. This deterioration may signal a mechanical issue with some machinery or a hole in a high efficiency particulate air (HEPA) filter, as examples.

It could be assumed that if there is a high particle count then there is chance to obtain a corresponding high viable count, but it may or may not be. Moreover, the presence of microorganisms may not be shown through the viable counting methods outlined in Chapter 6 because these methods are measuring different things and have different metrologies. Essentially the pharmaceutical and healthcare sectors have relatively sensitive total particle counters at its disposal, yet, on the other side the microbiological monitoring methods are relatively poor. In the ideal world, the two sets of data should be comparable to understand the sterility assurance of aspects like aseptic processing; but in the actual monitoring systems we cannot compare data and the microbiological monitoring can also see massive contamination of our processes. Some inroads have been made with spectrophotometric particle counters, as outlined in Chapter 9.

A further variable is the relationship between the concentrations of particles in the air to the risk of these particles settling out onto a surface; where surfaces are "critical" (such as close to exposed medicinal products), then this risk rises. Ascertaining the likelihood of this depends on the adequacy of the cleanroom design and whether the airflow is disrupted, such as the appearance of a new object or through the activities of people. Under unidirectional airflows the risk is lessened through the very fast velocities and directional airflow. Within cleanrooms, where the air is nonunidirectional (generally turbulent), an influencing factor is the air distribution which is a product of the type of air diffuser (a four-way diffuser, for instance, is generally superior to other types). Other variables, as shown through computational fluid dynamics, include the air inlet supply velocity, temperature difference between air supply and the room, and the release position of contamination also influenced the local airborne cleanliness (Whyte, Hejab, Whyte, & Green, 2010).

The particle deposition rate is also a factor of the relative size of the particles, with larger particles being more likely to settle due to gravitational forces ("gravitational sedimentation") and the position of the airstream relative to a surface (air velocity slows down the closer the air is to a given surface) (Whyte, Agricola, & Derks, 2016; Whyte, Whyte, & Eaton, 2012).

The type of surface is also influential if the surface charge differs to the particle charger; here electrostatic attraction forces occur (Whyte, Agricola, & Derks, 2015).

PARTICLE COUNTERS: OPERATION BASICS

Particle counting is performed using a discrete particle counter. This is a device that measures the size and number of airborne particles (some of which will be viable and many more which will be nonviable). The particle counter is a device which draws air in using a pump at a controlled flow rate. The air is passed into a sensor area and through a light beam created by a laser diode. The amount of light reflected from each particle is measured electronically (as an electronic pulse). The larger the particle, then the larger the amount of reflected light (the greater the height of the light pulse). This allows the particle counter to "count" the number of particles in a given volume of air (as the number of light pulses) and to assess the size of the particles counted (Fig. 1).

There are five components that make up a laser particle counter:

1. A laser or high intensity light source.
2. Reflector.
3. Electronic photo detectors.
4. Vacuum pump.
5. Digital counting electronics.

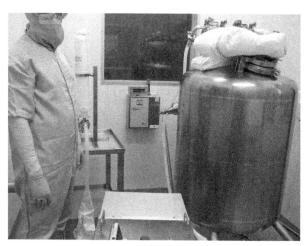

■ **FIG. 1** Particle counting in a cleanroom. *(Image courtesy Tim Sandle.)*

Particle counting is performed using a discrete particle counter. This is a device that measures the size and number of airborne particles (some of which will be viable and many more which will be nonviable). There are five components that make up a laser particle counter:

1. A laser or high intensity light source.
2. Reflector.
3. Electronic photo detectors.
4. Vacuum pump.
5. Digital counting electronics.

Particle counters size particles by matching a signal response generated by the contaminant particle to an equivalent size of polystyrene latex sphere. The counter works by having a photodiode which detects light scattered by single particles passing through a laser, sited within the sensing zone. Light scattering is made up of:

a. Reflected light—when a light hits a particle and is angularly deflected;
b. Refracted light—when a light goes through the particle and its direction of travel is changed;
c. Diffracted light—where light comes close to the particle and is bent around it.

The scattered light from the laser is then concentrated by a lens system and converted into electrical pulses by the photodiode. The amplitude of the pulses is proportional to the particle size and by measuring the height of the signal and referencing it to the calibration curve the counter can determine the size of the particle, and by counting the number of pulses produced by the photodiode the number of particle counts can be determined.

In operation, the particle counter compares the response it is getting from the particle signal to the calibration curve generated with latex spheres. What particle counters typically do is compare the response from the interaction of that particle and the laser light and then relating that, not to some irregular particle of unknown morphology, but to a latex sphere in a background of air. So the instrument itself is not counting and sizing particles, it is counting and sizing flashes of light and relating them to a similar response from latex in air. Therefore particles with different scattering responses will size either smaller or larger relative to the latex standard.

Different particle counters have different flow rates. The flow rate is the rate at which air is drawn into a particle counter, and thus the time taken for the counter to measure a fixed volume of air. The long-standing flow rate has been 1.0 cubic feet per minute (equivalent to 28.3 L/min). This flow rate is the baseline for cleanroom certification.

Counters should be fitted with isokinetic probes, when used in EU GMP Grade A/ISO 14644 Class 5 environments for sterile manufacturing, in order to ensure that the air velocity entering the counter is the same as the speed of the air within the clean zone. A similar requirement appears in the sterile products guidance issued by the US Food and Drug Administration (FDA, 2004).

LIMITATIONS OF PARTICLE COUNTERS

Particle counters, as with other types of instruments used for environmental monitoring, have limitations. The accuracy of the measured size distribution is dependent upon the response of the counter, which is affected by the refractive index and shape of the particles as well as by the optical design of the instrument, including the light source used (Liu, Szymanski, & Ahn, 1985). It is recognized that particle counters, calibrated ISO 21501, are verified to have a counting efficiency of ±50% based on the smallest size measured as part of the calibration exercise, and with the particle size at 1.5 times the smallest size having a counting accuracy of ±20%. Instruments that conform to the relevant part of ISO 21501 (Part 4) (ISO, n.d.) are used for the classification of air cleanliness in cleanrooms and associated controlled environments in accordance with ISO 14644-1 (see later).

Particle counters count different colored particles at different levels of efficiency. The darker the particle, then the less accurate the count will be. This is because the counters count using laser optics. Very black particles may not be counted. It also stands that the recording of large particles may not actually indicate large particles at all. Sometimes smaller particles "clump" together in a way that leads to a large particle being recorded (Gebhart & Anselm, 1988).

It is recognized that most particle counters will give occasional "false" readings, particularly for the 5.0 μm particle count, due to "electronic noise," stray light, or due to a sudden release of particles (Cbannell & Hanna, 1963). What is important, when assessing 5.0 μm particles, is the trend and whether such particles occur regularly. In such circumstances the event is less likely to be "noise" and more likely an indication of a problem.

Counters are also prone to contamination. For example, counters can become contaminated when operated outside of cleanrooms or where disinfectant has been spayed into the counter, among other factors. If a counter is suspected of being contaminated, contamination often resides within the tubing. A flick of the tubing can sometimes indicate contamination. Where there is doubt, the tubing should be changed. Due to particle counters being prone to contamination (such as from disinfectant sprays) it is recommended that counters are capped when not in use and also when disinfection is taking place within the vicinity of the counter.

OPERATIONAL ISSUES WITH PARTICLE COUNTERS

There are several aspects of particle counter operation which need to be considered. These considerations include counting modes, sample volumes, sample sizes, counter positioning, and so on.

With counting parameters, particle counts can be set for one of two counting modes (Akey, 2005):

a. Cumulative count: where the counter is set to count the number of particles for the selected size and greater. For example, if a counter is set to count 0.5 μm particles, it will count all particles at the 0.5 μm and greater (such as 0.5, 0.7, 1.0, 5.0, and 10.0, depending upon the number of available channels on the counter).

> Where two channels are used routinely, the monitoring requirement is:
> - 0.5 μm, which is particles $\geq 0.5\,\mu m \leq 4.9\,\mu m$
> - 5.0 μm, which is particles $\geq 5.0\,\mu m \leq 9.9\,\mu m$

b. Differential mode: where the counter is set to only count the number of particles of the selected size. For example, if a counter is set to count 0.5 μm particles, it will only count particles of the 0.5 μm size. This setting is sometimes used for investigative work, but it is not used for routine cleanroom assessments.

For assessing particle counts according to the EU GMP guide a sample size of 1 cubic meter of air is required (cleanroom classification differs as discussed later) (Eudralex, 2015). This is equivalent to 1000 L. ISO 14644 Part 1 sets out the required sample volumes for cleanroom classification (ISO, 2015a). For continuous particle counting of batch filling, routine spot check sampling and for assessing rooms following maintenance or shutdown, a good policy is to sample one cubic meter. There are times when it is not possible to sample a cubic meter due to a short activity or where an activity is curtailed (such as the end of a product fill, when continuous sampling is being conducted).

Where a full cubic meter cannot be taken it is not good practice to extrapolate the data. This is because particle counts, in a given volume of air and when sampled over a period of time, are not normally or homogenously distributed (Chen, Zhang, & Barber, 1995). The distribution of particles is a probability distribution for the speed of a particle within the air—the magnitude of its velocity. The distribution also depends on the temperature of the system and the mass of the particle. In physics, particularly statistical mechanics, the Maxwell–Boltzmann distribution or Maxwell speed distribution describes particle speeds in idealized gases where the particles move freely inside a stationary container without interacting with one another, except for very brief collisions in which they exchange energy and momentum with each other or with their thermal environment (Laurendeau, 2005). Mass distribution, or distribution of mass with respect to particle size, is the most important particle distribution as far as indoor air quality is concerned. As opposed to extrapolation it is preferable to set a limit based on historical data.

Similarly with some control over sample volume, with particle counters, samples of a size of $<$1 min should not be taken. These are statistically unrepresentative. If a counter is stopped part-way through a 1 min sample (as might occur with the continuous monitoring), the fraction of the minute should be disregarded and data collected up to the last whole minute assessed. This is the reason why, when taking a cubic meter, using a counter counting at one cubic foot per minute, a 36 min sample is taken. With this, sample run times vary according to the design and model of the particle counter. To sample 1 cubic meter using a particle counter that counts at 1 cubic foot per minute takes 36 min (there are 35.2 cubic feet per cubic meter). Likewise, for a counter counting at 2 cubic feet per minute then one 18 min sample is required, and so on.

Another important consideration is with the positioning of the counter. Particle counting should normally be conducted at the working height. This may vary from room to room and between operations. With room locations, for both classification and routine monitoring, the counter is located according to risk assessment. The optimal approach is to locate a counter close to the main activities in the room (such as high personnel presence or where equipment is operating, since this represents the areas of greatest potential contamination risk).

Before using mobile particle counters it is typical for the counters to be purged in the dynamic state. This is in order to assess that the counter is operating satisfactorily and that any high value recorded particles relate to a source other than the particle counter.

Particles can remain inside a particle counter and collect on the laser diode and mirror. The act of regularly "purging" a particle counter assists in keeping the sensor area free from particles and ensures that the measured counts are the "true" counts.

As indicated before, for the monitoring of unidirectional airflows (as required for Grade A/Class 5 environments), an isokinetic probe is required to be fitted to the counter inlet. An isokinetic probe is simply a cup or funnel-shaped inlet accessory specifically designed to gather a representative sample of the area being tested. Its dimensions are based on the volume of the sampled air through the particle counter and the velocity of the sample air as it approaches the probe. When used in turbulent or laminar flow air, the isokinetic probe provides a superior method to terminate sample tubing.

For most environments the particle counter tubing is of importance, to allow a probe to be positioned in the optimal location. The two key considerations are the type of tubing and the length. The tubing should be a type of thermoplastic tubing, either Bev-A-Line tubing or Tygon (these are coextruded tubing consisting of a PVC exterior and a Hytrel interior); polyurethane; or alternatively stainless steel (which can be applied to the measurement of high temperature devices like hot air ovens). In terms of size, the tubing is typically of 13 mm diameter with a bend radius not <100 mm, to avoid particles getting stuck in the tubing. To avoid the phenomena of "drop out," which is a particular problem for 5 μm particles; tubing should be 1 m or less in length (as recommended by the international standard ISO 14644). A related factor is with the tubing diameter for particle loss can also occur due to too great a tubing diameter. The recommended internal diameter of tubing for particle counters, by particle counter manufactures, is 0.6 cm (quarter of one inch). This may vary depending upon the flow rate of the counter.

LIMITS SETTING

For particle counting of controlled environments, the recommendation is that the action level is the recommended guideline from the EU GMP Guide for Grade A and B areas. This guideline is approximately the same as the clean room limits in the ISO 14644 series. Where EU GMP is not appropriate, then ISO 14644 maximum concentrations can be used as the action levels. The user may also elect to set an alert level; this is typically assessed on a review of historical data with the proviso that is remains sufficiently below the action level as to be sufficiently sensitive.

The comparison between EU GMP and ISO 14644 Part 1 is not straightforward since cleanrooms have different limits depending upon whether they are in the "at rest" (static) or "in use" (dynamic) state. Tables 1 and 2 shows some equivalency values.

Table 1 Static or "at rest" state

EU GMP Grade/ISO 14644 Class	Standard			
	EU GMP		ISO 14644	
	0.5 μm counts per cubic meter	5.0 μm counts per cubic meter	0.5 μm counts per cubic meter	5.0 μm counts per cubic meter
A/5	3,520	20	3,520	N/A
B/6	3,520	29	3,520	N/A
C/7	352,000	2,900	352,000	2,930
D/8	3,520,000	29,000	3,520,000	29,300

Table 2 Dynamic or "in operation" state

EU GMP Grade	Standard			
	EU GMP		ISO 14644	
	0.5 μm counts per cubic meter	5.0 μm counts per cubic meter	0.5 μm counts per cubic meter	5.0 μm counts per cubic meter
A/5	3,520	20	3,520	N/A
B/7	352,000	2,900	352,000	2,930
C/8	3,520,000	29,000	3,520,000	29,300
D/9	Not specified	Not specified	35,200,000	293,000

FREQUENCY OF PARTICLE COUNTING

During aseptic batch filling, the EU GMP Guide (Annex 1) requires continuous particle counting (in the dynamic state). For other areas of manufacturing and for nonsterile processing the microbiologist will need to determine the frequency using appropriate risk assessment tools. Particles are measured as counts per cubic meter. Further particle counting should be performed at rest (or in the static state).

An important consideration is the positioning of the particle counter. The location of a particle counter could be determined from:

- The results of the particle count classification study, if one location was "worst case"
- By means of examining the process flow and selecting representative tests of the operation
- By means of risk assessment. For example, does the operation in question impinge on a neighboring cleanroom (perhaps one of a different grade)? In such an example a particle counter may be required to

be placed in the adjacent area. The distance of the particle counter sampling probe from the main activity to be monitored should also be determined.

CLEANROOM CLASSIFICATION

As well as ongoing assessments of pharmaceutical manufacturing areas, particle counters are also used to classify cleanrooms. The common standard is ISO 14644 (most importantly Parts 1 and 2, last updated in December 2015). Here cleanrooms and isolators are classified, according to the appropriate class, as either "as built," "at rest," or "in operation" (Sandle, 2016). Classification is the process of qualifying the cleanroom environment by the number of particles using a standard method. The end result of the activity is that cleanroom x is assigned ISO Class y. Importantly classification is distinct from routine environmental monitoring and distinct from process monitoring, such as the requirement in EU GMP Annex 1 for continuous monitoring of aseptic filling.

The ISO 14644 standard is applicable to cleanrooms used across a range of industries (including semiconductors and other electronics); it therefore needs to be interpreted in relation to its applicability to biocontamination control. Some specific areas are highlighted later (drawn from Part 1 of the standard, with Part 2 providing information about the monitoring required to maintain compliance) (ISO, 2015b).

Particle Sizes

Cleanroom users can elect to look at one or more particle sizes. With GMP, for classification purposes, cleanroom managers need to look for particles equal to or $>0.5\ \mu m$. This means that classification differs from routine monitoring for sterile products (here, as indicated before, EU GMP requires particles of equal to or $>0.5\ \mu m$ and equal to or $>5.0\ \mu m$ to be assessed).

Number of Locations

Earlier versions of the ISO 14644 standard required the user to calculate the surface area of the cleanroom in square meters (Schicht, 2003). From this the square root was taken and the number generated provided the number of particle counter locations. These are then placed at equidistant intervals within the cleanroom. With the 2015 revision, the method changed and became one based on a look-up table. The table uses a range of cleanroom sizes and provides the number of locations required (if the exact room size is not listed, the user selects the next largest room size and picks the

Table 3 Illustration of number of particle count measurements required for different size cleanrooms

Cleanroom	Room size	Number of locations
A	200 m^2	23
B	36 m^2	9
C	8 m^2	4

appropriate number of locations). These numbers are based on a statistical method called hypergeometric distribution. This is very different to the square root approach, which was based on binominal distribution. Without going into statistical detail, the former approach assumed that in each location a particle counter was placed, the particles in the cleanroom were normally distributed. In contrast, the revised approach is based on particles not being normally distributed. The new approach allows each location to be treated independently.

As an example, consider three cleanrooms coded A, B, and C (Table 3).

Location of Particle Counters

Once the number of locations has been selected, the room is divided up into sectors and a particle counter placed in each sector. With the previous standard, these sectors were equal in size and a counter placed in approximate center. With the 2015 standard, the position where the counter is placed within each sector is determined by the user. The standard allows counters always to be placed at the same point within the sector, randomly placed within the sector, or evenly distributed, or selected by risk. The risk-based approach would be the best one to adopt. A risk-based decision could be based on variables like room layout, equipment type, airflow patterns, position of air supply and return vents, air change rates, and room activities. The reason for not selecting the center of the location relates back to the issue of particle distribution: particle counts no longer assumed to be homogenous within a sector.

Furthermore, additional locations can be added at the discretion of the facility. This might arise from the room-by-room risk assessment.

Air Volumes to be Sampled

The volume of air sampled needs to be sufficient to detect at least 20 particles of the largest particle size selected. The standard supplies a formula to be used. The outcome is the number of liters that need to be sampled in each location. The standard requires a minimum of 2 L per location; the application of the formula can result in this being higher. Generally the lower the particle count limit, the greater the volume to be sampled (so a larger volume is taken from an EU GMP Grade B room compared with a Grade C room).

Results Assessment

For assessing results from cleanroom classification exercises, the following approach may prove useful:

1. Recording the results for each location.
2. Convert the results to a cubic meter sample per room.
3. This is set out using the formula published in the standard.
4. It should be noted that the formula states "number of particles at each location or average." This is because an option exists to add more than one particle count location per sector. When this occurs the results are averaged and the average used as the number to proceed with the previous calculation. Individual results may fall outside of the class, provided that the mean is within.
5. Although assessment is based on an average, each individual result must be within limits. Those out of limits need to be investigated.

SUMMARY

The use of particle counters for cleanroom and controlled environment monitoring forms an essential part of the biocontamination control program. Particle counters can be used for continuous monitoring (as is required for aseptic processing); event specific monitoring; and for assessing cleanroom performance, such as air change effectiveness indices used to evaluate the ventilation effectiveness of the cleanroom's air supply. This chapter has outlined the importance of such monitoring activities, drawing out the risks of particles (including microbial carrying particles) being deposited out of the airstream and onto cleanroom surfaces (through forces like gravitational settling, turbulent deposition, and electrostatic attraction). The chapter has discussed the main mechanism for assessing airborne particulates, through the use of optical particle counters, presenting their design features and operational limitations.

The chapter has also focused on the use of appropriate limits and the key requirements for cleanroom classification based on airborne particulate classification.

REFERENCES

Akey, J. (2005). Info overload: What do my particle counts mean? *Indoor Environment Connections, 6*(11), 1–2.

Cbannell, J. K., & Hanna, R. J. (1963). Experience with light scattering particle counters. *Archives of Environmental Health: An International Journal, 6*(3), 386–400.

Chen, Y., Zhang, Y., & Barber, E. M. (1995). A new mathematical model of particle size distribution for swine building dust. *Transactions of American Society of Heating, Refrigerating and Air-Conditioning Engineers, 101*(2), 1169–1178.

De Abreu, C., Pinto, T., & Oliveira, D. (2004). Environmental monitoring: a correlation study between viable and nonviable particles in clean rooms. *Journal of Pharmaceutical Science and Technology, 58*(1), 45–53.

Ensor, D., Donovan, R., & Locke, B. (1987). Particle size distributions in clean rooms. *The Journal of Environmental Sciences, 30*(6), 44–49.

Eudralex. The rules governing medicinal products in the European Community, Annex 1, published by the European Commission, Brussels, Belgium, 2015.

FDA. Guidance for industry sterile drug products produced by aseptic processing–current good manufacturing practice, FDA, Rockville, MD, 2004.

Gebhart, J., & Anselm, A. (1988). Effect of particle shape on the response of single particle optical counters. In G. Gouesbet, & G. Gréhan (Eds.), *Optical particle sizing* (pp. 393–409). Boston, MA: Springer.

Halls, N. (2004). Microbiological environmental monitoring. In N. Halls (Ed.), *Microbiological contamination control in pharmaceutical clean rooms* (pp. 23–52). Boca Raton, FL: CRC Press.

ISO ISO 14644-1, Cleanrooms and associated controlled environments—Part 1: Classification of air cleanliness, ISO, Geneva, Switzerland, 2015a.

ISO ISO 14644-2 Cleanrooms and associated controlled environments—Part 2: Monitoring to provide evidence of cleanroom performance related to air cleanliness by particle concentration, ISO, Geneva, Switzerland, 2015b.

ISO ISO 21501-4:2007, Determination of particle size distribution—single particle light interaction methods—Part 4: Light scattering airborne particle counter for clean spaces, ISO, Geneva, Switzerland.

Laurendeau, N. M. (2005). *Statistical thermodynamics: Fundamentals and applications*: (p. 434). Cambridge: Cambridge University Press.

Liu, B., Szymanski, W., & Ahn, K.-H. (1985). On aerosol size distribution measurement by laser and white light optical particle counters. *The Journal of Environmental Sciences, 28*(3), 19–24.

Ljungqvist, B., & Reinmuller, B. (1996). Some observations on environmental monitoring of cleanrooms. *European Journal of Parenteral Science, 1*, 9–13.

Raval, J. S., Koch, E., & Donnenberg, A. D. (2012). Real-time monitoring of non-viable airborne particles correlates with airborne colonies and represents an acceptable surrogate for daily assessment of cell-processing cleanroom performance. *Cytotherapy, 14*(9), 1144.

Sandle, T. (2012). Introduction to particle monitoring. *Pharmig News, 48*, 6–9.

Sandle, T. (2016). ISO 14644 Parts 1 and 2—The revised cleanroom standard and contamination control. In: R. E. Madsen, & J. Moldenhaurer (Eds.), *Vol. 4. Contamination control in healthcare product manufacturing* (pp. 3–32). River Grove, IL: DHI.

Schicht, H. H. (2003). The ISO contamination control standards—a tool for implementing regulatory requirements. *European Journal of Parenteral and Pharmaceutical Sciences, 8*(2), 37–42.

Whitby, K. T., & Vomela, R. A. (1967). Response of single particle optical counters to nonideal particles. *Environmental Science & Technology, 1*(10), 801–814.

Whyte, W., Agricola, K., & Derks, M. (2015). Airborne particle deposition in cleanrooms: deposition mechanisms. *Clean Air and Containment Review, 24*, 4–9.

Whyte, W., Agricola, K., & Derks, M. (2016). Airborne particle deposition in cleanrooms: relationship between deposition rate and airborne concentration. *Clean Air and Containment Review, 25*(1), 4–10.

Whyte, W., & Bailey, P. (1989). Particle dispersion in relation to clothing. *The Journal of Environmental Sciences, 32*(2), 43–49.

Whyte, W., & Hejab, M. (2007). Particle and microbial airborne dispersion from people. *European Journal of Parenteral and Pharmaceutical Sciences, 12*(2), 39–46.

Whyte, W., Hejab, M., Whyte, W. M., & Green, G. (2010). Experimental and CFD airflow studies of a cleanroom with special respect to air supply inlets. *International Journal of Ventilation, 9*(3), 197–209.

Whyte, W., Whyte, W. M., & Eaton, T. (2012). The application of the ventilation equations to cleanrooms. Part 1: The equations. *Clean Air and Containment Review, 12*, 4–8.

Chapter 9

Rapid and Alterative Microbiological Methods

CHAPTER OUTLINE

Introduction   141
Developments With Pharmaceutical Microbiology   142
Benefits of Rapid and Alternative Microbiological Methods   144
Regulatory Acceptance of Rapid Methods   145
Classes of Rapid Microbiological Methods   146
    Growth-Based Methods   146
    Direct Measurement   146
    Cell Component Analysis   147
    Optical Spectroscopy   147
    Nucleic Acid Amplification   147
    Micro-Electrical-Mechanical Systems   147
Guidance for Selecting Rapid Microbiological Methods   148
    Key Considerations   149
    Internal Company Obstacles   150
    Validation   151
    Method Transfer   154
    Training   154
    Expectations From the Vendor   155
Summary   155
References   156

INTRODUCTION

Conventional microbiological methods, such as the types established in the European and US pharmacopeia, have served microbiologists for decades and have helped to ensure the production of microbiologically safe products. As technology has advanced and scientific understanding has improved, conventional methods have been recognized as having many limitations. Hence rapid microbial methods have become a prevalent topic in microbiology quality control, particularly among QC laboratories with lean or

Biocontamination Control for Pharmaceuticals and Healthcare. https://doi.org/10.1016/B978-0-12-814911-9.00009-2

paperless initiatives, especially through automation, or which seek to improve detection or accuracy in results recovery as part of a contamination control program. Rapid and alternative microbiological method technologies aim to provide more sensitive, accurate, precise, and reproducible test results when compared with conventional, growth-based methods.

The use of rapid and alternative microbiological methods fits with the pharmaceutical industry concerns with risk assessment and the use of real-time monitoring. Quality risk management, for example, is about the adoption of science-based decision making where improved knowledge helps with the quality management of pharmaceutical manufacturing. Quality risk management is a systematic process for the assessment, control, communication, and review of risk to the quality of drug product across the product life cycle. Associated with risk-based pharmaceutical quality assessment systems are the development and implementation of new technologies that fit with the process analytical technology (PAT) approach. PAT seeks to facilitate continuous manufacturing improvements via implementation of an effective quality system.

The adoption of methods is not necessarily a one-size-fits-all proposition for every facility or process. Furthermore, in highly regulated industries such as pharmaceutical manufacturing, it can be difficult to sway the industry away from the tried and true traditional methods.

In general, rapid methods can be grouped into three distinctive categories in accordance with their application. These categories include qualitative, quantitative, and identification methods. Qualitative rapid methods provide a presence or absence result that indicates microbial contamination in a sample. Quantitative methods provide a numerical result that indicates the total number of microbes present in the sample. Identification methods provide us with a species or genus name for the microbial contaminant in a sample. This chapter, while looking at these broad classes and in addressing some of the emerging technologies, is not so much about the different rapid microbiological methods that are available; it is more concerned with some of the considerations that need to be considered for their selection. As such, the chapter provides some advice for the microbiologist to consider when drawing up a rationale for the selection of a rapid or alternative microbiological method.

DEVELOPMENTS WITH PHARMACEUTICAL MICROBIOLOGY

Conventional microbiological methods, including those long-established and described in the European, Japanese, and US Pharmacopeia, have served microbiologists well over the past century and have helped to ensure the production of microbiologically safe products. For example, a wide range of microbiological methods have been successfully verified using plate count methods to enumerate and identify microorganisms (within an accepted margin of error (Sutton, 2011)). However, conventional methods have the limitations. These limitations include the time taken to produce a result and the inability of many methods to recover all of the microorganisms that might be present in a sample.

Considering these issues further, with the time taken to produce a result this relates to the incubation period required for conventional methods that rely on agar as a growth medium. Such methods are relatively slow and results are only available after an incubation period (somewhere between 2 and 10 days, depending on the application) (Gray et al., 2010).

A further limitation is culturability and the issue of "viable but nonculturable (VNBC)" microorganisms. Many bacteria, although maintaining metabolic activity, are nonculturable due to their physiology, fastidiousness, or mechanisms for adaptation to the environment. Some research suggests, for example, that <10% of bacteria found in cleanrooms are culturable (Sandle, 2011). Thus it stands that some rapid microbiological methods (RMMs), especially those that do not rely on growth, may provide a higher recovery count as compared with traditional methods. With rapid methods that do not directly "grow" microorganisms, such as those that detect metabolic activity, it is possible to correlate the new measurements, such as a fluorescing unit, with the old measurement (i.e., the "colony forming unit") and establish new acceptance levels.

These concerns with limitations of conventional methods, as well as the possibilities afforded by technological advances, led to a new generation of rapid and alternative microbiological methods emerging. Rapid microbiological methods (RMM) and alternative microbiological methods include any microbiological technique or process which increases the speed or efficiency of isolating, culturing, or identifying microorganisms when compared with conventional methods (Duguid, Balkovic, & Moulin, 2011).

As to what rapid methods are, according to FDA (FDA, 2008):

> *"RMMs are based on technologies which can be growth-based, viability-based, or surrogate-based cellular markers for a microorganism (i.e., nucleic acid-based, fatty acid-based). RMMs are frequently automated, and many have been utilized in clinical laboratories to detect viable microorganisms in patient specimens. These methods reportedly possess increased sensitivity in detecting changes in the sample matrix (e.g., by-products of microbial metabolism), under conditions that favor the growth of microorganisms."*

Although the use of the word "rapid" is often used to describe the range of techniques employed, some of the methods included within this collective do not give a more rapid result but instead provide a more accurate, precise, or detailed result (and thus the term "alternative" is employed).

RMMs can be applied to a range of microbiological test including raw materials, water, intermediate products, final products, and environmental monitoring. There are a sufficient range of RMMS as to provide an assessment of the microbiological quality throughout an entire production operation. RMMs may also be used by Research and Development. For example, in understanding formulations better in terms of microbial robustness, the support of marketing claims and communicating product benefits to consumers.

RMMs are essentially used as alternatives to four major types of conventional microbiological determinations (Miller, 2005; Moldenhauer, 2008; Noble & Weisberg, 2005):

1. Qualitative tests for the presence or absence of microorganisms (e.g., enrichment turbidity measurements of growth). For example, to determine if *Escherichia coli* is in a sample of water.
2. Quantitative tests for enumeration of microorganisms (e.g., plate count methods, to determine the bioburden of a sample).
3. Quantitative tests for Potency or Toxicity (e.g., what level of endotoxin is in the sample?)
4. Identification tests (e.g., biochemical and morphological characterization)

BENEFITS OF RAPID AND ALTERNATIVE MICROBIOLOGICAL METHODS

Looking at some of the advantages afforded by rapid methods further, aside from the time to result, another important area is area is throughput. Most rapid systems allow for higher volumes than the traditional method. In environments with considerable volumes of raw ingredients, in-process batches and final products to test, a high throughput can confer an important advantage for maintaining manufacturing uptime and moving inventory as quickly as possible.

Furthermore, RMMs can assist with:

- Designing more robust processes that could reduce the opportunities for contamination (fitting in with some quality-by-design objectives),
- Developing a more efficient corrective and preventative action process,
- Confirming that the process is in a continuous state of microbiological control through "real-time" monitoring (that meets some process analytical test objectives),

- Assisting with continuous process and product improvement.

Other advantages include labor efficiency and error reduction. Reducing errors is one of the greatest potential benefits of rapid enumeration. While some methods require extra human intervention—and thus create greater potential for mistakes—others automate the most error-prone processes. Given the right equipment, microbial counting, incubation changeovers, and data entry can all become far more reliable.

Arguably, RMMs enable a proactive approach to be taken to instances of microbial contamination, especially in relation to out-of-specification results. Here RMMs enable quicker responses to out-of-trend situations through providing real-time or near real-time results. This allows for corrective actions to be taken earlier.

Furthermore, when considering a RMM, the new method must offer a higher level of quality assurance. There needs to be a clear and demonstrable benefit in adopting the alternative method. Examples of this include:

- The ability to make critical business decisions more quickly.
- The prevention of recalls through greater method sensitivity to microorganisms.
- The detection of "objectionable" microorganisms.
- Recovery of higher or more accurate microbial numbers.
- Potential reduced stock holding through faster release times.
- Improvement in manufacturing efficiency.
- More proactive than reactive decision making.

It is because of these advantages that RMMs are areas of considerable investment by vendors and attract interest from microbiologists.

REGULATORY ACCEPTANCE OF RAPID METHODS

RMMs are accepted by the major global regulatory agencies. For example, in 2011 the FDA published their new strategic plan entitled "Advancing regulatory science at FDA" (FDA, 2011). In section 0 the FDA undertakes to "Support new approaches to improve product manufacturing and quality." With regard to control and reduction of microbial contamination in products the FDA supports those who:

- Develop sensitive, high-throughput methods for the detection, identification, and enumeration of microbial contaminants and validate their utility in assessing product sterility;
- Develop and evaluate methods for microbial inactivation/removal from pharmaceutical products that are not amenable to conventional methods of sterilization;

- Evaluate the impact of specific manufacturing processes on microbial contamination; and
- Develop reference materials for use by industry and academia to evaluate and validate novel methods for detecting microbial contamination.

CLASSES OF RAPID MICROBIOLOGICAL METHODS

Rapid or alternative methods can be categorized in different ways. On way is based on technology or application. Here, based on the pharmacopeia, the RMMS can be grouped into six categories.

Growth-Based Methods

Growth-based methods, where a detectable signal is usually achieved following a period of subculture (e.g., electrochemical methods). These methods generally involve the measurement of biochemical or physiological parameters that reflect the growth of microorganisms. These methods aim to decrease the time at which we can detect actively growing microorganisms. The methods continue to use conventional liquid or agar media. In summary they include:

- Impedance microbiology (measurable electrical threshold during microbial growth),
- The detection of carbon dioxide (CO_2),
- The utilization of biochemical and carbohydrate substrates,
- The use of digital imaging and autofluorescence for the rapid detection and counting of micro-colonies,
- Fluorescent staining and enumeration of micro-colonies by laser excitation,
- Selective media for the rapid detection of specific microorganisms.

Direct Measurement

Direct measurement, where individual cells are differentiated and visualized (e.g., flow cytometry). These methods generally use viability stains and laser excitation for the detection and quantification of microorganisms without the need for cellular growth. These methods include:

- Direct labeling of individual cells with viability stains or fluorescent markers has been demonstrated with no requirement for cellular growth.
- Flow cytometry (individual chapters are counted as they pass through a laser beam),
- Solid-phase cytometry (staining and laser excitation method).

Cell Component Analysis

Cell component analysis, where the expression of specific cell components offers an indirect measure of microbial presence (e.g., genotypic methods). These methods generally involve the detection and analysis of specific portions of the microbial cell, including ATP, endotoxin, proteins, and surface macromolecules. The methods include:

- ATP bioluminescence (the generation of light by a biological process),
- Endotoxin testing (LAL),
- Fatty acid analysis (methods that utilize fatty acid profiles to provide a fingerprint for microorganism identification),
- Matrix-assisted laser desorption ionization—time of flight (MALDI-TOF) mass spectrometry (microbial identification).

Optical Spectroscopy

Optical spectroscopy methods utilize light scattering and other optical techniques to detect, enumerate, and identify microorganisms (e.g., "real time" airborne pchapter counters). These methods include:

- Real-time and continuous detection, sizing and enumeration of airborne microorganisms and total pchapters. These methods are applied to the monitoring of cleanrooms.

Nucleic Acid Amplification

Nucleic acid amplification technologies such as PCR-DNA amplification, RNA-based reverse-transcriptase amplification, 16S rRNA typing, gene sequencing, and other novel techniques. These methods include:

- Riboprinting: 16S sequence of rRNA is highly conserved at the genus and species level.
- PCR methods for targeting specific microorganisms (millions of copies of the target DNA in a short period of time).
- Gene sequencing (specific dye labeling).

Micro-Electrical-Mechanical Systems

Micro-Electrical-Mechanical Systems (MEMS) utilize microarrays, biosensors, and nanotechnology, to provide miniaturized technology platforms. These methods include:

- Microarrays (DNA chips), evolved from Southern blot technology to measure gene expression (e.g., mycoplasma detection).

The reader should note that many rapid microbiological method signals that are significantly different from the colony-forming unit (cfu)—the mainstay of conventional, growth-based microbiology. Where data is generated by non-cfu rapid microbiological methods, alternative ways of reporting and evaluating the data are required. Moreover, other rapid microbiological methods will produce organism counts (by detecting and quantifying viable cells) that cannot be effectively detected using conventional methods, media, or incubation parameters. These higher recoveries can also prove challenging, especially in the context of defined compendial or regulatory limits.

GUIDANCE FOR SELECTING RAPID MICROBIOLOGICAL METHODS

It is important that care is taken in choosing a rapid or alternative method for a particular application. The method must determine a product's critical quality attribute and adhere to appropriate good manufacturing practice principles and validation requirements (Denoya, Colgan, & du Moulin, 2006).

In some ways, the process of applying introducing a rapid or alternative method does not differ significantly when compared with implementing a conventional method. The key points of ensuring the method is validated and shows acceptable recovery rates or accurate identification does not differ whether rapid or conventional methods are used (Griffiths, 1997).

When choosing to implement a RMM it is important to ensure the new method is appropriate for the company's formulations, facilities, and personnel. For example, the introduction of a method with a higher level of sensitivity needs to be aligned with the existing bioburden in raw materials, environment, and finished products.

Guidance for the implementation of rapid methods is available from both the US Pharmacopeia (USP) and the European Pharmacopoeia (Ph. Eur.):

- USP <1223> "Validation of alternative microbiological methods" (USP, 2011),
- Ph. Eur. 5.1.6. "Alternative methods for control of microbiological quality" (Ph. Eur., 2011a),
- Ph. Eur. 2.6.27 "Microbiological control of cellular products" (Ph. Eur., 2011b).

The Japanese Pharmacopoeia also contains a chapter on rapid method validation (The Japanese Pharmacopoeia, n.d.). The chapter states: "Although it is important in principle that a new method should have an equal or greater capability than the conventional method, a new method may be used after verifying their validity, even in the absence of equivalence to conventional methods." The comment here about not needing to confirm that the new (rapid method) is at least equivalent to the existing compendial method is out of keeping with the Ph. Eur. or USP approaches.

In addition, the FDA (US Food and Drug Administration) has published Guidance for Industry defining validation criteria for growth-based rapid or alternative microbiological methods. From an industry perspective, the PDA publishes a useful guide for implementation (PDA, 2013).

There are several considerations to be made and steps to be taken for the implementation of rapid microbiological methods. These are discussed as follows.

Key Considerations

An important consideration is to decide what is wanted from a rapid method and to consider this alongside a cost–benefit analysis. The first step is to consider the following questions:

- What do I want to achieve?
- How much budget do I have?
- Which technologies are available?
- Which technologies are "mature"? (who else is using them?)
- How "rapid" is the rapid method?
- What papers have been published? (are these "independent"?)
- What have regulators said?

The above can form part of a risk–benefit consideration. Risk–benefit analysis should focus on (Cundell, 2006):

- The defined purpose for the test method,
- The type and depth of information required,
- The limitations of the conventional method and what the rapid method might be able to offer.

Next a more detailed assessment should be undertaken. This includes considering such factors as time, accuracy, and automation.

With time, factors to consider are as follows:

- Time taken to prepare the test: is the rapid method faster, equivalent, or slower?
- Time taken to conduct the test,

- Sample throughout,
- Time to result,
- Whether there is a reduction in the time taken to conduct complementary tests,
- Whether more or less time is required for data analysis,
- Whether results reporting is simplified or more efficient?

With accuracy, issues to consider include:

- If the rapid method will lead to a reduction in human error
- If there is a reduction in subjectivity
- Whether the alternative method will detect more accurately in comparison to a conventional method?
- Whether there is a need for the rapid method to detect what a cultural method cannot?

Other considerations include:

- If there is a need for the electronic capture of data?
- Whether the method needs to be automation?
- If there is a need for connecting apparatus or linking the method to a laboratory information management system (LIMS)?

Internal Company Obstacles

The conventional microbiological methods currently used are, generally, already approved and provide meaningful data. Consequently, there may be reluctance within companies to change procedures and adopt RMMs. Thus arguments relating to the benefits of implementing RMMs may need to be explored.

Furthermore, there may be reluctance to adopt RMMs because of the capital investment in equipment, training, and possible adaption of current manufacturing processes, as well as the time and cost of the important validation required before use. The financial implications are naturally important considerations, and it is recommended that discussions on whether or not to employ new RMMs should involve multidisciplinary personnel, for example, senior management, quality unit, microbiology, production, business development, finance, members of supply chain. With business issues, one of the key concerns is return on investment. This can be assessed by considering the following:

- Operating costs of the conventional method,
- Operating and investment costs of the rapid method,
- Cost savings and cost avoidances of the rapid method.

The following questions can help with this step:

- How much will the validation cost?
- How long will the validation take?
- How many personnel will the validation require?
- How many tests will I need to run for the validation?
- Does the validation require a comparison with another (existing) method?
- How will the data be analyzed and reported?

The cost of implementation should not be considered in isolation as the cost–benefit to the business in terms of higher quality assurance, reduced stock inventory, and quicker release of product may generate cost reduction to the business in excess of the cost of implementation. Capital outlay and running costs will depend upon the RMM chosen and the equipment purchased.

Other aspects that can support a business case include:

- Online/at line systems can result in reduced microbiology testing and finished product release cycle times.
- RMMs can assist in more immediate decisions on in-process material.
- Reduced repeat testing and investigations.
- Maximizing warehousing efficiencies by way of reduced inventory holding.
- Reduction in plant downtime/return from shut downs.
- Increased production yield—shift to continuous manufacturing.
- Maximizing analyst output by eliminating waste activity.

Validation

When choosing an RMM consideration should be given to how it is going to be validated. Any methods that are being adopted need to yield results equivalent to or better than the method currently used which already gives an acceptable level of assurance. In addition, the RMM and the method currently used should be run in parallel for a designated time period as a condition of approval.

Validation will be centered on two key aspects: the assessment of the equipment and an assessment of the materials that the rapid method will assess (to demonstrate that microorganisms can be recovered from the material under test) (Sutton, 2005).

The validation strategy should reflect the RMM selected. Some methods that are based on analytical chemistry will suit validation criteria that include accuracy and precision, specificity, limit of detection, limit of quantification, linearity and range, ruggedness, and robustness. However, microbiology methods do not necessarily lend themselves to this approach to validation (in that not all of these criteria will be applicable), as the FDA indicate (Riley, 2011):

> *"While it is important for each validation parameter to be addressed, it may not be necessary for the user to do all of the work themselves. For some validation parameters, it is much easier for the RMM vendor to perform the validation experiments."*

Therefore the following validation strategy is recommended:

- Define the characteristic of the current test that the RMM is to replace.
- Determine the relevant measures that establish equivalence of the RMM to the current method. This may require statistical analysis.
- Demonstrate the equivalence of the RMM to the current method in the absence of the product sample.
- Demonstrate the equivalence of the RMM to the established method in the presence of the test sample.

More specifically, with certain groups of methods these various validation considerations can be interpreted as:

a. Qualitative methods
- Accuracy and precision, a presence absence test = low number of positives of a low microbial count (<10 cfu)
- Specificity = growth promotion test.
- Limit of detection = inoculate at <5 cfu in both the pharmacopeia method and the rapid method to be tested, over several replicates.
- Robustness = different variations of the normal test conditions, for example, different analysts, different instruments, and different reagent lots.

b. Quantitative methods
- Accuracy = suspensions at the upper end of the expected range and then serially diluted down and testing alongside the compendial method. The level of agreement should not be $<70\%$ compared with the compendia test.
- Precision = a statistically significant number of replicates should be used. The level of variance should generally be within the 10%–15% and should not be larger than that found with the pharmacopeia method.
- Specificity = carried out using a range of microorganisms.

- Limit of quantification = the lowest number of microorganisms which can be reliably counted.
- Linearity a directly proportional relationship between the concentration of microorganisms used and those expressed in the rapid method.
- Range = the results found in precision, accuracy, and linearity can be used here in order to determine the upper and lower limits of the rapid method's detection.
- Robustness = different variations of the normal test conditions, for example, different analysts, different instruments, and different reagent lots.

During the course of validation, deviations from the established criteria may occur. The implications of these will depend upon the seriousness of the issue and the degree of drift from established parameters. The deviation may or may not lead to recommencing the validation after an appropriate change has been made. In the most serious cases the deviation can lead to the abandonment of the qualification and the rejection of the equipment or system. All deviations require a deviation report to be generated. Deviation reports must be reviewed by a competent expert and be accepted by qualify assurance.

With the equipment qualification aspect, validation normally begins with the validation plan (VP). The VP is a document that describes how and when the validation program will be executed in a facility. The VP document will cover some or all of the following subjects:

- Introduction
- Plan origin and approval.
- Derivation.
- Scope of validation activities.
- Validation objectives.
- Validation plan review.
- Roles and responsibilities.
- An overview of activities.
- Division of responsibilities.
- System description.
- Overview of system.
- Overview of process.
- Validation approach.
- Site activities.
- Documentation and procedures.

- Scope of documentation.
- Validation schedule of activities.
- Project master schedule.
- References

From this plan, equipment validation is normally achieved through appropriate installation qualification, operational qualification, and performance qualification (IQ, OQ, PQ, respectively) (Miller, 2010). Here:

- IQ provides documented evidence that the equipment has been provided and installed in accordance with its specification. The IQ demonstrates that the process or equipment meets all specifications, is installed correctly, and all required components and documentation needed for continued operation are installed and in place
- OQ provides documented evidence that the installed equipment operates within predetermined limits when used in accordance with its operational procedures.
- PQ provides documented evidence that the equipment, as installed and operated in accordance with operational procedures, consistently performs in accordance with predetermined criteria and thereby yields correct results for the method.

Method Transfer

If a validated method is transferred to another laboratory (including third parties) appropriate change management should be in place. Full validation of the equipment (IQ, OQ, PQ) will need to be carried out. Full validation of the method may not be required but as a minimum it needs to be demonstrated that the method gives equivalent or comparable results to the original laboratory. Any changes to formulations need to be assessed to determine if full or partial revalidation of the method is required.

Training

It is important that when RMMs are introduced, sufficient training is provided to ensure a successful and complete implementation of the new methods. This should include the microbiologists and other personnel involved in the running of the tests and should also take account of the laboratory or manufacturing facilities. Different rapid methods may also require different steps for sample preparation. Rapid methods that require different preparation steps than traditional methods will require additional training and SOP updates.

Qualified microbiologists will still be required to interpret and manage the data, continue to develop the method, and to ensure that correct decisions are made. This should form part of the overall Microbial Quality Management system.

Expectations From the Vendor

Outside of the suitability of the technology there are a number of points that need to be satisfied in considering a specific technology most notably the experience of the vendor itself. The following points can be useful:

- What is the vendor's expertise to date?
- Is the vendor in a position to support your validation process?
- Does the vendor have the relevant QMS procedures in place?
- What stage is the vendor at in terms of development? For example, is the company financially sound?
- Is the technology known to regulators?
- Has the vendor made any product filings to regulators?
- Does the vendor supply relevant documentation with the technology (e.g., design of documents, providing material standards, and so forth?)
- Does the vendor provide training to analysts?
- Is the vendor in a position to react with a reasonable response time to technical issues?
- How often does the vendor envisage system/software updates and how will these be handled?

SUMMARY

Effective monitoring of pharmaceutical manufacturing processes can ensure that a state of control is being maintained (both in terms of the capability of processes and the effectiveness of controls designed to meet product quality). Here more accurate and sensitive microbiological methods play an important part. Moreover, such methods can help a manufacturer to focus on those areas for continual improvement (such as with understanding and reducing process variability). Furthermore, process and product understanding can be enhanced through increased knowledge. Furthermore, the use of advanced methods fits in with quality risk management approach and the central concerns of a biocontamination control strategy. This includes improving process design to prevent contamination or improving the data available to help to investigate a contamination event, and for providing corrective and preventative actions (Sandle, 2015).

The types of rapid microbiological methods discussed in this chapter have been classed as growth-based methods (rely on the measurement of biochemical or physiological parameters that reflect the growth of microorganisms), viability-based methods (viability stains and laser excitation for the detection and quantification of microorganisms without the need for cellular growth), cellular component methods (detection and analysis of specific portions of the microbial cell), and so on. This array highlights the richness and different types of methods available.

This chapter has outlined some of the key considerations to be made when deciding whether to adopt a rapid method and then subsequently for selecting between the different types of rapid methods that are available. The chapter did not set out to differentiate between different technologies (this itself is a rapidly developing field), but more to offer general advice to those tasked with making the selection and undertaking the work required to qualify the method so that it is available for the laboratory or process area to use.

REFERENCES

Cundell, A. M. (2006). Opportunities for rapid microbial methods. *European Pharmaceutical Review, 1*, 64–70.

Denoya, C., Colgan, S., & du Moulin, G. C. (2006). Alternative microbiological methods in the pharmaceutical industry: the need for a new microbiology curriculum. *American Pharmaceutical Review, 9*, 10–18.

Duguid, J., Balkovic, E., du Moulin, G.C. (2011). Rapid microbiological methods: where are they now?, American Pharmaceutical Review, November 2011: http://www.americanpharmaceuticalreview.com/Featured-Chapters/37220-Rapid-Microbiological-Methods-Where-Are-They-Now/.

FDA (2008). Guidance for industry validation of growth-based rapid microbiological methods for sterility testing of cellular and gene therapy products, FDA, Bethesda, MD.

FDA (2011). Strategic plan for regulatory science, FDA, Bethesda: MD, http://www.fda.gov/downloads/ScienceResearch/SpecialTopics/RegulatoryScience/UCM268225.pdf.

Gray, J. C., Staerk, A., Berchtold, M., Hecker, W., Neuhaus, G., & Wirth, A. (2010). Growth promoting properties of different solid nutrient media evaluated with stressed and unstressed micro-organisms: Prestudy for the validation of a rapid sterility test. *PDA Journal of Pharmaceutical Science and Technology, 64*, 249–263.

Griffiths, M. W. (1997). Rapid microbiological methods with hazard analysis critical control point. *Journal of AOAC International, 80*(6), 1143–1150.

Miller, M. (2010). The implementation of rapid microbiological methods. *European Pharmaceutical Review*, (2), 24–26.

Miller, M.J. (2005) Encyclopedia of rapid microbiological methods. Parenteral drug association and Davis, Healthcare International Publishing, LLC, Bethesda, MD, p. 103–35.

Moldenhauer, J. (2008). Overview of rapid microbiological methods. In M. Zourob, S. Elwary, & A. Turner (Eds.), *Principles of bacterial detection: Biosensors, recognition receptors and microsystems* (pp. 49–79).

Noble, R. T., & Weisberg, S. B. (2005). A review of technologies for rapid detection of bacteria. *Journal of Water and Health, 3*, 381–391.

PDA 2013. Technical Report No. 33, Revised 2013 (TR 33) Evaluation, validation and implementation of alternative and rapid microbiological methods.

Ph. Eur. (2011a). Alternative methods for control of microbiological quality. In *European Pharmacopoeia*. (7th ed.). Strasbourg, France: European Directorate for the Quality of Medicines. Section 5.1.6.

Ph. Eur. (2011b). Microbiological control of cellular products. In *European Pharmacopoeia*. (7th ed.). Strasbourg, France: European Directorate for the Quality of Medicines. Section 2.6.27.

Riley, B. (2011). A regulators view of rapid microbiology methods. *European Pharmaceutical Review*, *16*(5), 3–5.

Sandle, T. (2011). A review of cleanroom microflora: types, trends, and patterns. *PDA Journal of Pharmaceutical Science and Technology*, *65*(4), 392–403.

Sandle, T. (2015). Approaching microbiological method validation. *Journal of GXP Compliance*, *19*(4), 1–15.

Sutton, S. (2005). Validation of alternative microbiology methods for product testing quantitative and qualitative assays. *Pharmaceutical Technology*, 118–122. April 2005.

Sutton, S. (2011). Accuracy of plate counts. *Journal of Validation Technology*, *17*(3), 42–46.

The Japanese Pharmacopoeia, Seventeenth Edition (JP17). http://jpdb.nihs.go.jp/jp17e/.

USP (2011). USP <1223> Validation of alternative microbiological methods. In *United States Pharmacopeia* (34th ed.). Rockville, MD: The United States Pharmacopeial Convention.

Designing and Implementing an Environmental Monitoring Program

CHAPTER OUTLINE

Introduction   159
Frequency of Monitoring   161
   A Risk-Based Approach   163
Time of Monitoring   167
Duration of Monitoring   168
Locations for Monitoring   169
Monitoring Methods   171
Cleanrooms in Different Operating States   172
   Newly Built Cleanrooms   172
   In-use Cleanrooms   172
   Other Considerations   173
Assessing Cleaning and Disinfection Effectiveness   174
Data Review   174
Monitoring for Particulates   175
Staff Training   176
Written Program   176
Summary   177
References   177

INTRODUCTION

An environmental monitoring program is of great importance, as Chapters 4 and 5 indicate, to the overall biocontamination control strategy and is a regulatory expectation. However, such a monitoring program will only yield good information if it is designed properly. Despite such importance there is little information available in the literature and little in the pharmacopoeia when it comes to constructing the program (the USP gives some information for sterile manufacturing and there is a little in relation to bioburden control; the European Pharmacopeia makes no reference). Some information is

Biocontamination Control for Pharmaceuticals and Healthcare. https://doi.org/10.1016/B978-0-12-814911-9.00010-9

provided in ISO 14698, but for the most part the program needs to be constructed by the site microbiologist (Sandle, 2012a).

In order to establish a program, it is necessary to assess the process areas, especially those at a higher risk for potential microbial contamination. This information will be useful not only to determine the extent of the program, types, and frequency of testing, but also the levels.

The purpose of the microbiological environmental program can be summarized as follows:

- Provide crucial information on the quality of processing environment during manufacturing.
- Prevent future microbial contamination by detecting and reacting to adverse trends.
- Prevent the release of a potentially contaminated batch if the appropriate standards are not fulfilled.
- Prevent the risk of contamination of the dosage form to the recipient of the pharmaceutical product.
- Ensure the environmental controls in the production areas.
- Provide a profile of the microbial cleanliness of the manufacturing environment and serve as a tool for assessing sanitation procedures.

The design of an environmental monitoring program does not differ greatly between a sterile and nonsterile manufacturing site in terms of the overall design. The differences that emerge relate to the limits applied, the frequency, and the intensity of the monitoring (Dell, 1979).

Therefore in terms of assigning monitoring locations and frequencies, both sterile and nonsterile manufacturing need to be based on a scientific rationale. The key issue to consider is that each manufacturing facility is unique (Reich, Miller, & Patterson, 2003). Many variations exist and there can be no perspective program imposed. Variations include the process technology, room sizes, number of personnel present for a given activity, the overall design, and so on. This adds a degree of complexity to the monitoring program.

The complexity leads to different factors to be accounted for in designing a monitoring program. The following important aspects must be considered (Jimenez, 2004):

i. How frequent should the monitoring be?
ii. How long should the monitoring last for?
iii. How should the locations for monitoring be selected? (sample site rationale)

iv. Include site maps
v. How should the monitoring program react to cleaning and disinfection practices?
vi. Describe the sampling procedure
vii. Describe sample handling
viii. Describe the sample incubation regime
ix. Outline the methods for data analysis (statistical data trending)
x. Outline the investigative responses to exceeded action levels
xi. Include detail about the establishment of alert and action levels
xii. Describe the execution responsibilities

These issues need to be considered for both viable and nonviable contaminants. In doing so, the core purpose of environmental monitoring must be borne in mind (Moldenhauer, 2008):

- To demonstrate that environment quality is consistently within specified levels.
- To provide a timely and sensitive warning if the environmental quality or its control is becoming or have become unacceptable.
- To initiate a timely, comprehensive planed course of action whenever environmental monitoring results are indicative of unacceptable environmental quality or control (i.e., an "excursion" or an out-of-limits event).

Each of the earlier issues is examined in this chapter. Generally, the discussion relates to viable monitoring (with the methods outlined in Chapter 6 of this book). Particle counting is addressed in a separate chapter (Chapter 8).

FREQUENCY OF MONITORING

The frequency of environmental monitoring is a complex issue. A manufacturer will need to consider the risk of not monitoring a process step against the amount of resources available. Generally, for sterile manufacturing, environmental monitoring should be performed during each operation during batch filling and at a set frequency for other areas in relation to the manufacturing process (such as weekly for Grade C areas and perhaps monthly for Grade D areas) (Sandle, 2012b).

Hence, for sterile areas, a typical regime is:

- Monitoring performed for each operating shift in the Grade A/ISO Class 5 zone and for those Grade B/ISO Class 7 cleanrooms which are part of the batch fill or are associated with the batch fill. Each operating shift is defined as the duration of the batch fill and to cover all staff involved with the filling process. It is important to monitor staff shift "change-overs" and to note when this occurs in relation to the data any trends that emerge.

- Other Grade B areas daily.
- Grade C/ISO 14644 Class 8 (in operation) weekly.
- Grade D monthly.

For aseptic processing samples of air are taken at defined time intervals during the fill, and surfaces samples are taken at the end of the fill. This is because the latter are disruptive and the risk of personnel intervention is too great during filling. Furthermore, samples from each individual present in the fill should be monitored. A pragmatic approach could be adopted where there are two or more batches being filled during the same working day, where the rooms which support the batch fill operations (e.g., freeze-drying) will only be sampled once (Hertroys, Vught, & Donk, 1997).

For those Grade B/ISO Class 7 rooms, which are captive to an aseptic filling suite, but are not related to a batch fill, the sampling frequency would normally be weekly, fortnightly, or monthly depending upon the room use. This would be justified on the basis that these rooms have no direct bearing on the quality of the filling environment, but the rooms still require a high level of monitoring because of their being part of the aseptic filling suite and as indicators of contamination build up to the most critical area. Because this monitoring is not related to a specific filling activity and there is a high probability of personnel not being present, very often, the monitoring program will be biased toward surface sampling methods (Sandle, 2017).

In addition to batch- and process-related manufacturing, additional sampling sessions may be performed in response to particular events, such as immediately after cleaning and sanitization so that the effectiveness of the sanitization can be assessed and following maintenance to the cleanroom physical design (such as following the replacement of HEPA filters). Further reasons for monitoring may include routine sweeps using selective agars (such as during times of the year where fungi may be a concern, such as, the autumnal months) (Sandle, 2015).

When establishing the environmental monitoring program the tendency would be to err on the side of oversampling. At first glance, this seems like an easy solution but for many manufacturers it is simply not feasible from a cost or personnel perspective. Environmental monitoring is something to which considerable resources can be thrown and thousands of results produced. This can be both a wasteful and meaningless exercise unless the monitoring has been thoughtfully targeted and the data correctly interpreted to ascertain the "true" trends. The expense associated with purchasing, validating, and maintaining sampling equipment, supplies, and training personnel is often prohibitive. The best way forwards is based on a detailed examination of the process and the use of a risk-based assessment (Sutton, 2010).

For nonsterile production the common approach is to undertake risk assessment; routine dynamic monitoring of the "clean" environment and operations is important to ensure that modes of bioburden introduction are under control.

A Risk-Based Approach

As with many aspects of pharmaceutical microbiology, when establishing the frequency of environmental monitoring using a risk-based scheme, there is no clear right or wrong approach. The process of risk management includes the identification of risks, the assessment of risks, the prioritization of risks, the development of risk responses, and risk monitoring (and it should be remembered, when assessing pharmaceutical facilities, that environmental monitoring is but a small part of overall risk management and that environmental monitoring is not a risk-prevention tool, but a risk-monitoring tool).

When formulating a risk-based approach to environmental monitoring the areas of monitoring can be divided up based on their criticality to the process. As the process becomes more "critical" the level of risk is deemed to rise and the frequency of environmental monitoring and the number of samples in a given area increases. An example of this is illustrated in the following process flow diagram. The diagram depicts an aseptic manufacturing, where raw materials are handled in a Grade D/ISO Class 9 area and through to the formulated product is filled under Grade A/ISO Class 5 conditions.

The approach is relatively simple in that monitoring frequencies increase the "cleaner" the cleanroom becomes and arguably the risk to contamination to the product rises.

The previous approach can be expanded by dividing each area into sub-zones. For example, taking the aseptic filling of a pharmaceutical product:

Critical Areas in Aseptic Filling

1a—Area of aseptic processing where product is exposed (e.g., exposed vials bring filled);
1b—Area where product vials are closed (e.g., immediately after stoppering);
1c—Support areas under UDAF for aseptic processing (e.g., stopper bowls).

By focusing down on each process step, the microbiologist can direct the level of monitoring where the risk is greatest. Here the greatest risk befalls the exposed vials (step 1a, earlier) as opposed to where the product vials have been stoppered (step 1b, earlier). Although steps 1a to 1c each are important, and each requires monitoring, contamination at 1a could lead to an automatic batch rejection, whereas a case could be made to release where contamination occurs at steps 1b or 1c through risk assessment. This process will depend upon the type of product being manufactured and other circumstances.

Where different types of products are manufactured within the same facility, the frequencies of monitoring can be revised depending upon the type of product. Here aseptically filled products are at a far greater risk and demand a greater level of control than tablets, given that the former must be theoretically free of all microorganisms whereas the latter can have a low level of bioburden provided the product is free from objectionable microorganisms. In response to this difference, as per Table 1.

For supporting rooms and lower grade cleanrooms, the frequencies of monitoring for both sterile and nonsterile manufacturing can be approached by examining the operation taking place in each room within the facility.

For example, establishing the appropriate viable monitoring frequencies, for routine operations could be based on a review of the following factors:

1 Room activity such as process, storage, office/administration, washing, sterilizing, such as autoclave operation, sterile filtration, and sterile filling. The key questions to consider are as follows:
    - What is going on?
    - When is it taking place?

Table 1 Different frequencies of monitoring based on the type of product manufactured

Area	Frequency of monitoring
Parenteral solutions (aseptically filled)	HIGH
Ophthalmic solutions	
Inhalation solutions	
Aerosol inhalants	
Nasal sprays	MEDIUM
Vaginal and rectal suppositories	
Topicals	
Oral liquids	
Oral tablets and capsules	LOW

- What type of equipment is involved?
- How many personnel are involved?

2 Exposure risk.
- For how long is the product exposed?
- Is open processing involved? If so, for how long? (such as none, enclosed, open momentarily but mostly enclosed, open plant assembly, e.g., the difference between the operation of centrifuges as opposed to processing open product).

3 Room temperature.
- Cold, warm, or ambient? The difference here would be between a cold storage area and an autoclave preparation room.

4 Process stage.
- Raw material processing, intermediate manufacturing or final formulation?

5 Duration of process activities.
- Short, medium, or long term relative to all operations? For example, short may be <30 min, medium 1–4 h, long >4 h.

6 Water exposure.
- Is this high, medium, or low relative to all operations? This could be absence; medium may relate to water outlets being present in room or floor likely to be wet; and high could be a washup area).

This approach to the frequency of viable microbiological monitoring can lead to the construction of what is sometimes referred to as a "criticality assessment" of the cleanrooms.

Criticality Factors

The criticality assessment approach can be used to construct so-called criticality factors, where a given factor determines a given frequency of environmental monitoring. Given a large cleanroom facility it is not possible, without considerable time and cost, to monitor all areas to a high frequency. The author's own experience has involved a suite of 215 cleanrooms and a staff of three! In such circumstances monitoring needs to be rationalized by establishing a criticality scheme on which monitoring frequencies are based. Under this approach the final formulation process would receive more monitoring than an early stage of the manufacturing campaign that has a relatively closed process.

An example of monitoring frequencies under such a scheme could be, as per Table 2.

Each controlled area would need to be evaluated against set criteria and, with the use of a series of guiding questions, the monitoring frequency

Table 2 Examples of monitoring frequencies presented as criticality factors

Criticality factor	Frequency of monitoring
1	Daily/each batch
2	Weekly
3	Fortnightly
4	Monthly
5	Three-monthly
6	Six-monthly

Note: Generally, the frequency of monitoring increases the further the production process moves toward bulk product. Each cleanroom would be evaluated against set criteria and, with the use of a decision tree, the monitoring frequency would be determined.

would be determined. Decision criteria include considerations in two category areas: areas of higher weighting and areas of higher monitoring frequency. Examples of these categories could include:

Giving higher weighting to:

- "Dirtier" activity performed in a room adjacent to a clean activity, even if the clean activity represents later processing
- Areas that have a higher level of personnel transit (given that people are the main microbiological contamination source). This may include corridors and changing rooms.
- Routes of transfer
- Areas that receive incoming goods
- Component preparation activities and sites
- Duration of activity (such as a lower criticality for a 30-min process compared to a 6-h operation).

Having higher monitoring frequencies for:

- Warm or ambient areas as opposed to cold rooms
- Areas with water or sinks as opposed to dry, ambient areas
- Open processing or open plant assembly compared to processing that is open momentarily or to closed processing (where product risk exposure time is examined)
- Final formulation, purification, secondary packaging, product filling, and so on.

The decisions for each cleanroom should be reviewed at regular intervals. This may invoke changes to a rooms status (and hence its monitoring frequency) or to changes for different sample types within the room. For example, it maybe, that after reviewing data for 1 year, that surface samples produce higher results than air samples for a series of rooms. In this event the microbiologist may elect to vary the frequency of monitoring and take surface samples more often than air samples. There should also be an increased focus on cleaning and disinfection practices and frequencies based on such results (Denny, Kopis, & Marsik, 1999).

There are other reasons for varying the frequency of monitoring surface samples with respect to air samples. This is because air samples are direct indicator of the quality of the process and assign a level of control to the process, whereas surface samples indicate cleaning and disinfection. Air samples should generally be targeted toward an actual event taking place (such as key process step that might generate viable microorganisms, such as product mixing in an open can). In contrast, surface monitoring tends to be directed toward either a pre- or a postclean time, depending on the actual data required. If the results of surface samples are generally satisfactory, as indicated by trend analysis, then either the number of samples or the frequency at which they are taken can be reduced. If subsequent data showed an increase in counts the monitoring frequency could easily be restored. Indeed, all types of monitoring frequencies may increase as part of an investigation as appropriate.

Surface monitoring can also be further differentiated between floors and other surfaces, and between surfaces at working height. Surfaces at working height generally have tighter limits and are considered to be more critical as they are in closer proximity to the product. Surfaces at working are often horizontal surfaces. The differentiation between floors and surfaces using different monitoring limits is justified because no product touches the floor.

In summary, floor monitoring is generally a check of cleaning and basic hygiene; working height monitoring is designed to test the surface conditions close to the product processing steps, reagent preparation, and so on.

TIME OF MONITORING

Connected with the overall frequencies of monitoring is a consideration for the time of monitoring. It could be assumed that under dynamic conditions that worst-case times are the same as equal case times (i.e., any time of monitoring is equivalent to any other when the process is ongoing in terms of giving the "true" picture of contamination, and that trend analysis is the only way to measure true changes). This may or may not be the case and this issue can only be unraveled through a thorough understanding of the facility (Cundell & Bean, 1998).

Some parts of processing may be very specific and it may be important to direct monitoring toward certain events (such as air sample monitoring when a centrifuge is operating). Again, the consideration of the risk to the product is the key factor to weigh up. Example of specific events could include:

- Filling machine strip down;
- Loading freeze driers;
- Loading autoclaves and Isolators;
- Operation of centrifuges and C-I-P units (especially in relation to particle count generation).

There are other time-based events for consideration (Cundell, Bean, Massimor, & Maier, 1998). If a facility has been nonoperational for a few days (such as a bank holiday weekend) or over a shutdown it may be prudent to begin sampling a few days prior to production start-up in order to establish a base line. For sterile manufacturing areas, as part of the start-up program of cleaning and disinfection, facilities should always be monitored prior to any activity taking place. Where sufficient data has been gathered the facility may be used "at risk" based on good historical data and the data collected on the same day as processing begins. This will be necessary for the firm to decide how to approach this by way of a rationale and the degree of risk that is deemed acceptable.

DURATION OF MONITORING

Following on from considerations of the frequency of monitoring, the next logical question concerns for how long monitoring should take place for? This is relatively straightforward for viable monitoring for batch filling operations (within the Grade A/ISO Class 5 zone and the Grade B/ISO Class 7 room in which the fill takes place). This must be at intervals during the entire duration of the fill (the intervals will be at a random time during the fill for active air samples; and for the entire duration of the filling operation using settle plates alongside continuous particle counting). If it can be considered that no specific time represents "worst case," based on the discussion before, and therefore any given time is "equal case," so random sampling is justified. For the types of samples previously discussed, typical sampling regimen is:

- Settle plates are exposed for the duration of a fill (additional settle plates may need to be used if the fill exceeds the validated plate exposure time).

- Active air samples will be taken at the (near) start, (near) middle, and (near) end of the fill.
- Finger plates will be taken immediately after a:
  - Connection activity, for any persons present during the fill at a random time during the fill;
  - After a Grade A/ISO Class 5 zone intervention;
  - After any item of critical equipment is inadvertently touched;
  - When some activity has taken place by which aseptic technique or practice could be compromised.
- Plates should also be taken at any other time a microbiologist believes it to be necessary (random personnel sampling is often encouraged by the FDA).
- Surface monitoring (direct contact samples) will take place immediately at the end of the fill. This should not be performed during filling due to the invasive and disruptive nature of the techniques.
- Contact plates of gowns will be taken from all personnel immediately before they exit the Grade B/ISO Class 7 area (Aseptic Filling Suite).

For Grade C/ISO Class 8 and D process areas and in nonsterile manufacturing, other viable monitoring should be for a defined periods of time during an event or a process. Active air samples should be run so that one cubic meter of air is sampled and settle plates must be exposed for more than 1 h where possible (and extrapolated to express results as colony-forming units per 4 h). Exceptions to this include activities that are of a short duration where number of colony-forming units per event might be a preferable expression of the result to number of colony-forming units per 4-h exposure.

Surface monitoring should be performed at some point during the dynamic state. Again, if it is not considered that any given time represents "worst case," then any randomly sampled time represents "equal case" for a sample taken during the process.

LOCATIONS FOR MONITORING

Before considering the appropriate locations for microbiological monitoring it is an appropriate juncture to pause to consider the phenomena of microbial attachment to surfaces as this is a critical consideration for surface sampling.

Microorganisms will move around a clean area depending upon the design of the facility and the effectiveness of HVAC operational parameters such as the number of air changes per hour. The dispersal of microorganisms in non-laminar flow zones occurs relatively easily. Eventually any microorganisms present are either removed from a clean area or they are deposited onto a surface. There is no surface that will be totally free from the possibility of microbial attachment, although the design of surfaces can minimize the possibility.

Microbial adhesion is a complex and significant event in pharmaceutical cleanrooms and hospital pharmacies. There are several mechanisms by which microorganisms colonize a surface. The four common steps involved are transport, initial adhesion, bioattachment, and colonization. However, in general bacterial adhesion to a material surface can be described as a two-phase process including an initial instantaneous and reversible physical phase (phase one) followed by a time-dependent and irreversible molecular and cellular phase (phase two) (An & Friedman, 1997).

The transportation of a microbial cell to a surface is either by direct physical contact or as a result of gravity, convection, or diffusion. Once contact has been made with a surface the microbial cell can adhere to the surface either "reversibly" (i.e., temporarily) or "irreversibly" (i.e., permanently) through a combination of chemical or electrostatic forces. Irreversible attachment is more commonly associated with water systems in relation to the secretion of glycocalyx and the formation of biofilm communities5. This is outside the scope of this module.

Reversible attachment can be for a matter of a few seconds as microorganisms are dispersed around a facility or for longer time period whereby the microorganism could be dislodged from the sediment at a later date. Particles on the floor that are not completely contained or trapped to a surface will eventually, through air movement and vortices, become resuspended into the air. The level of resuspension could potentially impact upon product quality through greater opportunities for transmission. This poses problems for dealing with contamination control and the risk of transfer or redispersal into clean areas. Various studies have shown that transfer of contamination by people walking across floors has one of the highest redispersal factors.

There are a number of variables that affect the nature of microbial attachment to surfaces. These include surface type, bacterial species, moisture level, pressure, and friction. In some circumstances microorganisms can be very resilient to removal and hard to destroy by disinfection. For example, the phenomena of attachment can be enhanced for those bacteria possessing fimbriae as these are more difficult to dislodge. A second example is that transfer from moist surfaces is easier than for dry surfaces. These examples highlight the difficulties and complexities associated with the relationship between microorganisms and surfaces.

As indicated earlier, there is naturally a concern with the number of microorganisms and the ease of dispersal in critical areas. The risk from microorganisms is the contamination of personnel clothing and equipment, and the transfer to critical areas and potentially to product. There are different ways to avoid such contamination. Assuming that people are the source of contamination (i.e., all physical aspects of a cleanroom are operating satisfactorily) then there are four possible approaches to consider for the minimizing of contamination risk. The first approach would be concerned with preventing contamination from entering the critical area in the first place. The second would be focused on the physical removal of contamination, the third with the reduction of viability, and the fourth with destruction. Any microbiological monitoring program will need to consider which combinations are likely and which should be monitored and thus comprise part of the routine program.

In summary, a number of factors need to be considered when selecting sample sites to be included in the monitoring program:

- What is the level of activity and is it variable?
- Is there site product contact?
- Can microbial growth occur during production or between cleaning and disinfection of the site?
- Is the site inaccessible or difficult to clean and disinfect?
- Can activity in the area or the item itself contribute to the spread of contamination?
- Can sampling interfere with the manufacturing process and increase the risk of product contamination (as with aseptic filling)?
  - Open processing requires more frequent monitoring.
- Is the site wet or dry?
  - Wet areas are at greater risk of contamination.
- Is there any environmental monitoring history?
  - Sites with a troubled history will require more monitoring.

MONITORING METHODS

Monitoring methods are neither precise or absolute, which is the case for the majority of microbiological tests. These methods are relatively capable of recovering environmental contaminants under the conditions of the test and capable of showing a change in the normal flora. Industry experience of environmental monitoring data would indicate that this is generally the case—it is doubtful whether there is any manufacturer that has not had to investigate a result that exceeded their acceptance criteria.

The main monitoring methods are active air sampling, settle plates, surface samples (swabs and contact plates), and samples taken from personnel.

The sampling methods should be appropriate in relation to the types of contamination sources (and a comprehensive monitoring program should assess each of the main contamination sources). Chapter 6 looks at these in greater detail, together with the required choices over agars, incubation time, and incubation temperature. Rapid method alternatives are described in Chapter 9.

CLEANROOMS IN DIFFERENT OPERATING STATES

The amount of environmental monitoring undertaken and the number and selection of monitoring locations will vary for newly built and established cleanrooms (as will the frequency of monitoring). This difference is examined later.

Newly Built Cleanrooms

During initial start-up or commissioning of a cleanroom or other controlled environment, the locations for air and surface sampling should be determined. This normally takes the form of saturation monitoring and extensive room simulations in order to establish a "baseline" of the cleanroom's operating ability. Consideration should be given to the proximity to the product and whether air and surfaces might be in contact with a product or sensitive surfaces of container-closure systems. Such areas should be considered critical areas requiring more monitoring than nonproduct contact areas. In parenteral vial filling operations, these areas would typically include the container-closure supply and product exposure areas. The frequency of sampling will depend on the criticality of the specified sites and the subsequent treatment received by the product after it has been aseptically processed. The rationale for the relative importance of routine microbiological monitoring is based on the nature of the product being manufactured and the nature of the process involved. As manual interventions during the manufacturing operations increase, and as the potential for personnel contact with the product increases the relative importance of the environmental monitoring program increases. Following commissioning it is appropriate to increase or decrease sampling based on this program.

In-use Cleanrooms

The number of environmental monitoring locations will depend upon the size of the cleanroom and the activities taking place. This involves a study of the room or process, as such monitoring sites will vary for different activities.

The locations selected should be representative of the cleanroom and each site should be justified as to why it has been selected. In taking into account locations for monitoring the main areas of risk should be considered. According to Ackers, these are: "personnel working … [using] gloves are the most likely source [of contamination]." The monitoring program should acknowledge that people are the primary source of contamination cleanrooms. Other sources include equipment, when particles can be generated; process steps where aerosols may be generated; wet areas and wash bays; and routine equipment transfer.

To these risks, for sterile manufacturing, the filling or testing zone should be added. Other areas can be chosen based on where there is potential for direct product impact, where microbial contamination would affect product quality and where contamination could spread through movement of samples, equipment, or personnel.

Locations will include the air in the environment, critical surfaces and equipment, floors and walls, and from personnel. The program should be based on risk assessment (see later). This will bias monitoring to areas like routes of human traffic; areas which might become more heavily contaminated, such as door handles; where contamination is likely to spread or proliferate and transit routes; or focusing the program on checking areas prone to be neglected like cleaning regimes. Sometimes the most appropriate location, during activities like aseptic filling, will not be sampled because the act of sampling itself could cause contamination. In such cases this should be detailed in a rationale. In Grade A environments, further supporting evidence for the selected locations can be obtained from airflow studies.

One decision to be made is whether to rotate sampling locations or not. The argument in favor of this is that various areas of a cleanroom will be monitored, giving the data more range. The argument against this is that not rotating locations allow for greater consistency when the data is examined for long-term trends. Once established the locations for monitoring should be justified in a report and indicated on a sampling map so that sampling is consistent and reproducible.

Other Considerations

Other considerations for establishing monitoring locations can be brought to the fore through studying the process and developing a process flow schematic (such as that used when establishing the locations for monitoring). For example, it is important to take into account the following:

- Critical surfaces and equipment;
- Floors and walls;
- Personnel and personnel garments;
- For active air samplers it is important to locate these in areas that minimize any disruption of the airflow which might impinge upon operations.

To address this a risk-centric approach like hazard analysis critical control points (HACCP) can be very useful. Simplistically HACCP, or any risk assessment, identifies potential hazards, then identifies and puts in place controls to prevent the hazard occurring. In the context of pharmaceuticals and healthcare, the focus is with the product, both the level and type of contamination. Assessment of the critical control points (CCPs) will be based on which steps eliminate or reduce contamination to an acceptable level. For aseptic processing, for example, the target is elimination, even if this cannot necessarily be absolutely demonstrated (Jahnke & Kuhn, 2003).

This method is widely used in the food industry, where it is a requirement, and also in the cosmetic and toiletries industry. It can prove very useful for selecting appropriate monitoring sites.

ASSESSING CLEANING AND DISINFECTION EFFECTIVENESS

It is important that the monitoring program has some link to cleaning and disinfection practices. Thus it is important that the environmental monitoring program has some link to cleaning and disinfection practices. Data from the environmental monitoring program is important in measuring the effectiveness of cleaning and sanitization procedures, rotation of disinfectants, in-use concentrations, and so on, and should be used to make changes to the cleaning program as necessary. OOL investigations should consider factors like cleaning and disinfection frequencies, rotation, types of sanitizers, room use, numbers of personnel present, room activity, and so on. If a resistant microorganism is suspected, then this may necessitate a change of disinfectant type. However, it may be necessary to culture the resistant microorganism and perform a challenge test to the disinfectant based on the quantitative suspension or the surface (carrier) test. This will give some idea of the true nature of the resistance of the isolate to the disinfectant.

DATA REVIEW

Trend analysis is an important aspect of the monitoring program since data originating from single samples are often not significant. Data graphs, histograms, and statistical process control charts are examples of the tools that can be used and should be applied. The tool used will often depend on the volume of data to be analyzed. Graphical representation of individual data points is not a useful tool when dealing with copious volumes of data, in some cases many thousands of data points; in this scenario histograms (or similar) where the data plotted are grouped and the frequency of occurrence is plotted are more useful (Caputo & Huffman, 2004). Chapter 14 looks at data handling and review in greater detail.

Environmental monitoring results which exceed the action level; or where there is an upward trend relating to excursions of the alert level; or where the frequency of incidents exceeds a predetermined cutoff value, represent scenarios which should be investigated. This is the subject of Chapter 19.

MONITORING FOR PARTICULATES

Particle counting for contaminants as part of the routine monitoring program is a separate activity to cleanroom classification. Ongoing particle monitoring examines the quantity of airborne particles in the air. In Europe this is for particle cutoff sizes 5.0 μm and 0.5 μm using specialized particle counters. For USP conformance monitoring for the 0.5 μm cutoff size, in the dynamic (or in operation) state, is recommended, whereas both sizes are required for EU GMP and most manufacturers will monitor for both sizes of particles. Although monitoring determines the level of nonviable particles such monitoring gives a level of assurance regarding the presence of microorganisms. A high level of particles may imply corresponding levels of microorganisms (although this has never been determined, Ljungqvist and Reinmuller (1996), consider the relationship to be 10^5 particles: 1 microorganism). Therefore a rise in particle counts may correspond to a proportional rise in viable contamination. If a relationship can be determined then particle counting, generated as "real time" data, can be very useful in alerting a supervisor to a potential problem, which could be more quickly addressed, or to an increase in risk.

For sites with an Aseptic Filling Suite the common approach is for continued monitoring throughout the filling activity for the Grade A/ISO Class 5 filling zone and the Grade B/ISO Class 7 cleanroom or Grade A/ISO Class 5 isolator (as per the EU GMP Guide). Furthermore, rooms associated with the fill, such as areas where product vials are located and the loading of freeze-dryers are also monitored. Monitoring should also note events like shift changes and filling line interventions.

For Grade C/ISO Class 8 and D areas things can be more problematic. Given a large facility with many different operations being performed the organization will need to select those activities considered critical to its operations for dynamic state monitoring and construct a rationale around it. Chapter 8 addresses particle monitoring and cleanroom classification in greater detail.

STAFF TRAINING

It is important not to neglect the importance of personnel undertaking environmental monitoring and the need to ensure that they are suitably trained in sampling techniques and are familiar with the layout of the facility. Before commencing training, all staff must have:

- A training folder in which to record the outcome of training (i.e., all training is documented);
- In addition, training must be against an agreed procedure;
- Training must be delivered by staff that are competent to do so.

In designing a training scheme, a consistent approach is desirable. This will allow processes to be completed and to allow staff to understand what is involved.

WRITTEN PROGRAM

The environmental monitoring program should be captured as a policy or rationale, supported by method SOPs. It is the function of the policy to ensure that the thought processes behind the program are adequately captured.

As a minimum it is recommended that an approved procedure defines the following:

- Transfer of media and equipment into the cleanroom.
- Who is responsible for monitoring?
- The sites monitored.
- The frequency of monitoring.
- The techniques and methods used.
- The incubation conditions.
- How to report the samples taken.
- How to report results and by whom.
- Who is responsible for reviewing the results?
- The limits against which the results will be assessed.
- Interpretation of the results.
- The action to be taken in the event of an out of limit.
- The trend analysis tools to be used.
- Frequency of carrying out trend analysis and preparing trend reports.

In order to ensure the results are traceable to the sample, it is important to record pertinent information at the time of sampling, including:

- Sample site description.
- Date and time of sampling.
- Person who did the sampling.
- Activity at the time of sampling.
- Media type.
- Any deviations from the sampling plan.
- Transport/storage conditions and duration.

The later information is pertinent to an environmental monitoring SOP.

SUMMARY

Microbiological environmental monitoring is a means of demonstrating an acceptable microbiological quality in the controlled environment and detecting changes in a timely manner. It involves the collection of data relating to microbial numbers recovered from samples of air, surfaces, and people in a clean area. Such data enable the monitoring of trends over time, that is, the detection of upward and downward changes in that area. Besides running programs for monitoring numbers and types of microorganisms, particle counts (which may represent viable organisms on carriers or inert material) are also assessed as part of the program.

This needs to come together into a program, as this chapter has demonstrated. Hence the assessment of environments by environmental monitoring is undertaken through a defined environmental monitoring program. The program should be documented and detailed in a policy or rationale together with accompanying standard operating procedures.

REFERENCES

An, Y. H., & Friedman, R. J. (1997). Laboratory methods for studies of bacterial adhesion. *Journal of Microbiological Methods*, *30*, 141–152.

Caputo, R. A., & Huffman, A. (2004). Environmental monitoring: data trending using a frequency model. *PDA Journal of Pharmaceutical Science and Technology*, *58*(5), 254–260.

Cundell, A., & Bean, R. (1998). Statistical analysis of environmental monitoring data: does a worst case time for monitoring clean rooms exist. *Journal of Pharmaceutical Science and Technology*, *52*, 326–330.

Cundell, A., Bean, R., Massimor, L., & Maier, C. (1998). Statistical analysis of environmental monitoring data: does a worst case time for monitoring clean rooms exist? *PDA Journal of Pharmaceutical Science and Technology*, *52*(6), 326–330.

Dell, L. A. (1979). Aspects of microbiological monitoring for nonsterile and sterile manufacturing environments. *Pharmaceutical Technology*, 47–51. August 1979.

Denny, V. F., Kopis, E. M. and Marsik, J. (1999): Elements for a successful disinfection program in the pharmaceutical environment, PDA Journal of Pharmaceutical Science and Technology, Vol. 53, No.3, pp115–124.

Hertroys, R., Van Vught, P.A.M. and De Donk, H.J.M. (1997): Moving towards a (microbiological) environmental monitoring programme that can be used to release aseptically produced pharmaceuticals: a hypothesis, a practical programme, and some results, PDA Journal of Pharmaceutical Science and Technology, Vol. 51., No.1, pp 52–59.

Jahnke, M., & Kuhn, K.-D. (2003). Use of the hazard analysis and critical control points (HACCP) risk assessment on a medical device for parenteral application. *PDA Journal of Pharmaceutical Science and Technology*, 57(1), 32–34.

Jimenez, L. (2004): Environmental monitoring in Jimenez, L. (ed.) Microbial contamination control in the pharmaceutical industry, Marcel Dekker, New York, pp103–132.

Ljungqvist, B., & Reinmuller, B. (1996). Some observations on environmental monitoring of cleanrooms. *European Journal of Parenteral Science*, *1*, 9–13.

Moldenhauer, J. (2008). Environmental monitoring. In R. Prince (Ed.), *Microbiology in pharmaceutical manufacturing* (pp. 19–92). Bethesda, MD: Parenetral Drug Association.

Reich, R., Miller, M., & Patterson, H. (2003). Developing a viable environmental monitoring program for nonsterile pharmaceutical operations. *Pharmaceutical Technology*, 92–100. March 2003.

Sandle, T. (2012a). Environmental Monitoring: a practical approach In Moldenhauer, J. Environmental monitoring: A comprehensive handbook, Vol. 6, PDA/DHI: River Grove, IL, USA, pp 29–54.

Sandle, T. (2012b). Application of quality risk management to set viable environmental monitoring frequencies in biotechnology processing and support areas. *PDA Journal of Pharmaceutical Science and Technology*, *66*(6), 560–579.

Sandle, T. (2015). Cleanroom design. In J. Moldenhauer (Ed.), *Vol. 7. Environmental monitoring: A comprehensive handbook* (pp. 3–28).

Sandle, T. (2017) Environmental control and environmental monitoring in support of aseptic processing. In Sandle, T. and Tidswell, E. C. (Eds.) Aseptic and sterile processing: Control, compliance and future trends, DHI/PDA, Bethesda, MD, USA, ISBN: 9781942911128, pp 447–540.

Sutton, S. (2010). The environmental monitoring program in a GMP environment. *Journal of GXP Compliance*, *14*(3), 22–30.

Chapter **11**

Special Types of Environmental Monitoring

CHAPTER OUTLINE

Introduction   179
Monitoring to Support Parametric Release   180
The Need for Anaerobic Monitoring?   182
The Need for Psychrophilic Monitoring?   183
The Need for Thermophilic Monitoring?   186
Compressed Gas Monitoring   187
    Microbial Survival in Compressed Gases   189
    Microbiological Requirements   190
    Bacterial Endotoxin and Compressed Gases   192
Monitoring Sterility Test Environments   192
Monitoring Microbiology Laboratories   194
Test Controls   194
Summary   196
References   197

INTRODUCTION

The purpose of this chapter is to look at environmental monitoring, in support of biocontamination control, from a more applied perspective. This includes the use of parametric release, which can be used for terminally sterilized products. Parametric release is a sterility assurance release program where demonstrated control of the sterilization process enables an organization to use defined critical process controls, in lieu of the sterility test.

The chapter considers how the inclusion of test controls as part of the environmental monitoring regime can provide robustness as well as useful information should an out-of-limits result be obtained as to whether that result was or was not the consequence of laboratory error.

Biocontamination Control for Pharmaceuticals and Healthcare. https://doi.org/10.1016/B978-0-12-814911-9.00011-0

Among the "special" types of environmental monitoring performed the chapter looks at the end for (and more strongly the need against) monitoring for thermophilic and psychrophilic organisms. The case for monitoring (or otherwise) for anaerobic bacteria is also discussed. The chapter also discusses the particular requirements for the monitoring of compressed gases (including compressed air).

In assessing each of these "special" monitoring requirements the extent to which they are needed depends upon the particular facility and an understanding of any risks. If open processing is conducted in a cold room, for example, then a case might be made for some form of testing in the event that psychrophilic rather than psychrotolerant organisms are recovered. This is a key point with this chapter: the types of assessments discussed need to be considered to determine if they have a place in the contamination control strategy.

MONITORING TO SUPPORT PARAMETRIC RELEASE

A detailed examination of parametric release is outside the scope of this book. However, many pharmaceutical manufacturers will use environmental monitoring data as data of their parametric release procedures as a means to either assess the overall bioburden or as a means of considering the probable risk, in relation to terminally sterilized products. The approach is not suitable, in this author's opinion, for aseptically processed products.

European Organization for Quality defines parametric release as: "A system of release that gives the assurance that the product is of the intended quality based on information collected during the manufacturing process and on the compliance with specific GMP requirements related to Parametric Release."

Parametric release is based on evidence of successful validation of the manufacturing process and review of the documentation on process monitoring carried out during manufacturing to provide the desired assurance of quality of the product. It is a system of release that gives the assurance that the product is of the intended quality based on the information collected during the manufacturing process and on the compliance with specific requirements related to parametric release resulting in the elimination of certain specific tests of the finished product (Sandle, 2012).

Some of the types of things that need to be considered as part of parametric release are displayed in Fig. 1:

This means for products that are intended to be sterile that the microbiological quality of the batch of a medicinal product is stated by using the data

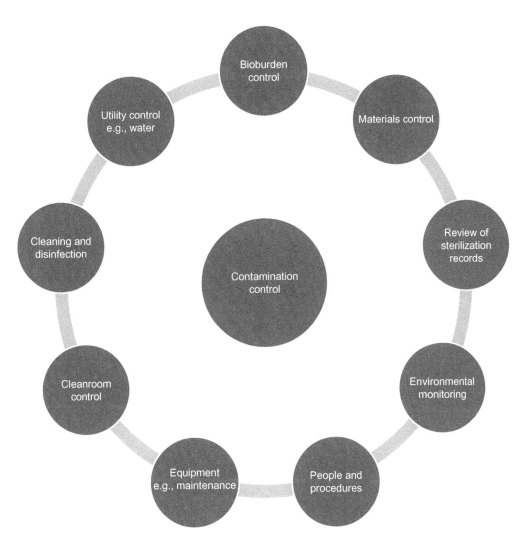

■ **FIG. 1** Key factors to consider for parametric release.

from environmental monitoring and process data (which includes other microbial test results from the examination of raw materials, water samples, and intermediate product). In particular, the procedures for quality control of starting materials, packaging materials, process water, and environmental monitoring are checked. Other aspects of importance are, for example, filtration procedures, equipment cleaning/sterilization procedures, maximum holding times for bulk solutions. In this context, a sterility test is not required in batch release. For assessing these sterile products, environmental monitoring data, especially when trended, provides a very useful picture concerning the probability and possibility of product contamination.

THE NEED FOR ANAEROBIC MONITORING?

Anaerobic environmental monitoring is rarely performed by pharmaceutical manufacturers and there is rarely any requirement for it to be performed. For nonsterile manufacturing there is little scientific reason whatsoever (except where certain products have been identified as at risk from certain toxins produced from organisms that can survive in the production process); for aseptic manufacturing there may be a requirement if particular gases are used with specialized filling machine equipment such as blow-fill technology (Jimenez, 2004). Blow-fill technology tends to use insert gases. When using inert gases (like nitrogen) or pressurized air in routine aseptic manufacturing process this has to be simulated during media fill. As the usage of nitrogen represents anaerobic conditions then it is arguable that sòme form of anaerobic monitoring should take place. The sterility of the inert gas has to be separately demonstrated by filtration procedure or by introduction of gas into the nutrient. Some manufacturers adopt to perform limited anaerobic monitoring during media simulation trials only.

An anaerobic organism or anaerobe is considered, in this context, to be any microorganism that does not require oxygen for growth. Different types of "anaerobes" can be considered thus:

- Obligate anaerobes (microorganisms that live and grow in the absence of molecular oxygen) will die when exposed to atmospheric levels of oxygen.
- Facultative anaerobes can use oxygen when it is present. Some examples of facultative anaerobic bacteria are Staphylococcus (Gram positive), *Escherichia coli* and *Shewanella oneidensis* (Gram negative), and Listeria (Gram positive).
- Aerotolerant organisms can survive in the presence of oxygen, but they are anaerobic because they do not use oxygen as a terminal electron acceptor;
- Microaerophiles are organisms that may use oxygen, but only at low concentrations (low micromolar range (~20% concentration)); their growth is inhibited by the normal oxygen concentration of air (approximately 200 micromolar) (e.g., *Campylobacter*);
- Nanaerobes are organisms that cannot grow in the presence of micromolar concentrations of oxygen, but can grow with and benefit from nanomolar concentrations of oxygen (e.g., *Bacteroides fragilis*).

Obligate anaerobes may use fermentation or anaerobic respiration. In the presence of oxygen, facultative anaerobes use aerobic respiration; without oxygen some of them ferment, some use anaerobic respiration. Aerotolerant organisms are strictly fermentative. Microaerophiles carry out aerobic respiration, and some of them can also do anaerobic respiration.

Where anaerobic monitoring is required the environmental monitoring samples are taken using standard agar (such as TSA). However, the samples are incubated using specialized cabinets or in gas jars. These systems are designed to cultivate anaerobic and microaerophilic organisms. Most gas jars are cylindrical jar and are composed of transparent and very thick, strong polycarbonate plastic. The jars typically hold anaerobic indicators and a gas-generation pack or even a second low-temperature catalyst. The catalysts are often palladium-coated ceramic beads which provide a large surface area for catalysis. And the object is to enable the rapid generation of an anaerobic atmosphere. Some catalysts require regeneration by dry heat; there will be a limit upon the number of cycles that a catalyst can be regenerated. The catalysts function to remove any residual oxygen in the jar to create a strictly anaerobic environment.

The frequency of anaerobic monitoring should be established by the microflora recovered or based on a consideration of probable risk. The level of risk is best established through an examination of historical data (Sandle, 2011).

THE NEED FOR PSYCHROPHILIC MONITORING?

Outside of the production of highly specialized medicinal products, most pharmaceutical cleanrooms, used for the preparation of tablets, creams, inhalers, and so on, are operated at temperatures suitable for personnel to work in (typically 18–25°C). In addition, common to many pharmaceutical facilities there are some areas which may become slightly warmer (such as where autoclaves are operated) and there are some areas which function as cold rooms. Cold rooms are used for product storage and conditioning and have become more widespread with the advent and growth of biotechnology products, where cold conditions are required for purification steps. To minimize the risk of contamination, cold rooms are required to be designed and operated as certifiable cleanrooms. Pharmaceutical process area cold rooms vary in their temperature of operation, with 1°C as the potential minima and the maxima, which is set anywhere between 10°C and 14°C. The cold rooms to which the case study outlined in this paper refers where operated between 2°C and 8°C.

Some medicines inspectors request monitoring data concerning microorganisms with optimal growth rates that fall outside of mesophilic conditions (what might be called extremophiles: microorganism requiring severe conditions for growth as defined by extremes of temperature, pH, chemical oxidizing agents, hypersalinity, or certain types of ultraviolet light) (Dutta & Paul, 2012). This regulatory approach has been noted with both US Food and Drug Administration (FDA) and European Medicines Agency (EMA), in relation to regulatory assessments of pharmaceutical process area cold rooms. Here, regulatory agencies have inquired about the possibility of microorganisms which can tolerate cold conditions (psychrotolerant) or which will only grow in cold conditions (psychrophilic) being present within cold room environments.

Psychrophiles or cryophiles are extremophilic organisms that are capable of growth and reproduction in cold temperatures. Such microorganisms can grow at temperatures lower than 15°C and most are found in the Arctic or in the sea (typically $T_{min} < 0°C$, to, $T_{max} > 15°C$). There are generally considered to be two groups of bacteria which can tolerate cold temperatures: obligate psychrophiles and facultative psychrophiles or psychrotrophs with relatively broad temperature ranges for growth. Obligate psychrophiles are those organisms having a growth temperature optimum of 15°C or lower and which cannot grow in a climate beyond a maximum temperature of 20°C. Psychrophiles are more often isolated from permanently cold habitats, whereas psychrotolerant microorganisms tend to dominate those environments that undergo thermal fluctuations (Thamdrup & Fleischer, 1998).

Obligate psychrophiles are adapted to their cold environment by having largely unsaturated fatty acids in their plasma membranes. Psychrophiles possess enzymes that continue to function, albeit at a reduced rate, at temperatures at or near 0°C. Psychrophile proteins do not function at the body temperatures of warm-blooded animals and they are unable to grow at even moderate temperatures. On the basis of risks in pharmaceutical processing, given most intended routes of administration, a psychrophilic contaminant would present only a low risk to the patient.

Facultative psychrophiles can survive at temperatures as low as 0°C up through approximately 40°C. These organisms exist in much larger numbers than obligate psychrophiles. They are generally not able to grow at cold temperatures (under 15°C), although they often maintain basic functioning. These organisms have evolved to tolerate cold conditions, where adaptation has required a vast array of sequence, structural, and physiological adjustments. Nonetheless, they are not as physiologically specialized as obligate psychrophiles and are usually not found in the very coldest of environments. Examples of such facultative psychrophiles are microorganisms that include

Listeria monocytogenes, Vibrio marinus, Pseudomonas fluorescens, and *Pseudomonas maltophilia.* These "cold tolerant" organisms are more often referred to as psychrotolerant microorganisms.

The basis of the regulatory concern is that such microorganisms may not, through their adaption to cold conditions, be detected due to an inability to grow, or only growing in reduced numbers, where mesophilic environmental monitoring is undertaken. Regulators have argued that under conditions of mesophilic monitoring, this leads to an underestimation of the numbers of microorganisms present in cleanrooms designed as cold rooms. Regulators further argue, perhaps more importantly, that the consequential failure to speciate those microorganisms which may present in cold areas means that the risk to the product cannot be fully understood (in that the microbial population in the cold area cannot be surveyed to determine if any of the microorganisms are objectionable in relation to the particular product and potential patient population that the product is intended for).

The counterargument to concerns about such psychrophilic microorganisms relates to their metabolic characteristics, that is, such organisms do not pose a risk to pharmaceutical processing because they cannot grow or reproduce in the product. A further argument is that "cold loving" microorganisms may be present, but they are found in such low numbers that do not pose a risk. From these two counterpositions, it can be contended that the focus should be upon risk assessment where any recovered objectionable microorganisms in pharmaceutical processing should be considered in relation to the question: does the particular microorganism, at a certain level, pose a risk to the patient should it contaminated a particular product?

To this question, it can be argued that although many pharmaceutical products are stored in cold areas, and assuming that product ingress could occur (however unlikely given product barrier safeguards), then the typical microorganisms found in pharmaceutical process cleanrooms would, given the environmental conditions of cold storage (10°C or lower), either not survive for long periods or would be in stasis and would therefore not proliferate. The exception to this would be if there was a microorganism that was specifically cold loving and was able to reproduce under such conditions. Here, the risk is compounded if the pharmaceutical manufacturer is not aware that such microorganisms are present. The potential risk arises, then, if there are some microorganisms present which will only reproduce at low temperatures and would not be detected by the standard environmental monitoring program (i.e., such organisms would not grow at the incubation regime currently applied and which is designed to capture "mesophilic" microorganisms) (Sandle & Skinner, 2013).

The way to approach this issue is either to develop a defensible rationale and state the case not to perform such monitoring, or to carry out regular monitoring, or to perform a one-off study. The answer should form part of the contamination control rationale.

THE NEED FOR THERMOPHILIC MONITORING?

There is no real case to be made for thermophilic monitoring, either in the cleanroom environment or within pharmaceutical water systems. A thermophile is a microorganism that lives at temperatures >45°C (and generally up ~70°C). Hyperthermophiles will grow at temperatures in excess of 70°C (Martinez, 2004).

With water systems, pharmaceutical water environments are extremely hostile environments. They are kept at high temperatures and have very low levels of organic materials, minerals, and salts and have a narrow pH range. It is therefore, scientifically, extremely unlikely that thermophilic (or any) microorganisms could live in hot water systems. Most objectionable microorganisms and human pathogens will not grow at temperatures >45°C.

With cleanrooms, some pharmaceutical manufacturers will examine prepared autoclave loads in using contact plates and swabs, or for other activities where heat is used (such as blow–fill–seal processes) (Poisson, Sinclair, & Tallentire, 2006). The purpose for performing the monitoring is to:

- Build up a library of the type of challenges posed to loads going into sterilizers;
- To react to any results that exceed preset action levels, either based on the counts obtained or the species identified.

Samples from the autoclave loads are commonly incubated at two temperature regimes:

- 20–25°C for a minimum of 3 days followed by 30–35°C for a minimum of 6 days, and
- 55–60°C for a minimum of 2 days.

The reason for performing the work at two different temperatures is to detect both mesophilic and thermophilic contamination. The reason for the thermophilic temperature is the autoclaves are superheat sterilization devices and thermophilic microorganisms may be, although this is theoretically unlikely, a specific cause for concern. Moreover, the chance of detecting thermophiles is low.

In both water systems and with cleanrooms, most extremophiles are anaerobic or microaerophilic chemolithoautotrophs. Because of their unique habitats, metabolism, and nutritional requirements, such organisms are not known to be or opportunistic pathogens, and they are not capable of colonizing a pharmaceutical area. Therefore there is little value in monitoring for such organisms.

COMPRESSED GAS MONITORING

Compressed gas is a general term for gas stored or held under pressure that is greater than atmosphere. Compressed gases are used at different stages of the pharmaceutical manufacturing process. Applications include weighing stations process line; use of gas to maintain an inert atmosphere above a liquid or powdered product inside a storage tank, silo, reactor, process equipment, or other vessel; use of liquid nitrogen for the preservation of biological samples; use of inert gas to pressurize new, repaired, or modified tanks, pipelines, and vessels; and use of inert gas to displace air and contaminants from storage tanks. Furthermore, compressed gases such as air, nitrogen, and carbon dioxide are deployed in operations involving purging or overlaying.

Compressed gas sampling for microorganisms is an important part of contamination control assessment (Sandle, 2013). While sampling is important, the method of sampling can be hindered by the design of the gas system, where sampling is not easily conducted in an aseptic manner, or by the design of the air sampling instrument. This section reviews the important aspects of compressed air sampling for microbiological assessment and looks at possible sources of contamination, should microorganisms be recovered.

Purity is a factor that needs to be maintained with compressed gas; hence the gas should be supplied oil free. Purity overall is achieved through a combination of filtration, purification, and separation. The process of creating the compressed gas can additionally introduce water vapor; thus a process must be in place to remove water vapor before the gas is expelled into a critical zone like a cleanroom. Compressed gas is typically discharged from the compressor hot and it will contain water vapor. Temperature is reduced by using a postcompressor cooler and, as the gas condenses, the water vapor and other impurities can be removed. The risk of water vapor is particularly high with compressed air, which is drawn into a compressor via the atmosphere. Atmospheric air contains a high proportion of water vapor (i.e., water in a gaseous form). Water removal is achieved through a combination of filtration and dehumidification.

Where air is drawn in from the outside, the process of drawing in air also introduces microorganisms, which require filtering out. The level of filtering depends upon whether "sterile" air is required (absence of viable microorganisms) or air with a low bioburden.

Compressed gas can be supplied at source either sterile or nonsterile. Sterility, where required such as with an inhalation product, is achieved through the use of a bacterial retentive membrane filter (0.2 μm pore size). Where a sterile-filtered gas is required it is important that the sterilizing grade filter is maintained dry for condensate in a gas filter that will most probably cause blockage or lead to microbial contamination. Risks of condensate are controlled by heating and use of hydrophobic filters (to prevent moisture residues in a gas supply system). Filters should also be changed periodically. As part of ongoing quality control, filters must be integrity tested at installation and at end of use.

Although national standards bodies have guidance documents for compressed air sampling, and reference is made within FDA and EU GMPs, the general approach and requirements for compressed gases are set out in a multipart ISO standard: ISO 8573. This standard consists of the following parts (ISO, n.d.):

- Part 1: Contaminants and purity classes,
- Part 2: Test methods for aerosol oil content,
- Part 3: Test methods for measurement of humidity,
- Part 4: Test methods for solid particle content,
- Part 5: Test methods for oil vapor and organic solvent content,
- Part 6: Test methods for gaseous contaminant content,
- Part 7: Test method for viable microbiological contaminant content,
- Part 8: Test methods for solid particle content by mass concentration,
- Part 9: Test methods for liquid water content.

Part 1 outlines the required purity classes based on the concentration of particles and level of impurities. The potential "impure" contaminants for compressed air, that can affect whether a required purity class is met, include:

- Particles (such as dirt, rust, pipe scale), with particles assessed by size. For example, as result of the mechanical compression process, additional impurities may be introduced into the air system. Generated contaminants include compressor lubricant, wear particles, and vaporized lubricant. Furthermore, fittings and accessories can contribute to particles.
- Water (in both vapor and liquid forms). Water is typically assessed by vapor pressure dew point. This is the temperature at which the air can no longer "hold" all of the water vapor which is mixed with).
- Oil (including aerosol, vapor, and liquid forms).

With purity, many parts of the pharmaceutical industry will use Class 1 compressed gas based on the maximum number of permitted particulates.

Microbial Survival in Compressed Gases

Although compressed gas and air systems are relatively harsh environments, they can aid microbial survival if there are available nutrients. The availability of nutrients is dependent upon the purity of the gas and airline. Nutrients suitable for metabolizing by microorganisms include water and oil droplets. Another factor that can affect survival is temperature, especially where temperatures are warmer (Stewart et al., 1995).

In addition to vegetative cells, bacterial spores are well equipped to survive the harsh environmental conditions. Spores are resistant to the types of temperature ranges and moisture levels found within compress gas lines. Another risk exists with biofilm, where microbial communities can potentially form and develop through attachment to air lines and tubing.

Although these risk factors exist, typically no microorganisms would be expected to be recovered from compressed gas lines. Research has shown that many microorganisms can survive and multiply in pressurized systems up to 10 bar and some are at least able to recover after being pressurized. However, at 160 bar pressure upwards, survival rates are very low. Where low level counts are recovered, these require investigation. More often the source is adventitious contamination, although a fault with the compressed air line cannot be ruled out.

Although microbial contamination of compressed air or gas is a rare event, incidents can occur. Sources of contamination include:

- *Source of the air or gas*: Contamination can arise from air intake from the surroundings (which can contain oil, dirt, dust, moisture, or microorganisms).
- *Piping distribution systems*: Piping distribution and air storage tanks, more prevalent in older systems, will have contaminant in the form of rust, pipe scale, mineral deposits, in addition to bacteria.
- *Bacterial retentive filter*: The filter may become blocked, lose its integrity, or become wet.
- *Compressor failure*: The compressor itself can create a contaminated environment. For example, the compressor's prefilters can become overloaded with dust and lint, causing the filter to cease functioning properly.
- *Sample valve*: The point-of-use sample valve may not be designed correctly or become faulty.

Microbiological Requirements

Microbial content itself does not influence the gas purity class assigned, although the standards recommend that microbial levels are assessed. Acceptable microbial numbers are subject to a separate assessment, with such assessment being based on an interpretation of GMP. A consensus is that the microbiological quality of the gas must be at least as good as the cleanroom air quality in which the process is taking place. Note that for EU GMP Grade A/ISO 14644 Class 5 areas, the microbial count would then be $<1\,cfu/m^3$ and the particle levels conform to the area at rest ≤3520 particles per m^3. Many companies, however, do not monitor gas or compressed air used in Grade A or B areas since these are sterile filtered as close as possible to the point of use. In such cases a filter integrity test is executed in lieu of microbiological monitoring.

Compressed air sampling should form part of an environmental monitoring program, along with cleanroom assessments. The program should take into account air points to be tested. This could be every point, points considered to be of greater risk (such as product contact), or representative points along a loop. The frequency of testing must also be considered, and this too would need to tie into risk.

While there is an argument, as set out here, for the testing of compressed air where there is product contact there is less of a consensus over the testing of nitrogen. While nitrogen gas can be used to dispense or transfer most fluids from storage, the ISO standard has no specific microbial testing requirements and very few microorganisms, of the types common to pharmaceutical manufacturing environments, would be likely to survive. On this basis a risk-based justification could be made not to perform nitrogen gas testing.

The user will need to determine whether each compressed gas line requires testing and the frequency of testing. Certainly all product contact compressed gases should be assessed. A sampling plan should also consider, and adapt to, the following:

- Cleanroom grade,
- Type of product manufactured,
- Increased or reduced production schedules,
- Seasonal changes,
- Equipment changes and modifications,
- Replacement of hardware or filters and dryers,
- Inactivity of system.

When sampling compressed air for microorganisms, it is important that the air is depressurized and that the flow rate is controlled. Control of the flow rate is important to ensure that a cubic meter of air is sampled within the required sampling time (this time will be instrument dependent). If the air sampler takes 36 min to capture a cubic meter of air, then it will be sampling at one cubic foot per minute. An external regulator will be needed to bring the flow rate down to the sampling rate of instrument. This is assessed using a flow meter. Pressure reduction to atmospheric conditions is of great importance and knowing the flow allows the agar exposure time to be assessed, so that one cubic meter of air is sampled (Sandle, 2010).

It is also important that isokinetic sampling of the air occurs and that air velocity is reduced until it is within the range of the sampler as identified by the manufacturer. This is not only necessary for obtaining the correct sample size but it also impacts on the possibility of microbial survival. The level of impact stress has been shown to affect microbial recovery on agar and be dependent upon the impaction velocity of the cells into the agar as well as the design and operating parameters. Due to the fact that any microorganisms present are transported under pressure and then suddenly released into atmospheric conditions, they may be damaged by the immediate expansion of the gas and the resulting shearing forces.

The head of the instrument and any attachments should ideally be sterile before use, to avoid contamination. The culture medium used with the instrument should have been tested for growth promotion and, as for environmental monitoring, has been validated as suitable for gas viable air monitoring. With most samplers the head will be autoclavable. Some users disinfect the tubes and hoses used to connect the sampler with a disinfectant like 70% isopropyl alcohol. This is mentioned as an option in the ISO standard, although this is erroneously described as "sterilization." Where a disinfectant is used it is important to run the air through the sampler without any agar plate in place; this is necessary to evaporate the disinfectant and to remove any residues. The presence of disinfectant could potentially lead to a "false negative."

With sampling, the sample inlet is connected to the compressed gas line and air is directed over an agar plate or strip. The method works by compressed gas, under reduced pressure, called "partial flow", is forced over the surface of an agar plate. Any microorganisms are impinged onto the surface of the agar.

The sampling time should be sufficient in order to sample one cubic meter of the agar. After sampling, the agar plate or strip is removed and incubated within a microbiology laboratory. At the end of incubation, the agar is examined for colony-forming units. Incubation can be for aerobic or anaerobic organisms, or both. The extent to which either is present should be based on initial validation and by taking into account whether such organisms pose a patient risk, should they end up being transferred into the end product.

The type of instrument recommended in the ISO standard is a "slit-sampler, a type of impaction air tester," although alternative samplers can be used, if justified. With a standard impactor sampler, air is drawn through a sampling head via a pump or fan and accelerated, usually through a perforated plate (sieve samplers), or through a narrow slit (slit samplers). This process creates a laminar flow through the sampler head. Hence, the air sampler should be fitted with a diffuser capable of maintaining laminar flow conditions. This is necessary so that particles pass through the sample head in a controlled flow.

An appropriate agar must be selected. An example is tryptone soya agar, which is a generally nutritious medium designed to recover a range of bacteria and fungi. A key factor to take into account is whether the process of sampling leads to undue desiccation of the agar, rendering any recovered microorganisms unable to grow on the agar due to depletion of growth nutrients. This will be affected by the flow rate, type of compressed gas, and the model of air sampler, together with the type of culture medium. A risk will remain that microbial cells will become damaged by mechanical stress during the sampling process and lose viability.

Bacterial Endotoxin and Compressed Gases

Some users elect to sample compressed air for bacterial endotoxin. Such testing remains relatively uncommon and it is only necessary should the compressed gas have a direct product contact and where there is a concern with Gram-negative bacteria. In most cases there should be no likelihood of endotoxin being present, especially in the context of nonsterile manufacturing.

The sampling method for bacterial endotoxin is tricky and inexact. Either colonies are examined for Gram-negative bacteria, and assessment is made about endotoxin risk; or the compressed is passed through pyrogen-free water.

MONITORING STERILITY TEST ENVIRONMENTS

Isolators used for sterility testing should be approached in a similar way as the monitoring of Grade A/ISO Class 5 areas. This section of the unit sets out the approach taken to environmental monitoring inside a half-suit isolator during sterility testing, at the author's laboratory.

The use of a sterility testing isolator in a regulated environment means that having reliable results for its sterility tests is essential, and although there is a history of confidence in the isolator system, having a microbiological environmental monitoring program is imperative. The reason for this is twofold: one, to demonstrate that if a product was to fail a sterility test then the reason for that failure could be attributed to the product alone and not as a factor of the isolator environment, and, two, to show that the overall background environment of the isolator is "in control" through trend analysis.

The microbiological environmental monitoring typically consists of air samples, settle plates, finger plates, and contact plates or swabs. A standard culture media is typically used, like tryptone soya agar (TSA), which is a nonselective, highly nutritious media. Preliminary work need to take place in order to confirm that the action of sanitizing the media into the isolator, using hydrogen peroxide or peracetic acid vapor, or alternative method, does not cause inhibition of the TSA's growth-promoting properties.

The microbiological environmental monitoring should be performed for each sterility test by the operator. This provides invaluable information in the event of a sterility test failure. Monitoring typically includes:

- *Settle plates*: uncovered TSA plates (9 cm diameter) exposed either side of the testing environment for the duration of the test. The final result should be converted to a number of colony-forming units (cfu) per 4 h.
- *Air sample*: there are pros and cons concerning the use of an air sampler inside an isolator. This debate centers on the disruption of the airflow that an air sampler may cause. The view here is that an air sample should be taken at each sterility test since having an assessment of the air quality outweighs any possible the effect on the airflow.
- *Finger plates*: at the end of the test, the operator should take finger plates ("dabs") of each gloved hand by imprinting his/her fingers onto an agar plate. It is important that the gel strength of the agar is suitable for this task.
- *Swabs or contact plates*: the last microbiological monitoring activity is the taking of surface samples at set locations.

Once all the monitoring had been completed, the isolator is cleaned with an appropriate disinfectant to remove residues, such as an isopropanol alcohol-based disinfectant.

Samples should be appropriately incubated (Chapter 7 discusses incubation regimes). The action limit applied to all samples should be 1 cfu, which matches the same environmental standard as a process environment. A result at or exceeding the "action level" implies an "out-of-specification" investigation of aspects like the isolator gloves and the overall integrity; the matter becomes more serious should an upward trend develop.

MONITORING MICROBIOLOGY LABORATORIES

Although there is no written regulatory requirement or guidance, it can be prudent to perform some level of environmental monitoring within the microbiology laboratory and associated incubators. The data gathered from such monitoring can be useful in assessing out-of-limits results especially when considering if contamination arose from the laboratory environment.

The data gathered from such exercises can be examined and trended in a similar way to that from nonsterile manufacturing facilities. Although there are no prescribed action levels or specifications, most laboratories should have monitoring levels below to EU GMP Grade D/ISO Class 9 specifications (Table 1).

Although there is no direct relationship to testing within the microbiology laboratory, the data gathered can be illuminating in terms of hygiene status and it could be useful should any test errors require root cause investigation.

TEST CONTROLS

Most microbiological tests should have a test control, in order to assess validity, especially in relation to adventitious contamination. This is normally a negative control, although positive controls are used in some specific laboratory tests. Such controls serve a number of purposes:

- To assess the aseptic technique of the tester.
- To test the quality of the media and reagents.

Table 1 Possible alert and action levels for monitoring microbiology laboratories

Sample type	Warning level (cfu)	Action level (cfu)
Active air	Not defined	200
Settle plate	Not defined	100
Contact plate	Not defined	50

Table 2 Example of viable microbiological environmental monitoring test controls

Test Method	Control	Purpose
Microbiological monitoring: swab	Negative	For plain swabs: swab is soaked in Ringer's solution and streaked out onto an agar plate, under a UDAF. This demonstrates that the Ringer's solution, swab, and agar are not contaminated. For transport swabs: a swab is tested as presented. This control tests the environment in which the swab was taken, sampled, stored, and transported and the Technician's technique in preparing and plating out swabs. *Performed once during each monitoring session.*
Microbiological monitoring: contact plate	None	Sterility of media checked through nutritive properties release procedure.
Microbiological monitoring: active air sampler	None	Sterility of media checked through nutritive properties release procedure.
Microbiological monitoring: finger plate	None	Sterility of media checked through nutritive properties release procedure.
Microbiological monitoring: settle plate	None	Sterility of media checked through nutritive properties release procedure.

- To test the "testing" environment.
- To demonstrate that samples are operating as expected.

Controls should be examined as part of out-of-specification or out-of-limits reporting. A control, which is OOS or OOL, should be recorded onto an OOS/L report form (or an electronic record) and assessed along with samples tested during the test session. For samples that are OOS/L, the control should be examined for contamination or to check that it operated as expected. Controls can also be used as part of training and as a check for ongoing assessment. Where a control is consistently overaction the preventative action can include retraining and assessment.

For viable environmental monitoring, test controls are normally negative controls. A *possible approach* to the use of controls is outlined in Table 2.

A second form of control is with growth promotion testing. This is addressed in Chapter 7 of this book. Growth promotion testing can additionally be used if there are doubts about the media (such as stored outside of standard incubation conditions or media that has gone beyond its expiry time, although of course the acceptability of using testing to mitigate poor practices needs to be understood within a given organization's quality system). An example of the growth promotion test is presented in Table 3.

These types of controls can provide useful information about the suitability of the media and its handling.

Table 3 Example of media growth promotion test controls

Test method	Control	Purpose
Growth promotion testing	Positive	To demonstrate that the challenge count to the media on test is within the acceptance range of <100 cfu.
	Comparative control	To show how the test media compares to a previously released lot of the same media type with respect to the test challenge.
	Sterility	Batches of media are incubated for a specified duration and inspected for contamination by the manufacturer. This demonstrates that the media has been prepared in a way that maintains sterility. The strains used to inoculate plates are visually checked for purity.
	Negative	Can assess whether media has become contaminated.

SUMMARY

Although there are some important fundamentals for the contamination control strategy, as discussed in many of the chapters in this book, there are other aspects that might need to be included depending upon the nature of the pharmaceutical or healthcare organization. This relates to certain types of organisms found in specific locales. Are anaerobes of concern, for example? If nitrogen is used as part of the manufacturing process then this may be so. These questions are best addressed through risk assessment. In doing so, the nature of the likely contaminants needs to be assessed. Undertaking additional monitoring for psychrophiles, for example, serves no purpose if the organisms recovered from process rooms operating at <10°C are all capable of being recovered from standard environmental monitoring conducted using mesophilic incubation temperatures.

The risk concept also applies to parametric release. This approach is not suitable for aseptically filled products but it can be applied to terminally sterilized products, with controls in place. Where environmental monitoring can assist is not only with the assessment of the absolute numbers recovered but also with the types of organisms recovered, in terms of their resistance to thermal destruction. Understanding the organisms is also something that needs to be factored into a risk assessment.

The chapter has additionally addressed compressed gas monitoring. This is important to have in place since compressed gases are generally viewed as critical utilities when either in direct product contact or directly entered into the cleanroom environment. The chapter has also looked at test controls and the monitoring of sterility test facilities and of microbiology laboratories, areas that are associated with the primary environmental monitoring program but which equally do not form a central part of the program.

The extent to which each area discussed here should be applied, of if it all, needs to be risk assessed, taking into account the nature of the process and the types of hazards that might occur.

REFERENCES

Dutta, C., & Paul, S. (2012). Microbial lifestyle and genome signatures. *Current Genomics*, *13*(2), 153–162.

ISO ISO 8573-1:2010, Compressed air contaminants and purity classes, ISO, Geneva, Switzerland.

Jimenez, L. (2004). Environmental Monitoring. In L. Jimenez (Ed.), *Microbial contamination control in the pharmaceutical industry* (pp. 103–132). New York: Marcel Dekker.

Martinez, J. (2004): Hyperthermophilic microorganisms and USP hot water systems, Pharmaceutical Technology, Vol. 6, No.7, February, pp 50–65.

Poisson, P., Sinclair, C., & Tallentire, A. (2006). Challenges to blow/fill/seal process with airborne microorganisms having different resistances to dry heat. *PDA Journal of Pharmaceutical Science and Technology*, *60*(5), 323–330.

Sandle, T. (2010). Selection of active air samplers. *European Journal of Parenteral and Pharmaceutical Sciences*, *15*(4), 119–124.

Sandle, T. (2011). Environmental monitoring. In M. R. Saghee, T. Sandle, & E. C. Tidswell (Eds.), *Microbiology and sterility assurance in pharmaceuticals and medical devices* (pp. 293–326). New Delhi: Business Horizons.

Sandle, T. (2012). Environmental Monitoring: a practical approach. In J. Moldenhauer (Ed.), *Vol. 6. Environmental monitoring: A comprehensive handbook* (pp. 29–54). River Grove, IL: PDA/DHI.

Sandle, T. (2013). Contamination control risk assessment. In R. E. Masden, & J. Moldenhauer (Eds.), *Vol. 1. Contamination control in healthcare product manufacturing* (pp. 423–474). River Grove, IL: DHI Publishing.

Sandle, T., & Skinner, K. (2013). Study of psychrophilic and psychrotolerant microorganisms isolated in cold rooms used for pharmaceutical processing. *Journal of Applied Microbiology*, *114*(4), 1166–1174.

Stewart, S. L., Grinshpun, S. A., Willeke, K., Terzieva, S., Ulevicius, V., & Donnelly, J. (1995). Effect of impact stress on microbial recovery on an agar surface. *Applied and Environmental Microbiology*, *61*, 1232–1239.

Thamdrup, R., & Fleischer, S. (1998). Temperature dependence of oxygen respiration, nitrogen mineralization, and nitrification in Arctic sediments. *Aquatic Microbial Ecology*, *15*, 191–199.

12

Cleanroom Microbiota

CHAPTER OUTLINE
Introduction 199
Growth Requirements of Microorganisms 200
Strategies for Microbial Survival in the Cleanroom
Environment 201
Effect of Survival Strategy on Microbial Identification 202
Types of Microorganisms Found in Cleanrooms
and Their Origins 203
    Personnel 203
    Air 204
    Surfaces (Equipment, Walls and Ceilings) 205
    Raw Materials 205
    Packaging Materials 206
    Water 207
Details of Cleanroom Microbiota 207
Viruses 210
Conclusion 210
References 211

INTRODUCTION

Examining the range, types, and patterns of microorganisms found in cleanrooms (sometimes described as the collective "microflora" or, more accurately, "microbiota") provides essential information for microbiologists in understanding cleanroom environments and for assisting with contamination control. Such benchmarking helps to establish a "norm" and provide a measure for trending purposes (such as noting the frequency of occurrence of isolates by genera or species over time and across cleanrooms or locations within cleanrooms) (Akers, 1997). Furthermore, establishing the normal microbial flora and using microbial identification can be used to assess the effectiveness of the cleaning and sanitization program and to investigate the source of microbial contamination, especially when environmental monitoring action levels are exceeded.

Biocontamination Control for Pharmaceuticals and Healthcare. https://doi.org/10.1016/B978-0-12-814911-9.00012-2

Notwithstanding the importance of such information, there have been very few studies of pharmaceutical cleanroom microbiota published in recent years. Despite the low number of published analyses, such studies can prove to be very useful for microbiologists in benchmarking the types and frequency of incidence of the more common microorganisms likely to occur in cleanrooms. This is an important feature of ensuring good microbiological control. Most importantly, examinations of the microbiota allow microbiologists to make comparisons with their own data against that collected from similar organizations.

GROWTH REQUIREMENTS OF MICROORGANISMS

Microorganisms on earth are widely distributed across different environmental habitats. They are present in water, air, sediments, and soil (Wilson, 1997). One of the reasons for the wide distribution of microorganisms in the environment is the great physiological diversity regarding the utilization of inorganic and organic compounds to sustain microbial viability, maintenance, reproduction, and growth. Although microbial populations are present in all types of habitats, there are several major limiting factors that affect microbial distribution, survival, and proliferation in the environment.

These factors are divided into two categories: first, the range of substrates, the consumables needed (concentration of organic and inorganic compounds) to support cell division; and second, the nature of the environment, that is, temperature, pH, osmotic pressure, and so forth.

Even within "ideal" chemical conditions, microbial growth will be slow, although it can be enhanced by the presence of trace elements and carbohydrates, fats, proteinaceous material, amino acids, sugars, and vitamins such as nicotinic acid, riboflavin, and thiamine. Notwithstanding the simple nutritional requirements of some organisms, others exhibit specific needs (these needs form the basis of selective and diagnostic culture media). The microbial cells degrade organic and inorganic compounds to sustain microbial metabolism. Some microbial species do not require high concentrations of organic or inorganic compounds to survive and grow. Microbial species such as *Pseudomonas* spp., *Acinetobacter* spp., *Burkholderia* spp., and *Stenotrophomonas* spp. exhibit a tremendous physiological versatility by using a wide variety of organic and inorganic compounds to support microbial metabolism. Microorganisms carry the energy needed for metabolic processes in the phosphate energy-rich molecule called adenosine triphosphate (ATP).

Microorganisms must be able to respond to variations in nutrient levels, and particularly to nutrient limitation, in order to survive. The growth of microorganisms also is greatly affected by the chemical and physical nature of their surroundings. An understanding of environmental influences aids in the control of microbial growth and the study of the ecological distribution of microorganisms. The ability of some microorganisms to adapt to extreme and inhospitable environments is truly remarkable. For example, *Bacillus infernus* is able to survive at a depth 1.5 miles below the Earth's surface, without oxygen and at temperatures above 60°C. Microorganisms that grow in such harsh conditions are termed "extremophiles."

In general, microbial growth is influenced by various environmental factors such as:

- Available water,
- Concentration of particulates in the air,
- Concentration of hydrogen ions (pH),
- Temperature,
- Redox potential (Eh),
- Pressure,
- Light intensity.

STRATEGIES FOR MICROBIAL SURVIVAL IN THE CLEANROOM ENVIRONMENT

Microbial ecology in pharmaceutical environments is controlled by various environmental factors such as temperature, pH, nutrient availability, pressure, and water availability. Microbial flora in cleanroom environments can be effectively controlled by adjusting different parameters (Hyde, 1998). Unlike microorganisms growing in culture, microorganisms within the pharmaceutical environment—the cleanroom—behave in different ways according to different environmental conditions.

How do microorganisms respond to different environmental fluctuations in the environment? Pharmaceutical manufacturing comprises physical processes such as blending, compression, filtration, heating, encapsulation, shearing, tableting, granulation, coating, and drying. These processes expose microbial cells to extensive environmental stresses. Microorganisms respond to the lack of nutrients and other environmental fluctuations by undertaking different survival strategies (Roszak & Colwell, 1987). Thus microorganisms recovered from production environments are stressed due to the fluctuations of parameters during manufacturing processes, lack of nutrients, low water activity, contact with chemicals, and temperature changes. With these strategies, microorganisms are not always metabolically active and reproducing.

Under conditions of limited supply of nutrition vegetative forms of certain bacteria, notably Gram-positive rods and Actinomycetes, form highly resistant and dehydrated forms which are called as endospores. Bacterial endospores can resist extreme conditions and survive for years in the absence of nutrients. However, when nutrients return, these spores can germinate and become growing cells (Setlow & Johnson, 2007). Bacterial spores are more resistant than fungal spores and yeasts, and considerably more resistant than vegetative bacteria to the actions of antiseptics and disinfectants (Russell & Furr, 1996).

Biofilm formation is another important survival strategy against environmental stress. A biofilm is a complex aggregation of microorganisms growing on solid substrate. A biofilm contains about 15% of microbial cells and 85% extra polymeric substance (EPS). EPS is composed of polysaccharides, proteins, other polymers, and water. Biofilms are characterized by structural heterogeneity, genetic diversity, and complex community interactions. A biofilm formation is often initiated by micro colonies from one type of organism. However, biofilms quickly become heterogeneous as mixed cultures of bacteria, as well as fungi, algae, and protozoa join the established structure and become intermixed. In fact, within a biofilm different types of microorganisms can coexist and form stable communities. It is resistant to phagocytic amoebae, and much more resistant than planktonic cells to antimicrobial agents. For example, chlorination of a biofilm is usually unsuccessful because the biocide only kills the bacteria in the outer layers of biofilm. The bacteria within the biofilm remain healthy and the biofilm can regrow. Repeated use of antimicrobial agents on biofilms can cause bacteria within the biofilm to develop an increased resistance to biocides. In the pharmaceutical environments, biofilms can develop on the product contact surfaces of equipment and interiors of water purification and distribution system, which leads to clogs, corrosion, and biological contamination of the system (Reidewald, 1997).

EFFECT OF SURVIVAL STRATEGY ON MICROBIAL IDENTIFICATION

When microbial populations adopt some of these survival strategies which, identification by standard methods is difficult and this can lead to erroneous conclusions. For instance, Gram-positive bacteria such as *Bacillus* spp. and *Clostridium* spp. develop dormant structures called spores (Underwood, 1998). Moreover, Gram-negative bacteria such as *Escherichia coli*, *Salmonella typhimurium*, and other Gram-negative rods can undergo a viable but nonculturable stage (Roszak & Colwell, 1987). Furthermore, bacterial cells that do not grow on plate media but retain their viability also move through the viable but nonculturable stage; however, such organisms are still capable of causing severe infections to humans. Similar responses have been reported by bacteria exposed to drug solutions where significant morphological and size changes have been observed (Whyte, Niven, & Bell, 1989). Bacterial cells challenged into different types of injectable products have been shown to undergo different changes in their metabolism, enzymatic profiles, and structural changes that have interfered with their identification using standard biochemical assays (Papapetropoulou & Papageorgakopoulou, 1994). Furthermore, some bacteria undergoing starvation survival periods are theoretically capable of penetrating 0.22 μm rated filters, which are designed to retain most bacterial species (Sundaram, Mallick, Eisenhuth, Howard, & Brandwein, 2001).

Therefore using biochemical identification tests, along with colony and cell morphology to discriminate and identify microorganisms from environmental samples might, in some cases, yield unknown profiles that will not provide any significant information on the microbial genera and species. Hence the development of better analytical methods has provided a more accurate and sensitive representation of the distribution and activity of microorganisms in the stressed environment. The better methods include genotyping, analysis of whole cell fatty acid methyl esters, mass spectrometry, and pyrolysis. This new information has supplemented the knowledge obtained using traditional culture and enrichment methods.

TYPES OF MICROORGANISMS FOUND IN CLEANROOMS AND THEIR ORIGINS

The commonly considered five main sources of microbial contamination in cleanrooms are (Halls, 2007) as follows:

1. Personnel.
2. Room air.
3. Surfaces (equipment, wall, floor).
4. Raw materials and packing materials which entered into the cleanroom.
5. Water (where applicable).

Personnel

Microorganisms may be transferred to pharmaceutical preparations from the process operator. This is undesirable for sterile products, as it could result in patient death; and in the case of tablets and powders such contamination may result in spoilage of solutions or suspensions. A level of protection is afforded by personnel wearing masks, gloves, and cleanroom suits and through protective airflow barriers from unidirectional airflow cabinets (Cundell, 2004).

Of the natural skin flora *Staphylococcus aureus* is perhaps the most undesirable for nonsterile products. It is common on the hands and face and, since it resides in the deep layers of the skin, is not eliminated by washing. Other bacteria present on skin are the Micrococci, other Staphylococci, *Sarcina* spp. and diphtheroids, but occasionally Gram-negative rods such as *Acinetobacter* spp. and *Alcaligenes* spp. achieve resident status (Somerville-Millar & Noble, 1974). In the fatty and waxy sections of the skin, lipophilic yeasts are often present, *Pityrosporum ovale* on the scalp and *P. orbiculare* on glabrous skin. Various dermatophyte fungi such as species of *Epidermophyton*, *Microsporum*, and *Trichophyton* may also be present. Ear secretions may also contain saprophytic bacteria. Additionally, the Human Microbiome Project has revealed a rich diversity of microorganisms carried on the human body (Wilder, Sandle, & Sutton, 2013).

Air

A second critical area is the air in the facility. Air ventilation systems in manufacturing facilities are built to minimize the survival, distribution, reproduction, and growth of microbes. This facility is provided with heating ventilation and air conditioning (HVAC), which controls these parameters (as set out in Chapter 5). The air is filtered through a filter to prevent the introduction into the facility of any particle larger than 0.3 μm. Microorganisms are commonly associated with particles in the air. Therefore the exclusion of these particles in the facility minimizes the chances of microbial distribution and contamination by air.

Airflow and pressure are controlled to exclude any nonviable and viable particle from entering critical areas. Humidity also controls the number of microorganisms in a room. The more humid is the room, the more chances there are for microorganisms to be carried by droplets of moisture. Therefore a dry room provides a more hostile condition for microbes to grow than a humid room. Additionally, ultraviolet light (UV) is applied to some contained devices to reduce microbial contamination by air, although the effectiveness of UV light remains a matter of conjecture.

Some of the microbial species commonly found in air samples in pharmaceutical environments are bacteria such as *Micrococcus* spp., *Bacillus* spp., *Staphylococcus* spp., *Corynebacterium* spp. Common mold species are *Aspergillus* spp. and *Penicillium* spp.

Surfaces (Equipment, Walls and Ceilings)

Unless equipment is cleaned and sanitized, there is always the risk of microbial contamination. However, cleaning and sanitization of the equipment must provide a hostile environment for microorganisms to survive and grow. With general cleanrooms, bacteria such as *Pseudomonas* spp., *Staphylococcus epidermidis*, *Bacillus* spp., and so on, are commonly found on surfaces and equipment. With aseptic processing areas, and areas where there are no water sources, microorganisms like *Pseudomonas* spp. would not be expected.

If any filters or straining bags made from natural materials such as canvas, muslin, or paper are used, then care must be taken to ensure that they are cleaned and sterilized regularly to prevent the growth of molds such as *Cladosporium* spp., *Stachybotrys* spp., and *Aureobasidium (Pullularia) pullulans*. These fungi can utilize cellulose and would thus impair the fibers (Underwood, 1998).

Molds are the most common flora of found on walls and ceilings and the species usually found are *Cladosporium* spp., *Aspergillus* spp. (in particular *A. niger* and *A. flavus*), *Penicillium* spp., and *Aureobasidium (Pullularia)* spp. Such fungi are particularly common in poorly ventilated buildings with painted walls. These fungi derive most of their nutrients from the plaster on to which the paint has been applied and a hard gloss finish is more resistant than a softer, matt one. The addition of up to 1% of a fungistat, such as pentachlorophenol, 8-hydroxyquinoline, or salicylanilide, can slowdown the rate of fungal growth. To reduce microbial growth, all walls and ceilings should be smooth, impervious, nonshedding, and washable and this requirement may be met by cladding with a laminated plastic (Underwood, 1998). Continuous sanitization and disinfection of floors, drains walls, and ceilings are advised to avoid the microbial colonization areas.

Raw Materials

Raw materials account for a high proportion of the microorganisms introduced during the manufacture of pharmaceuticals, and the selection of materials of a good microbiological quality aids in the control of contamination levels in both products and the environment. Different types of bacteria commonly found in pharmaceutical raw materials include *Lactobacillus* spp., *Pseudomonas* spp., *Bacillus* spp., *Escherichia* spp., *Streptococcus* spp., *Clostridium* spp., *Agrobacterium* spp., and so on, and molds such as *Cladosporium* spp. and *Fusarium* spp. The types of microorganisms will relate to the type of material and its point of origin. Some of the raw materials utilized for the development of pharmaceutical formulations are based upon natural products, and thus they can contain a high microbial load. For example Ku et al. (1994) reported crude Chinese drugs were contaminated with bacterial and fungal isolates. In a survey of 19 crude drugs, where a total of 119 samples were analyzed, it was found that 66% of samples contained coliforms, 59% *Bacillus cereus*, 1% *Salmonella* spp., and 3% *S. aureus*. The fungal flora of materials of plant origin such as gum acacia and tragacanth, agar, and starches may arise from that are indigenous to plants and may include molds such as species of *Cladosporium*, *Alternaria*, and *Fusarium* and nonmycelated yeasts.

To ensure the quality control of raw materials they are subject to bioburden tests, as described in the pharmacopeia (total aerobic microbial count and total yeast and mold count). For specific microorganisms, these are screened for presence or absence of indicator microorganisms. Therefore the absence of *E. coli*, *S. aureus*, *Pseudomonas aeruginosa*, and *S. typhimurium* is required before these types of raw materials can be used in pharmaceutical products. Some manufacturers also elect to screen for other types of "objectionable" microorganisms of relevance to the material, process, or finished product.

Packaging Materials

Packaging material has a dual role for it acts both to contain the product and to prevent the entry of microorganisms or moisture which may result in spoilage. It is therefore important that the source of contamination is not the packaging itself. The microbiota of packaging materials is dependent upon both its composition and storage conditions. This, and a consideration of the type of pharmaceutical product to be packed, determines whether a sterilization treatment is required (for aseptically filled products all primary packaging: vials, closures, and crimps must be sterile and pyrogen free). Glass containers are sterile on leaving the furnace but are often stored in dusty conditions and packed for transport in cardboard boxes. As a result, they may contain mold spores of species of *Penicillium*, *Aspergillus*, and bacteria such as *Bacillus* species.

Packaging materials which have a smooth, impervious surface, free from crevices or interstices, such as cellulose acetate, polyethylene, polypropylene, poly vinyl chloride, and metal foils and laminates, all have a low surface microbial count. Cardboard and paperboard, unless treated, carry mold spores of species of species of *Cladosporium*, *Aspergillus*, and *Penicillium* and bacteria such as *Bacillus* spp. and *Micrococcus* spp. The risk increases where cardboard becomes damp and as a result introducing cardboard into cleanrooms is avoided where possible.

Water

Water is often the major component of pharmaceutical preparations and it can be a very significant source of contamination. Water for pharmaceutical processes is further treated to minimize microbial numbers, endotoxin substances, and organic and inorganic compounds. The less organic compounds there are in the water, the fewer microorganisms to be found. Bacterial species such *Pseudomonas* spp., *Alcaligenes* spp., *Stenotrophomonas* spp., *Burkholderia cepacia*, *Burkholderia pickettii*, *Serratia* spp., and *Flavobacterium* spp. are commonly found in water samples. Other types of bacteria can also be present but when found, they indicate fecal sources of contamination. These bacteria are *E. coli*, *Enterobacter* spp., *Klebsiella* spp., *Salmonella* spp., *Shigella* spp., *Clostridium perfringens*, and *Enterococcus* spp. Product or environment contamination may arise directly from the process water, indirectly from cleaning operations, or by cross-contamination from the wet areas of floors, sinks, and drains to the processing equipment. To overcome this, water must be strictly controlled. For the most critical operations, Water for Injection (WFI) is used.

DETAILS OF CLEANROOM MICROBIOTA

Most common microorganisms in cleanrooms are Gram-positive bacteria (Hyde, 1998). These microorganisms often have a close phylogenetic affiliation as indicated by comparative analysis of partial 16S rRNA studies, such as between the *Micrococci* and *Staphylococci*. The most common species include species of *Micrococcus*, *Staphylococcus*, *Corynebacterium*, *Bacillus*, *Aspergillus*, and *Penicillium* (Wu & Liu, 2007). In addition, there are, in fewer numbers, certain fungi associated with cleanrooms.

With the genera *Staphylococcus* and *Micrococcus*, many of the species are indigenous to humans. Although Gram-positive microorganism are ubiquitous in cleanrooms and make up the overwhelming majority of isolates, there is little published work relating to the expected proportion of microorganisms found in cleanrooms, except that the majority isolated are Gram-positive cocci (Wilson, 1997; Wu & Liu, 2007). The vast majority of bacteria isolated from cleanrooms are mesophilic aerobic or facultatively aerobic bacteria.

Sandle (Sandle, 2011) reported that higher proportion of Gram-positive cocci are recovered from air samples than from surface samples, and this group remains the most commonly recovered from both sample types. This is consistent with the findings from the Grade B area and is consistent with the literature which indicates that personnel will shed such microorganisms

(Booth, 2006; Cundell, 2004). Gram-positive rods occur in slightly higher numbers for surface samples. This proportion is consistent with the theory that the majority of Gram-positive rods will be carried or deposited from footwear, especially through the transmission of soil or from incoming materials or equipment. A higher proportion of Gram-negative rods in the cleanroom will relate to the operation of wet areas and wash bays. Although water can remain on the floor, it is common for aerosols to be produced (either through equipment operation or by splashing). With cleanrooms without a water source, the characteristic microbial population identified in such controlled areas is composed of bacteria, such as *Staphylococcus* spp., *Micrococcus* spp., and *Bacillus* spp.

The top most common microorganisms present in cleanroom environment are Gram-positive organisms. Sandle (Sandle, 2011) reported that *Micrococcus luteus* and *Micrococcus lylae*—two obligate aerobes—were the most commonly represented microorganisms over the nine-year period of analysis done in various pharmaceutical establishments in England and Wales. The second most common are staphylococci. Staphylococci are the causative agents of many opportunistic human and animal infections and are considered among the most important pathogens isolated in the clinical microbiology laboratory. Here the most commonly occurring *Staphylococcus* species found in cleanrooms were *S. epidermidis*, *S. capitis*, *S. hominis*, and *S. haemolyticus*.

The second most common genera are species of *Bacillus* (and related genera) present in pharmaceutical cleanrooms. Bacteria of the *Bacillus* genus can adopt several strategies, including the formation of dormant, highly resistant entities called spores, to ensure their individual survival and, even more importantly, the survival of the population. For their resistance characteristics, bacterial spores have been defined as the stress "survival capsules." In fact, spore formers upon sporulation remain viable in the environment after long period of dormancy, with some reports placing this limit at 40–250 million years (Cano et al., 1994). Spore long-term survival could be explained by their dormancy, their high resistance to heat, desiccation, acid, radiation, chemicals, their persistence in the environment in terms of adhesion potential, and their phenotypic variability. Sandle (2011) reported that the common species of bacillus isolated from the pharmaceutical cleanroom are *Bacillus sphaericus* and *Bacillus fusiformis*. The numbers of Gram-positive rods are proportionately higher than for air and surface samples, which may suggest a tendency for personnel to touch surfaces.

According to the Sandle findings the numbers of Gram-positive rods are relatively higher in Grade C and D cleanrooms, indicating the greater opportunities for such microorganisms to be transported into cleanrooms. Unlike Grade A and B clean areas, where many items entering the cleanrooms would have been subject to some type of sterilization, equipment entering lower grade cleanrooms is often subject to less stringent controls. These microorganisms and their spores can be carried into clean areas on footwear or by equipment transfer; a low level is not unexpected.

Second to Bacillus species are *Corynebacterium* species, which occur commonly in nature in the soil, water, plants, and food product. The non-diphtheroid *Corynebacterium* species can even be found in the mucosa and normal skin flora of humans and animals. Some species are known for their pathogenic effects in humans and other animals. These organisms are nonspore formers. A species of similar appearance, also sometimes isolated from cleanrooms, are species of *Brevibacterium*.

The numbers of Gram-negative bacteria recovered from a cleanroom environment will be very low across air, surface, and personnel samples categories. A low number may be transferred from changing rooms or related to personnel hygiene issues (such as coughing or sneezing). Sandle (2011) reported that only 6% of Gram-negative rods found in samples and 4% in surface samples. Greater number of water sources found environment (sinks, wash bays) introduce Gram-negative bacterial contamination into the cleanrooms. The most commonly reported Gram-negative bacterial isolates are *P. aeruginosa* and other species of *Pseudomonas*, *Moraxella* and *Rhodococcus*. Other organisms identified by DNA-based methods are *Pantoea* spp., *Ralstonia pickettii*, *Enterobacter cancerogenus*, *Aeromonas hydrophila*, and so forth.

Fungi in pharmaceutical processing environments originate from air, water, personnel, and the material introduced into different facilities, where products are manufactured and tested. There is no published evidence of fungal contamination profile in pharmaceutical cleanrooms. Very few articles are available regarding mold contamination incidences from pharmaceutical cleanroom environments. Therefore it is very difficult to make comparison between the aerobiocontamination data across different regions.

Over the years, several mold issues associated with pharmaceutical cleanrooms, cold rooms, and controlled areas have been reported (Vijayakumar, Sandle, & Manoharan, 2012). Molds are ubiquitous in nature and therefore pose a risk to pharmaceutical manufacturing operations. Such molds are detected by effective environmental monitoring regimes by a range of air and surface monitoring techniques using appropriate microbiological culture media (Sandle, 2011). Several vaccine and pharmaceutical companies in Europe experienced an increase in mold contamination due to increase in ambient temperatures and issues with items brought into cleanrooms. Wet or damp areas are a further factor which can encourage fungal growth in cleanrooms. Typical cleanroom fungi are: *Aspergillus* spp., *Penicillium* spp., *Trichophyton* spp., *Penicillium* spp., and *Cladosporium* spp.

VIRUSES

While generally outside the scope of this book, viral contamination is common in biopharmaceutical sectors and, depending on the product, can be of concern. Viral contamination of pharmaceutical processes is a specialized area and falls outside the scope of this book. However, viral contamination of cell lines used for the production of biopharmaceuticals presents potential hazards to the process operators as well as the patient, and so a brief discussion is important. Viral contamination may originate from the cell line, the raw materials, or the process operators. Viruses may be found in contaminated water supplies such as Adenovirus, Enterovirus, Hepatitis A, Norwalk agent, Reovirus, Rotavirus, and Coxsackie Virus. To eliminate viruses, heat is the most reliable method of virus disinfection. Most human pathogenic viruses are inactivated following exposure at 60°C for 30 min. The virus of serum hepatitis can, however, survive this temperature for up to 4 h. Viruses are stable at low temperatures and are routinely stored at −40°C to −70°C. Some viruses are rapidly inactivated by drying; others survive well in a desiccated state. Ultraviolet light inactivates viruses by damaging their nucleic acid and has been used to prepare viral vaccines. For products that cannot be subject to heat, alternative viral removal steps include solvent–detergent and nanofiltration (Froud, Birch, McLean, Shepherd, & Smith, 1997).

CONCLUSION

This chapter has discussed the microorganisms found in cleanrooms. The chapter has considered the types of species found and the possible sources of their origins. While the number of published studies is limited, and comparators will be limited through variations relating to geography, cleanroom type, and variations in processing, the material presented in this chapter should act as useful reference for the cleanroom microbiologist. To enable an assessment of microbial trends, the microbiologist should regularly review and trend isolates from the environmental monitoring program.

Trends and reviews of cleanroom microbiota should be adaptable and focused on industry developments. Advances in identification methods, as well as reclassification of microorganisms through sequencing data, will produce more unusual species as well as regroupings; moreover, the results of the Human Microbiome Project suggest that people are host to richer and more diverse community of microorganisms than ever previously realized. However, while microbial taxonomy may change, the types and sources of microbial contamination within the cleanroom will not. For this, the discussion around microbial types, patterns, and contamination sources presented in this chapter should prove to be a valuable tool for those with an interest in cleanroom microbiology.

REFERENCES

Akers, J. E. (1997). Environmental monitoring and control: proposed standards, current practices, and future directions. *Journal of Pharmaceutical Science and Technology*, *51*(1), 36–47.

Booth, C. (2006). Microbe monitoring. *Cleanroom Technology*, 18–20.

Cano, R. J., Borucki, M. K., Higby-Schweitzer, M., Poinar, H. N., Poinar, G. O., et al. (1994). Bacillus DNA in fossil bees: an ancient symbiosis? *Applied and Environmental Microbiology*, *60*, 2164–2167.

Cundell, A. M. (2004). Microbial testing in support of aseptic processing. *Pharmaceutical Technology*, 56–66. June.

Froud, S. J., Birch, J. R., McLean, C., Shepherd, A. J., & Smith, K. T. (1997). Viral contaminants found in mouse cell lines used in the production of biological products. In M. J. T. Carondo, B. Griffiths, & J. L. P. Moreira (Eds.), *Animal cell technology* (pp. 681–686). Dordrecht, The Netherlands: Kluwer Academic Press.

Halls, N. (2007). Risk management: practicalities and problems in pharmaceutical manufacture. In N. Halls (Ed.), *Pharmaceutical contamination control* (pp. 171–204). Bethesda, MD: PDA/DHI.

Hyde, W. (1998). Origin of bacteria in the clean room and their growth requirements. *PDA Journal of Pharmaceutical Science and Technology*, *52*, 154–164.

Ku, Y. R., Chou, L. M., Jang, C. F., Liu, Y. C., Lin, J. H., & Wen, G. C. (1994). Study of microbial contamination in concentrated Chinese medicine. *Journal of Food Drug Analysis*, *1*, 49–62.

Papapetropoulou, M., & Papageorgakopoulou, N. (1994). Metabolic and structural changes in *Pseudomonas aeruginosa*, Achromobacter CDC, and Agrobacterium radiobacter cells injured in parenteral fluids. *PDA Journal of Pharmaceutical Science and Technology*, *48*, 299–303.

Reidewald, F. (1997). Biofilms in pharmaceutical waters. *Pharmaceutical Engineering*, 8–10. June.

Roszak, D. B., & Colwell, R. R. (1987). Survival strategies of bacteria in the natural environment. *Microbiological Reviews*, *51*, 365–379.

Russell, A. D., & Furr, J. R. (1996). Biocides: mechanisms of antifungal action and fungal resistance. *Science Progress*, *19*, 27–48.

Sandle, T. (2011). A review of cleanroom microbiota: types, trends and patterns. *PDA Journal of Pharmaceutical Science and Technology*, *65*(4), 392–403.

Setlow, P., & Johnson, E. A. (2007). Spores and their significance. In M. P. Doyle, & L. R. Beuchat (Eds.), *Food microbiology: Fundamentals and frontiers* (3rd ed., pp. 35–67). Washington, DC: ASM Press.

Somerville-Millar, D., & Noble, W. C. (1974). Resident and transient bacteria of the skin. *Journal of Cutaneous Pathology, 1*(6), 260–264.

Sundaram, S., Mallick, S., Eisenhuth, J., Howard, G., & Brandwein, H. (2001). Retention of water-borne bacteria by membrane filters. Part II: Scanning electron microscopy (SEM) and fatty acid methyl ester (FAME) characterization of bacterial species recovered downstream of 0.2/0.22 micron rated filters. *PDA Journal of Pharmaceutical Science and Technology, 55*, 87–113.

Underwood, E. (1998). Ecology of microorganisms as its affects the pharmaceutical industry. In W. B. Hugo, & A. B. Russell (Eds.), *Pharmaceutical microbiology* (6th ed., pp. 339–354). Oxford, England: Blackwell Science.

Vijayakumar, R., Sandle, T., & Manoharan, C. (2012). A review on fungal contamination in pharmaceutical products and phenotypic identification of contaminants by conventional methods. *European Journal for Parenteral and Pharmaceutical Sciences, 17*(1), 4–18.

Whyte, W., Niven, L., & Bell, N. D. (1989). Microbial growth in small-volume pharmaceuticals. *Journal of Parenteral Science and Technology, 43*, 208–212.

Wilder, C., Sandle, T., & Sutton, S. (2013). Implications of the human microbiome on pharmaceutical microbiology. *American Pharmaceutical Review, 16*(5), 17–21.

Wilson, J. D. (1997). Setting alert-action limits for environmental monitoring programs. *PDA Journal of Pharmaceutical Science and Technology, 51*, 161–162.

Wu, G. F., & Liu, X. H. (2007). Characterization of predominant bacteria isolates from clean rooms in a pharmaceutical production unit. *Journal of Zhejiang University Science B, 8*(9), 666–672.

Assessment of Pharmaceutical Water Systems

CHAPTER OUTLINE

Introduction   213
Use of Water in Pharmaceutical Manufacturing   214
   Potable Water   214
   Purified Water   215
   Water for Injections   215
   Sterile and Nonsterile Products   216
Endotoxin Risks and WFI   216
   Controlling Endotoxin Risks in WFI   217
Controlling Other Microbial Risks to Water Systems   218
Addressing Water System Contamination   219
Water System Monitoring: Sampling, Testing, and Reporting   220
   Total Aerobic Viable Counts   220
   Undesirable ("Objectionable") Microorganisms   222
   Test for Bacterial Endotoxin   222
   Sample-Related Contamination   223
Summary   223
References   223

INTRODUCTION

The pharmacopoeia deal with ingredient water as one of two categories: purified water and water for injection. Water for injection can be microbiologically defined as water complying with the requirements contained in the monograph for purified water with the addition of a limit of not >0.25 EU/mL and a tighter standard for microbial limits. Hence in relation to sterile products the pharmacopeial differences between WFI and Purified Water are clear; WFI has a restriction on endotoxin content and Purified Water has not, therefore only WFI may be used in as ingredient water for preparations which are also required to comply with endotoxin limits, namely, the parenteral products (Sandle, 2004a).

Biocontamination Control for Pharmaceuticals and Healthcare. https://doi.org/10.1016/B978-0-12-814911-9.00013-4

Purified Water may be prepared by distillation, ion exchange, or reverse osmosis. WFI, until 2017, to be compliant with Ph. Eur. was only permitted to be prepared by distillation. Lipopolysaccharide has a molecular weight of around 10^6, heavy enough to be left behind when water is rapidly boiled off as in a still. In 2017 the Ph. Eur. was updated to match the USP, and henceforth WFI may be prepared by distillation or reverse osmosis. The decision to expand WFI to include reverse osmosis was not supported by all, not least because of concerns that the application of reverse osmosis on endotoxin removal (ion exchange does not remove endotoxin from water). Distillation certainly removes endotoxin from water. Reverse osmosis at least in theory removes endotoxin from water by acting as a molecular sieve through which lipopolysaccharide cannot pass.

In addition to microbial control, there is a need for the chemical purification of water in order to prevent interaction with drug substances and/or other ingredients in the formulation. The combination of chemical and physical methods used to purify water is based on robust technology which can, in most cases, reduce the level of chemical "contaminants" to less than one part per million (ppm or $1:10^{-6}$), and assay sensitivity is frequently in the range of parts per billion (ppb or $1:10^{-9}$). The methods of chemical analysis generate answers quickly enough to ensure a rapid response to problems.

This chapter provides an overview of pharmaceutical grade water, with a focus on contamination control concerns.

USE OF WATER IN PHARMACEUTICAL MANUFACTURING

Different grades of water are suitable for use in various aspects of pharmaceutical manufacture. These systems should be appropriately designed and qualified (Sandle, 2017a). An important point is that when water is used in connection with something which comes into contact with a pharmaceutical preparation its final rinse in its cleaning must be done with water of the same grade as that used in the pharmaceutical preparation.

The different types of water are described in the following sections.

Potable Water

Potable water is, by definition, drinking water, and the starting material required by the regulatory authorities in both Europe and the United States for any pharmaceutical grade of purified water. The use of potable water in any final dosage form is not permitted. Potable water is sometimes referred to as mains or towns water.

Private water companies or municipalities supply potable water according to local quality requirements, which are, in principle, very similar and are designed to protect human health. Health protection is concerned with monitoring water quality, ensuring that levels of chemical pollutants remain within established safety criteria, and that waterborne diseases will not be transmitted. The microbial standard almost universally applied is a heterotrophic plate count of 500 cfu/mL or less and the absence of indicator microorganisms of fecal origin in samples of 100 mL. If the limits are exceeded the water supplier must take immediate action which usually involves additional chlorination.

Purified Water

Purified water is intended for use in formulation of medicines that are not intended to be sterile and apyrogenic. Purified water is widely used for oral and topical products and in granulation processes for tablets and capsules. It is also the feed water for the production of water for injection (WFI) and for pharmaceutical grade clean steam. Purified water is also used for the rinsing of equipment and for the preparation of cleaning solutions. The microbial action limit in Europe is 100 cfu/mL (equivalent to 10,000 cfu/100 mL, given that the main test method is by membrane filtration). In the United States, the compendia recommend that the limit is set by risk assessment.

Purified water is prepared by reverse osmosis. Reverse osmosis units use a semipermeable membrane and a substantial pressure differential to drive the water through the membrane to achieve chemical, microbial, and endotoxin quality improvements. The systems exist in multiple design formats and are often used in series. Reverse osmosis functions as a size-excluding filter operating under a highly pressurized condition.

Water for Injections

Water for injection (WFI) is the highest quality of water used by the pharmaceutical industry and it may be prepared either by reverse osmosis or distillation. Reverse osmosis is described before; with distillation, the process functions by turning water from a liquid to a vapor and then from vapor back to liquid. Endotoxin is removed by the rapid boiling which causes the water molecules to evaporate and the relatively larger endotoxin complex molecules to remain behind. Most models of distillation equipment are validated to achieve 2.5–3 log reductions in endotoxin concentration during distillation.

WFI is used for the preparation of parenteral medicines, dialysis, and irrigation solutions. Large volumes are also consumed by the biotechnology industry for the preparation of cell culture media. To meet the requirements in Europe, the microbial action limit is 10 cfu/100 mL, and the level of bacterial endotoxin must be <0.25 EU/mL. In the United States, the compendia recommend that the limits are set by risk assessment.

Sterile and Nonsterile Products

This quite simply means that for sterile parenteral products WFI should be used for:

- final rinse for cleaning product contact equipment and tools,
- final rinse for cleaning containers and closures,
- for diluting disinfectants.

In nonsterile pharmaceutical facilities, it is typical for purified water to be used for cleaning, disinfectant preparation, and product formulation.

WFI is not commonly used in hand wash sinks, and it is variable whether it is used for the final rinse in laundering sterile area garments (it is much more corrosive than "normal" softened water). Further with sterile manufacturing areas, water sources should not be permitted in EU GMP Grade B/ISO 14644 Class 7 (in operation) areas nor should there be drains. Never forget the humble drain. These are not permitted in Annex 1. Where water is required for cleaning in EU GMP Grade A/ISO 14644 Class 5, and Grade B areas it should be sterile filtered WFI. WFI should be used for diluting disinfectants and subsequently the dilutions should be sterile filtered into the Grade B area. Floors should be dried with sterilized squeegee mops.

ENDOTOXIN RISKS AND WFI

WFI as prepared by the pharmacopeially approved processes of distillation (or suitable reverse osmosis processes) will comply in terms of permitted bioburden and endotoxin levels (if sampled directly from the preparation point and not contaminated in sampling or testing). However, it is immediately fed to a storage tank and pumped round a distribution system where at least in theory microbiological contamination may be lurking and shedding endotoxin.

Endotoxin is the primary risk for WFI systems; only very poorly designed WFI systems will see a bioburden problem (here an atypical event, such as poor maintenance work where the system has been cut into, will see a contamination event leading to biofilm formation) (Hall-Stoodley, Costerton, & Stoodley, 2004).

To understand what endotoxin is, the bacterial cell structure needs to be considered. The structural rigidity of the bacterial cell wall is conferred by a material called peptidoglycan (also known as murein). It is a polymer consisting of sugars and amino acids that forms a mesh-like layer outside the plasma membrane of bacteria, forming the cell wall. In Gram-positive bacteria peptidoglycan is present as a thick layer which is outermost in the cell wall. In Gram-negative bacteria, the peptidoglycan is only a thin layer and it is not the outermost layer. Gram-negative bacteria are sometimes described as having a cell envelope rather than a cell wall. The term envelope better describes the loosely attached layer of material called lipopolysaccharide which is located outside a thin structural layer of peptidoglycan (Guy, 2003).

Although intimately associated with the cell envelope of Gram-negative bacteria, lipopolysaccharide is constantly shed by the bacteria into the environment, much like the shedding of the outer layers of human skin. When Gram-negative bacteria die and lyse, all of their lipopolysaccharide is shed into the environment. Furthermore, when bacterial cells are lysed by the immune system, fragments of membrane containing lipid A are released into the circulation, causing fever, diarrhea, and possible fatal endotoxic shock (also called septic shock).

Controlling Endotoxin Risks in WFI

When used in bulk for manufacturing purposes the Ph. Eur. applies a microbiological limit to WFI, this is not >10 cfu/100 mL. This microbiological limit for WFI does not tie in with the endotoxin specification. The amount of endotoxin associated with Gram-negative bacteria is thought to be around 10–15 g per bacterium. The first batch of reference standard endotoxin titrated at 1 EU $= 2 \times 10^{-10}$ g (Rudbach et al., n.d.). Therefore the endotoxin limit of 0.25 EU/mL for Water for Injections can be understood to correspond to 5×10^{-11} g/mL or about 10^4 bacteria/mL. Despite the fact that there is a great deal of uncertainty about these figures, and that Gram-negative bacteria not only have associated endotoxin but also shed endotoxin continuously, and that Gram-positive bacteria are generally not very endotoxic, it is apparent that water which meets the limit for endotoxin may exceed the limit for viable microorganisms (10 cfu/100 mL).

The means of controlling the development of Gram-negative (and other) microorganisms in water storage and distribution systems are (Sandle, 2017b) as follows:

1. *Smooth internal surfaces in tanks and in pipe work*: Microorganisms adhere less well to smooth surfaces than to rough surfaces. The reader should note that the degree of roughness and smoothness is a "micro" phenomenon, suitable and unsuitable internal finishes would not be discernible to the average triple blade shaver. Pipe joints can disrupt smoothness, as can welds.
2. *Continuous movement of the water in tanks and rapid flow in pipe work*: Where shear forces are involved microorganisms adhere poorly to

surfaces. Where there is no movement of the water there is no shear, shear increases with speed of flow.

3. *Avoidance of areas where water can remain stagnant*:
   - These include "dead legs"—water may stagnate in branch pipes branched from a circulating main if the length of the branch is too long to allow the turbulence of the flowing main to disturb the contents of the branch pipe. FDA has defined "dead legs" according to their dimensions in the 1993 Guide to Inspection of High Purity Water Systems but fundamentally the principle is to always minimize the length of branch pipes.
   - Water can also remain stagnant in valves, particularly at user points and even more particularly at user points which are not in frequent and regular use. This is counteracted by use of so-called hygienic or "zero dead leg" valves which although significantly better than the alternatives (say ball valves) should not lead to a sense of false security, as they can harbor endotoxin-shedding biofilms.
   - Ring mains should be sloped (have "drop") from point of origin to the point of return to ensure that systems are completely drainable.

4. *Avoidance of leakage*: Water leaks can cause bridging of water to the external environment through which bacteria may enter the system. Storage tanks should be equipped with filter on their air vents to prevent airborne microbiological ingress. They may even be held under a "blanket" of an inert gas such as nitrogen.

5. *High temperature storage and distribution*: The risks of endotoxin-shedding biofilms despite the best attempts at control above are thought to be so consequential that the regulatory bodies require the temperature of storage and distribution to be maintained higher than 75°C. It should however be considered that 75°C is too high a temperature for most pharmaceutical formulation purposes and scalds your hands too if they come into contact with it. This means that user points are generally equipped with some form of cooling—heat exchangers used for this purpose may be a source of endotoxin and bacterial contamination and may thus cancel out many of the benefits of high temperature circulation. There are alternative forms of cold water systems or systems where water is only periodically heated. This author has reservations about these types of systems.

CONTROLLING OTHER MICROBIAL RISKS TO WATER SYSTEMS

Generally Purified Water is found in EU GMP Grade C/ISO 146744 Class 8 areas (in operation), which serve as support areas for first stage cleaning purposes, or in nonsterile pharmaceutical facilities. With sterile manufacturing facilities, this is sufficiently far enough away from the aseptic core to avoid problems of transferred endotoxin contamination. Nonetheless care must be taken to ensure that these sources are contained in separated rooms preferably with closable and that personnel are properly equipped such that they do not transfer microorganisms from these water supplies and attendant floor drains to product–contact equipment.

Systems for purified water and highly purified water are not usually maintained at high temperature, instead use is made of ultraviolet light and inline filters to maintain microbial quality. Three important points to consider are (Sandle, 2013) as follows:

1. UV light is not a sterilant and its efficiency depends on path length, speed of flow, and age of the light source. It is very useful for catalyzing the breakdown of ozone or hydrogen peroxide used as sanitizing agents.
2. Filters are an ideal matrix for colonization; they need careful control by monitoring pressure differentials and frequent sanitization or changing. If a biofilm has formed on a filter, sanitization will kill the majority of microorganisms within the biofilm but will probably not remove the biofilm matrix which may be rapidly recolonized. In addition, the presence of highly resistant persister cells within the population will remain unaffected and subsequently regrow.
3. Bends in the pipework should be as gentle and as few as possible. Tap points should be kept to a minimum. Any disruption to the smooth flow of the water results in turbulence which assists biofilm formation by creating more opportunities for circulating microorganisms to impact onto colonizable surfaces.

Biofilm is a thin layer of material on walls of storage or distribution tubing. It is associated with the presence of Gram-negative bacteria and resulting bacterial endotoxins. Because bacteria control in storage and distribution systems is difficult when an established biofilm is present, the theory, mechanism, and microbial control factors are important.

ADDRESSING WATER SYSTEM CONTAMINATION

Water system contamination can be addressed through several means. These include (Sandle, 2014):

a. Chlorination.
b. Tap flushing techniques.
c. Holding water at high temperatures.
d. Point of use (terminal) filtration.

With the use of chlorination and high temperatures, engineering staff should aim to treat water system regularly. With chemical treatment (e.g., sodium hypochlorite, chloramine, or chlorine dioxide), the important aspects are the concentration of the chemical and ensuring that the chemical is left in place for a suitable contact time. One downside with chlorine is that it can cause corrosion and it produces some by-products which are difficult to remove and can be costly to dispose of. In some modern systems, ozonation and ultraviolet light are used as sanitization methods. These methods work particularly well in a recirculating system where water flows over a multiple lamp system. However, some weaknesses are that the penetration of ozone and UV light into water is small, and any dead bacteria present in the system will further hinder penetration.

With holding water at high temperatures in the distribution loop (such as 75°C) this prevents most microorganisms from surviving. In extreme cases some of the water systems can be 'superheated' by steam, bringing the distribution system to either 115°C or 121°C. Carrying out chemical treatment or heating can help to prevent biofilms from forming.

Tap flushing should be carried out by nursing and clinical staff and this is discussed later. With point-of-use filtration (0.22 μm porosity filters), this has facilitated beneficial hydrotherapy for burns and wound trauma patients in several hospitals. However, while filtration helps to remove contamination it does not address the cause of contamination.

With the risk of Legionnaires' disease the regular flushing of showers, the changing of shower heads, and maintaining water at a hot temperature can aid in the control and avoidance of the causative agent (outbreaks can be controlled by reelevating the hot water temperature to maintain levels of at least 50°C close to the point of use, ensuring that the water is cooled sufficiently for the patient to use) (Wadowsky, Yee, Mezmar, Wing, & Dowling, 1982).

As a last resort, sections of pipework believed to contain a biofilm can be removed and replaced. This, however, is a time-consuming, costly activity.

WATER SYSTEM MONITORING: SAMPLING, TESTING, AND REPORTING

It is important that samples for microbiological analysis are taken appropriately in order to assess water system control.

Total Aerobic Viable Counts

Within Europe monographs for WFI, purified water and highly purified water require R2A to be used as the culture medium for conducting the bioburden test. With the USP no medium is recommended and the selection of the most appropriate culture medium rests with the site microbiologist (and ideally through a validation study). The widespread use of Reasoner's 2A medium (R2A) is because it has long been recognized that total aerobic counts performed on water samples using low nutrient media (and preferably low 20–25°C incubation temperatures) give much higher results (Reasoner & Geldrich, 1985).

With water system monitoring, it is important to understand that whatever cultural technique is used, it will only show a fraction of the microbial population in the sample (Sandle & Skinner, 2005). For that reason the specifications for water counts are described as action limits; they are not considered to be pass/fail limits. If an action limit is exceeded, its impact on the product must be evaluated. In terms of test methods, the method of choice is membrane filtration. This is because a larger sample size is tested and more representative data generated.

Alternatively, rapid microbiological methods can be used, especially those that can increase accuracy of counting or which can shorten the incubation time required for detection, or better still, to replace colony formation as the detection signal and obtain results in "real time." In recent years different approaches have been developed. These approaches include ATP bioluminescence and the direct counting of fluorescently labeled microbial cells.

For the monitoring of water systems appropriate alert and action levels should be set for both bioburden assessment, types of microorganisms, and for levels of bacterial endotoxins (Sandle, 2015). Action levels, where appropriate, are typically drawn from the pharmacopeia or national water standards, whereas alert levels are assessed by the pharmaceutical organization, based on a review of historical data. Due to the complexity and dynamics of water monitoring an action limit is not a pass/fail specification. What it does mean is that if an action limit has been exceeded the impact on the product(s) involved needs to be carefully investigated and evaluated. The investigation should be designed to establish the cause of the excursion, and if possible, eliminate it. The evaluation should examine the impact on the product and its ability to withstand microbial challenge, as well as the patient group and their susceptibility to infection (this assessment additionally assumes knowledge of the contaminating microorganism and thus identification may be important). With action limit excursions the investigation and evaluation should be carefully documented and a justification for product release or rejection should be prepared. In addition, to fully understand the performance of a water system over time, the results from the system should be trended (Sandle, 2004b).

Undesirable ("Objectionable") Microorganisms

An 'objectionable' microorganism is any microorganism that can cause infections when the drug product is used as directed or any microorganisms capable of growth in the drug product. In most situations this can be translated to the absence of *Pseudomonas aeruginosa* and the absence of any *Pseudomonas* spp. in nonsterile ophthalmic preparations. However, it is going to be the responsibility of every pharmaceutical manufacturer to make their own judgments on objectionable microorganisms. The rationale of judgment will have to be based on product application and patient group vulnerability.

Test for Bacterial Endotoxin

Bacterial endotoxins test (BET) is the generic term used for the detection and quantitation of endotoxin. BET assays are described in the Japanese Pharmacopoeia, European Pharmacopoeia, and United States Pharmacopeia. The primary method is the LAL (*Limulus* Amebocyte Lysate) test, using a reagent sourced from the North American Horseshoe Crab: *Limulus polyphemus* (Cooper, Levin, & Wagner, 1971). Hence LAL is an aqueous extract obtained after lysis of blood cells (amoebocytes) from certain species of horseshoe crab.

The LAL method uses lysate and that the lysate detects endotoxin produced from the lysis of Gram-negative bacteria. This detection is based on the natural biochemical clotting mechanism which occurs within the horseshoe crab as part of its natural defense against microorganism infection. Here, when endotoxin comes into contact with LAL it initiates a series of enzymatic reactions that result in the activation of a pathway to the production of at least three serine protease zymogens (Factor C, Factor B, and proclotting enzyme). This pathway alters amoebocyte coagulogen (an invertebrate fibrinogen-like clottable protein) to form coagulin gel.

Some reagents do not rely on the collection of blood from the horseshoe crab, but they are designed to work in a similar manner. These reagents are recombinant versions of the Factor C, the activation of which is the first step in the LAL reaction cascade.

Alternative tests for endotoxin, and other pyrogenic substances, are the rabbit test (Seibert, 1925) (which is little used, due to it insensitivity), and the monocyte activation test (MAT). Using whole human blood (cryoblood or fresh blood), the MAT imitates the innate immune response to a fever reaction caused by pyrogens. It simulates the human fever reaction better than the rabbit-based pyrogen test (Perdomo-Morales, Pardo-Ruiz, Spreitzer, Lagarto, & Montag, 2011).

Sample-Related Contamination

Contamination issues can also arise with water system sampling. These can arise via personnel or through poorly maintained equipment. In particular, the hoses and tubes used to supply water from sink outlets can be a source of contamination. Studies suggest that flexible water hoses (such as those made of a synthetic rubber-based component) are more likely to become contaminated and hold microbial communities than flexible hoses made from alternative materials with standard rigid plumbing or components.

SUMMARY

Pharmaceutical grade water is a critical utility in any facility. An excursion in system operation may affect product water quality, which in turn may affect patient and product. These effects may cause significant loss of revenue to the organization. Personnel responsible for pharmaceutical water systems operation and oversight must be cognizant of the issues discussed herein and must be proactive in their prevention.

This chapter has looked at the microbiology of water systems and it has provided an overview of different types of pharmaceutical grade water. The chapter has additionally considered contamination control measures for water systems, from aspects of water system design to measures to consider when contamination occurs.

REFERENCES

Cooper, J. F., Levin, J., & Wagner, H. N. (1971). Quantitative comparison and in vitro and in vivo methods for the detection of endotoxin. *Journal of Laboratory and Clinical Medicine, 78*(13).

Guy, D. (2003). Endotoxins and depyrogenation. In N. Hodges, & G. Hanlon (Eds.), *Industrial pharmaceutical microbiology: Standards and controls* (pp. 12.1–12.15). Passfield: Euromed Communications.

Hall-Stoodley, L., Costerton, J. W., & Stoodley, P. (2004). Bacterial biofilms: from the natural environment to infectious diseases. *Nature Reviews. Microbiology, 2*(2), 95–108.

Perdomo-Morales, R., Pardo-Ruiz, Z., Spreitzer, I., Lagarto, A., & Montag, T. (2011). Monocyte activation test (MAT) reliably detects pyrogens in parenteral formulations of human serum albumin. *ALTEX, 28*(3), 227–235.

Reasoner, D., & Geldrich, E. (1985). A new medium for the enumeration and subculture of bacteria from potable water. *Applied Environmental Microbiology, 49*, 1–7.

Rudbach, J. A., Akiya, F. I., Elin, R. J., Hochstein, H. D., Luoma, M. K., Milner, C. B., et al. (1976). Preparation and properties of a national reference endotoxin. *Journal of Clinical Microbiology, 3*(1), 21–25.

Sandle, T. (2004a). Three aspects of LAL testing: glucans, depyrogenation and water system qualification. *PharMIG News*, (16), 3–12. June/July.

Sandle, T. (2004b). An approach for the reporting of microbiological results from water systems. *PDA Journal of Pharmaceutical Science and Technology*, 58(4), 231–237.

Sandle, T. (2013). Avoiding contamination of water systems. *The Clinical Services Journal*, 12(9), 33–36.

Sandle, T. (2014). Microbiology of pharmaceutical grade water. In G. Handlon, & T. Sandle (Eds.), *Industrial pharmaceutical microbiology: Standards and controls* (pp. 10.1–10.19). Passfield: Euromed Communications.

Sandle, T. (2015). Characterizing the microbiota of a pharmaceutical water system—a metadata study. *SOJ Microbiology & Infectious Diseases*, 3(2), 1–8.

Sandle, T. (2017a). Design and control of pharmaceutical water systems to minimize microbial contamination. *Pharmaceutical Engineering*, 37(4), 44–48.

Sandle, T. (2017b). Microbiological monitoring of pharmaceutical water systems. *European Pharmaceutical Review*, 22(2), 25–27.

Sandle, T., & Skinner, K. (2005). Examination of the optimal cultural conditions for the microbiological analysis of a cold demineralised water system in a pharmaceutical manufacturing facility. *European Journal of Parenteral and Pharmaceutical Sciences*, 10(1), 9–14.

Seibert, F. B. (1925). The cause of many febrile reactions following intravenous injection. *American Journal of Physiology*, 71, 621–651.

Wadowsky, R. M., Yee, R. B., Mezmar, L., Wing, E. J., & Dowling, J. N. (1982). Hot water systems as sources of *Legionella pneumophila* in hospital and nonhospital plumbing fixtures. *Applied and Environmental Microbiology*, 43(5), 1104–1110.

Chapter 14

Data Handling and Trend Analysis

CHAPTER OUTLINE

Introduction   225

Microbial Data Variations   226

Distribution of Microbial Data   227

Trending Microbial Data   229

Histograms   229

Control Charts   230

What Control Charts Can Indicate   230

Common Causes   231

Special Causes   231

Setting Up Control Charts   233

Shewhart Charts   233

Cumulative Sum Charts   237

Other Charts   239

Frequency of Trending   239

Investigating Out of Trend   241

Tracking Microorganisms   242

Alert and Action Levels   244

Setting Alert and Action Levels   244

Data Integrity   245

Summary   246

References   246

INTRODUCTION

Statistical interpretation of microbial data can be very useful, especially in making sense of the thousands of results that pass through the typical healthcare or pharmaceutical microbiology laboratory. However, knowledge of statistics and the application for microbial data are often lacking from curricula and there are often misunderstandings when data is reviewed in the laboratory. The application need not be overly complex. Descriptive statistics allow microbiologists to summarize large amounts of data to more understandable levels using numerical descriptors (such as mean, mode, median, or standard deviation). Graphical methods or frequency tables

Biocontamination Control for Pharmaceuticals and Healthcare. https://doi.org/10.1016/B978-0-12-814911-9.00014-6

are very useful for trending data, and inferential statistics allow microbiologists to make generalizations and predictions or to estimate the relationship between variables using incomplete information (Lorowitz, Saxon, Sondossi, & Nakaova, 2005). In this context, statistics are often needed to help summarize considerable volumes of generated data.

Where a high count is obtained, such as from a filling needle in relation to aseptic processing, the consequences are clear: potential nonsterile product and the need for investigation. With a larger amass of quantitative data, however, the significance is often less clear. Microbiological data is affected by variability, with variability arising from sample variation, population variation, and assay variation. Data is also affected by the variations of the culture media used or where an alternative "unit" is used to represent microbial activity (as with many rapid microbiological methods); added to this are concerns with data integrity (Tidswell & Sandle, 2018), such as differing interpretations when samples are read, and colonies counted. For this reason, there is a need for trend analysis. Indeed, it can be argued that environmental monitoring data cannot be made sense of without trending (Hertroys, Van Vught, & Van De Donk, 1997).

A third area where statistical analysis is required is with the setting and review of alert and action levels. Another area, related to but outside the scope of this book, is with experimental design, such as to support microbiological method validation. Statistics help to define the experimental problem, with experimental design, considering the weight of evidence, assessing statistical power, and identifying sources of variation, scope of inference, measurement scale, scale transformation (McArthur & Tuckfield, 2016).

This chapter considers variations in microbial data (which connects with data integrity) and looks at where data handling and trend analysis are required to support the biocontamination control program, such as with limits setting and trend analysis.

MICROBIAL DATA VARIATIONS

Microbial data variations are affected by method and by distribution. Taking inherent method variability first, with a common method like the use of active air samplers, for example, each sampler will only detect 50% of a given particle size cutoff; and event here not all of the collected organisms will be culturable. With all plate counts, as would be used for bioburden determinations, plate count data yield large variations when the average of the counts is small (Eisenhart & Wilson, 1943). There are several factors that affect the accuracy of plate counts, which Sutton has described

(Sutton, 2011). These variations extend to directing plating and to membrane filtration techniques (Clark, Geldreich, Jeter, & Karbler, 1951). Colonies can be difficult to count for several reasons (Chang, Hwang, Grinshpun, Macher, & Willeke, 1994):

- The act of colony counting is not only repetitious but it can also lead to errors and thus problems of data integrity.
- In low count assays minor counting errors will have significant effects.
- A related error is when numbers of cfus on a plate can lead to false results due to overcrowding of bacteria.
- Indistinguishable colony overlap (i.e., masking).
- Assessing colonies near the plate periphery.
- Increased density of collected culturable microorganisms.

Some of the variations can be overcome through rapid microbiological methods, or enhancements that support traditional methods like automated colony counters, which have the additional advantages of counting consistency, reducing the incubation time, and improving data capture and integrity (Jones & Cundell, 2018).

Even where such methods are verified there are often differences between the types of studies conducted in the laboratory, where microbial strains adapted to highly nutritious growth media are used, compared with the attempt to recover microorganisms from the environment, where the species types are more diverse, where the bacteria have undergone environmental adaptation (which means they may not find transfer to highly nutritious media the optimal starting point for initiating binary fission), and where the organisms may be damaged or in a "stressed" state.

Distribution of Microbial Data

It is necessary to understand the distribution of microbial data as a prerequisite to most analyses. Certainly, it is important, before discussing trending systems, to consider the distribution of microbial counts. This has a considerable impact upon the trend charts and on the techniques for the calculation of alert and action levels. Microbial counts in the environment rarely resemble normal distribution (where a classical bell-shaped curve or binomial pattern is obtained, where the area under the curve is divided into two symmetrical halves). Normal distribution is a phenomenon found in many aspects of physical and biological science (from measurements like human height). Normal distribution is displayed, at its most simples, as a histogram (Sandle, 2014).

In practice, the distribution of microorganisms and microbial counts shows either Poisson distribution (such as from a water system where microorganisms are distributed randomly) or show a marked "skewness." In the following graph (Fig. 1), the distribution of the data can be considered as skewed (i.e., it displays a lack of symmetry). This is typical of the counts obtained from an EU GMP Grade B/ISO Class 7 cleanroom where there are many results with zero count or counts of one or two colony-forming units (cfu), and relatively few at the higher numbers. The long, thin tail toward the left of the graph can be described as negative skewness or negative exponential distribution.

With Poisson distribution the frequency of counting "events" over "time" is more random. Thus the phenomena of Poisson distribution accounts for events where a sample from a water system may, for example, exceed an action level on one day, be below the action level for another two days, and then be above action on the fourth day. This type of distribution is more common to pharmaceutical water systems.

The lack of normality and seeming randomness of the distribution is of importance when using control charts. Before constructing a control chart the collected data should be examined to see if it follows normal distribution. Although, as stated earlier, it is improbable that the distribution of microorganisms as indicated by "counts" from environmental monitoring will follow normal distribution, any statistical analysis that is based on normal distribution remains the more accurate approach. Therefore it is incumbent upon the user to demonstrate if there is normal distribution (Tang, 1998).

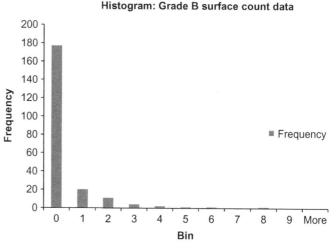

■ **FIG. 1** Grade B/ISO Class 7 surface count data.

Where data does not follow normal distribution, data can be *transformed* into an approximation of normal distribution and thereby plotted onto a control chart. There are no preset "rules" for data transformation. A common approach, as outlined by Sokal and Rohlf (1995), is to transform *low count* data (such as that obtained from a EU GMP Grade A/ISO Class 5 environment) by taking the square root of each datum and to transform data with *higher counts* by converting each datum to its logarithm at base 10 ($\log_{10}$) (Sokal & Rohlf, 1995). In performing $\log_{10}$ transformations, in the event that a count is zero, this requires the addition of a value of "1" to each value of zero. So that this does not distort relationships with other results, a value of "1" is added to *each* datum in the data set.

TRENDING MICROBIAL DATA

Many of the types of samples discussed in this book reveal only partial information as single data points; more is revealed when data is contextualized and examined across time (and space, where samples from a process or adjacent cleanrooms should be compared with each other). In the context of environmental monitoring in particular, a single high count of say 10 cfu will reveal less meaningful information than, say, a cluster of five samples recording 1 colony. It also stands that it is often very difficult to determine assignable cause of a single microbiological excursion.

Hence, data coming from a single sample are often not significant and given further that microbiological monitoring techniques often have a high degree of variability (which is certainly the case with the "classic" methods for environmental monitoring), there needs to be a greater emphasis upon trending data. In this context, graphic or statistical presentations of results collected over a period of time can prove useful in distinguishing sampling variation from trends, or in indicating that a significant change has occurred with the data collected (Caputo & Huffman, 2004). This helps put out-of-limits results in context and enables patterns to be discerned even though the results fall within the specified limits.

At its simplest, trend analysis involves plotting data values, for which a target value can be established, against values for time, production lot number, or some other identifiable parameter. One means to achieve this is with control charts.

Histograms

The histogram approach, as illustrated in Fig. 1, has other uses. It is useful when reviewing the locations for environmental monitoring, for instance. Suppose, for example, that three active air samples are taken within a cleanroom. If the microbiologist wished to remove one of the air samples in order to save time and money, by constructing a histogram with all three samples and then constructing a histogram with one sample removed allows a comparison to be made. If the proportion of zero results does not significantly alter then there could be a case to be made for removing one of the air samples.

Histograms also help with displaying data to look for incidents of contamination, such as for reviewing the frequencies of incidences above zero against historical data. This enables "frequency of incident" comparisons to be performed on a regular basis in order to examine cleanrooms for trends.

Control Charts

Control chart methods may be applied to provide an objective and statistically valid means, to assess the quality of the risk zones and are particularly applicable to monitoring. In the verification step, sampling for batch acceptance purposes can be applied as another quality control technique. Charting by means of Shewhart control charts, control charts "based on range," or "cumulative sum charts" may also be appropriate to measure the deviation from usual random spread and to highlight out-of-limits results (Sandle, 2004).

As to what constitutes a variation in trend, there are control chart rule to drawn upon. The important thing is to study the data. Single excursions may be notable in that they may be part of a trend, for example, a repeated individual excursion always seen on Fridays may be indicative of a repeating problem with environmental control.

There are four major types of control chart for variables data, each of which will be useful for different applications (Hayes, Scallan, & Wong, 1997):

1. The x chart, based on the average result;
2. The R chart, based on the range of the results;

The previous two charts use the average and range of values determined on a set of samples to monitor the process location and process variation.

3. The s chart, based on the sample standard distribution; and
4. The x chart, based on individual results.

What Control Charts Can Indicate

If the chart indicates that the process being monitored is not in control, analysis of the chart can help us to determine the sources of variation, which can then be eliminated to bring the process back into control. For processes that are *not* in a state of statistical control, the charts will:

a. Show excessive variations;
b. Exhibit variations that change with time.

When such conditions arise, control charts can be used to differentiate between such variations, to show:

a. Those variations that are normally expected of the process due to chance or common causes. These should be expected, to an extent;
b. Those variations that change over time due to assignable or special causes. These often require some form of action.

The difference between *common causes* (a common cause variation is the "noise" within the system) and *special causes* (new, unanticipated, emergent, or previously neglected phenomena within the system) is important in determining what action to take for a follow-up investigation. There is no consensus as to what a common cause is and what a special cause is. Some tentative examples include:

Common Causes

- Inappropriate procedures
- Poor design
- Poor maintenance of machines
- Lack of clearly defined standing operating procedures
- Poor working conditions, for example, lighting, noise, dirt, temperature, ventilation
- Substandard materials
- Ambient temperature and humidity
- With machinery (such as particle count generation from a filling machine): normal wear and tear or variability in machine settings
- Seasonal variations with data

Special Causes

- Poor adjustment of equipment
- Poor batch of raw material
- Power surges
- Change of process staff
- Change of culture media

This necessary investigative step will not be expanded upon in this chapter, but it does relate to discussions about corrective and preventative actions examined elsewhere in this module.

Control charts have three basic components:

- A center line (usually the mathematical average of the entire samples plotted).
- Upper and lower statistical control limits. These are three standard deviations (or standard errors from the center line).
- The data plotted over a time period.

Thus, to start with, control charts require a target value. The target values used in the examples in this chapter related to data collected during the previous year. Hence the previous year was used to establish the "norm" for future samples in a given room. Using control chart terminology this was necessary to establish what the common variability of the environment was. This approach could be unrepresentative if the previous year did not represent a typical year. For the purposes of this chapter the reader will need to assume the use of the collected data as a benchmark was the correct approach to take.

Control charts use upper and lower control limits and warning limits, in addition to a straight line at the center of the graph (which is the mean). Data is plotted against the central line. For most microbiological monitoring, normally only the upper levels are of concern (the upper control level: UCL, and the upper warning level: UWL, respectively). These monitoring levels alert the chart user to react to major changes in trend. When limits are set using historical data it is expected that a certain percentage of results will fall outside the limits when plotted. The UCL and UWL can determine the probability (or "chance") that future counts will fall outside (Kourti & MacGregor, 1996).

In this context, *warning limits* represent approximately a 0.025 or 2.5% chance. Alternatively, sometimes a 5% chance is employed. The choice here is in reaching a balance between the probability of false alarm and the earlier detection of a possible problem. *Control limits* (or *action limits*) represent an approximate 0.001 or 0.1% chance and this is an approximation of three standard deviations from the mean. By employing upper limits set at three standard deviations, these are wide enough to avoid taking unnecessary action for what would otherwise prove to be "statistical noise" (or the small rise and drop in low level microbial counts).

The detection of data rising above the UCL rise is theoretically rare (if the control chart has been set up correctly) and any results that would exceed it would indicate that:

a. The variation is due to an assignable cause
b. The process is out-of-statistical control (which may or may not be the same as out-of-microbiological control).
When a meaningful amount of data is plotted (such as 1 year or more of data), several points rising above the UCL are indicative of an out-of-control situation (and thereby this requires some form of corrective action). In contrast, a single point outside of the control levels would be regarded as "statistical noise."

Setting Up Control Charts

Assessing data distribution is important since results to be plotted in a control chart, when the process is known to be "in control" should be normally, or nearly normally, distributed. Where this is not the case then the data must be "normalized" by an appropriate mathematical transformation. It is also important that during the initial setting up of the charts it is essential that the process be operated in a stable and controlled manner, so that the data values used to establish the operational parameters of the SPC procedure are normally distributed. A general "rule of thumb" stipulates at least 20 sets of individual results to compute the mean, standard deviation, and other summary statistics in order to estimate the distribution of the results and construct control limits and target value.

To illustrate different types of control charts, two are examined as follows: cumulative sum (or "cusum") charts and Shewhart charts. In terms of selecting between these two types of chart, cusum charts are more sensitive to small process shifts; however, large, abrupt shifts are not detected as fast as in a Shewhart chart. With Shewhart charts, systematic shifts are easily detected; however, the probability of detecting small shifts fast is rather small. Hence, the cusum chart might be better suited for Grade A/ISO Class 5 data or Grade B/ISO Class 7 data; and the Shewhart chart for higher count data.

Shewhart Charts

The concepts underlying the control chart are that the natural variability in any process can be quantified with a set of control limits and that the variation exceeding these limits signals a change in the process. Shewhart charts either measure variables when the quality characteristic of a process is measured on a continuous scale (as in the examples used in this chapter) or they are used for attributes when the quality characteristic of a process is measured by counting the number of nonconformities (defects or high counts) in an item or the number of nonconforming (defective or high counts) items in a sample (this is the "classic" statistical process control chart). It should be noted that the underlying assumption is that the data is normally distributed. Therefore it is important to understand (and to transform if necessary) the microbiological data before using control charts.

Charts typically consist of (Wheeler & Chambers, 1992):

- Points representing a statistic (e.g., a mean, range, proportion) of measurements of a quality characteristic in samples taken from the process at different times [the data].
- The mean of this statistic using all the samples is calculated (e.g., the mean of the means, mean of the ranges, mean of the proportions).
- A center line is drawn at the value of the mean of the statistic.
- The standard error (e.g., standard deviation/sqrt (n) for the mean) of the statistic is also calculated using all the samples.
- Upper and lower control limits (sometimes called "natural process limits") that indicate the threshold at which the process output is considered statistically "unlikely" are drawn typically at three standard errors from the center line.

The power of Shewhart charts is that they can be studied for unusual events or patterns in the data. Applications include:

- Gaining an understanding of the variability of the process,
- Being able to mark changes,
- To determine if improved reactions occur following any changes,
- To demonstrate effectiveness of any actions taken.

Various events can be marked on the charts and the charts can be studied for changes in direction and for different "movements." Such movements and events include:

I. A point lying beyond the control limits
II. 2 consecutive points lying beyond the warning limits
III. 7 or more consecutive points lying on one side of the mean (this is an important issue because the 7th point is regarded as no longer being random)
IV. 5 or 6 consecutive points going in the same direction (indicates a trend)

Shewhart charts are particularly useful in distinguishing variation due to *special causes* from variation due to *common causes*.

In the context of environmental monitoring, special causes are local, sporadic problems such as the poor management of a particular water outlet in a process area or an air sample count. In general, they are:

- Localized.
- Exceptions to the system.
- Considered abnormalities.
- Specific to a:
  - Certain process;
  - Certain outlet or sampling site;
  - Certain method of sanitization, and so on;
  - Sampling technique;
  - Equipment malfunction, for example, filling machine pumps;
  - Cross-contamination in laboratory;
  - Engineering work;
  - Sanitization frequencies.

Whereas common causes are problems inherent in the manufacturing system, such as a problem with the operation of a breakdown of the HVAC system where particle count control in a cleanroom has been lost. In general, they are:

- Inherent to the process because of:
  - The nature of a system.
  - The way a system is managed.
  - The way a process is organized and operated.

They can only be corrected by:

- Making modifications to a process.
- Changing a process for an alternative.

Once the special causes have been identified and eliminated, the process is said to be in *statistical control (or statistically stable)*. When statistical control has been established, Shewhart charts can be used to monitor the process for the occurrence of future special causes and to measure and reduce the effects of common causes.

Care needs to be taken in not confusing between common causes and special causes. To do so could result in a Type I or Type II error being made. A Type I error is to treat as a special cause any outcome when it actually came from a common cause. Whereas, with a Type II error something is to attribute a common cause to any outcome when it came from a special cause.

Once changes have been made the aim of monitoring using a Shewhart chart is to reduce variation in the plotted data.

Shewhart charts have control limits. Data is plotted against the control limits, where the center line in the chart is the *grand average*. Shewhart charts also have an upper warning level and an upper control level, and corresponding lower levels, which are established around the process mean. The upper and lower control levels are approximations of three standard deviations from the process mean. There are different ways to calculate the control levels.

In the following example these were also based on the benchmarked data, where it was expected that no more than 2.5% of the data would exceed the upper warning level and that no more than 0.1% of the data would exceed the upper control level. These represent an *approximation* for the microbial data because the assumption behind Shewhart charts is that the data is normally distributed, and the data employed in the charts has been transformed (as previously discussed).

The target value for the Shewhart charts used in the following example was set based on 10% of the current action level. This was because the action level is statistically set so that approximately 10% of results are above the limit and 90% are as follows.

As an example, the following chart (Fig. 2) displays some Grade B active air sample data.

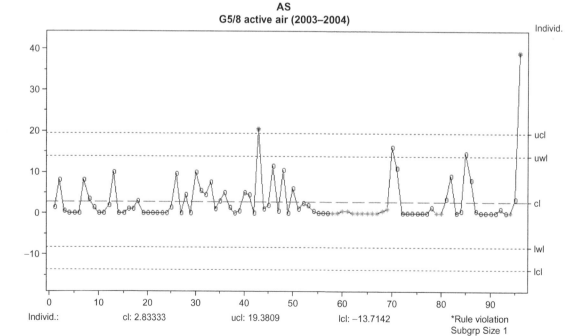

FIG. 2 Example control chart for air sample data.

The example chart (Fig. 2) indicates the counts during the latter part of the chart were satisfactory with most results clustered along the central line. Excursions above the upper warning limit were not sustained and no adverse trend developed. The final count for was very high and exceeded the upper control limit. However, there is no indication—based on the previous trend—that this would develop into a series of adverse counts.

Cumulative Sum Charts

Cumulative sum charts ("cusum") chart is one example of a type of control chart. These charts are used to decide whether a process is in statistical control by detecting a shift in the process mean. The cumulative sum chart is particularly useful for studying the gradual influence of time. Where there is no time trend, the cusum is flat. A change in the level over time is reflected in a change in the slope of the cusum.

Cusums function by displaying cumulative sums of the deviations of measurements or subgroup means from a target value. This can be an increase or a decrease away from the target. Cusum charts are theoretically more sensitive to shifts in the process mean than Shewhart charts. Cusums will show (Grigg, Farewell, & Spiegelhalter, 2003):

- If changes have taken place;
- Approximately when the change has taken place.

Cusum charts plot the cumulative sum of the deviations between each data point (a sample average) and a reference value, T (for target). Each point on a cusum chart is based on information from all samples (measurements) up to and including the current sample (measurement). Cusums measure the degree of variation from a target value.

When studying a cusum chart the main focus is with the slope of the plotted line, not just the distance between plotted points and the centerline. Significant variations from the target value are described as "steps." These can be in an upward or a downward direction. The concern for the type of data examined in this report is for upward steps because increasing microbial counts are of concern; for other applications, outside of reviewing microbial counts, the downward direction of charts maybe of interest also. It should be noted that the direction of the cusum can wander from the mean even when the data is generally on target.

Significant upward steps are when two out of the three values, from a subgroup that is plotted as a mean (one point on the graph), are outside of the target range. When this situation occurs the statistical software used here indicates this with a "*" sign to indicate a change in the trend (this can be an improvement or a potential out-of-control situation). These are descriptions of more significant events than simple upward steps.

The power of cusums can be increased through the use of V-masks. A V-mask is, unsurprisingly, in the shape of a V and is placed sidewise (>) with the vertex placed at a fixed distance from the last plotted point. If the cusum graph is outside or moving outside of the V-mask, then the chart can be considered as going out of statistical control, whereas if the data falls within the V-mask branches it can be described as being within statistical control. If this movement is in a downward direction below the target line, this is indicative of the data having very low counts and being satisfactory. If the movement is in an upward direction and is above the target line, this is indicative of the data having a series of high counts and is unsatisfactory. The importance of V-masks is that one cusum can be compared to another, for the same data set, at different time periods. If the V-mask has shifted then an indication of the trend can be derived.

Consider, for example, a plot of surface contact plates (Fig. 3).

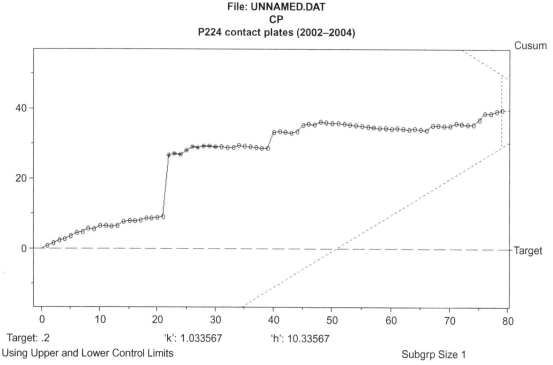

File: UNNAMED.DAT 26/4/105
File: UNNAMED.DAT
CP
P224 contact plates (2002–2004)

Target: .2   'k': 1.033567   'h': 10.33567

Using Upper and Lower Control Limits   Subgrp Size 1

■ **FIG. 3** Example cusum chart for surface contact plate data.

The chart (Fig. 3) shows that two step upward trends have taken place: one during the first quarter of the chart and one during the middle portion. The first upward step was of more significance, as indicated by the "*" symbol on the chart. This is indicative of seven or greater plotted points being of the same trend. However, the data then proceeded not to show any significant upward trend and remains in control, as indicated by the relation of the points to the V-mask.

Other Charts

Sometimes microbiological data can be simply plotted onto a standard X–Y chart, with an action (and/or an alert) level added. Depending on the pattern of data it might be prudent to transform the data. Consider some Grade B/ISO Class 7 particle counts (Fig. 4).

The pattern is distorted due to some high counts. Fig. 5 uses the same data set which has been used. This time the data has been converted to log_{10}. The data is easier to track.

FREQUENCY OF TRENDING

Whichever method of reporting is selecting, environmental monitoring data must be presented, interpreted, and summarized so that senior management can understand the trend and the "big picture" (Hussong & Madsen, 2004). This data needs to be presented at the correct frequencies (i.e., not too often or too infrequently). There is no right or wrong way to present data. However, a clear and simple approach is often the most useful. This can include:

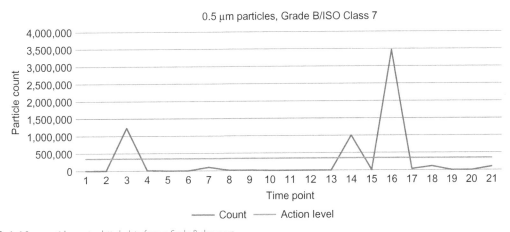

■ **FIG. 4** 0.5 µm particle counts plotted, data from a Grade B cleanroom.

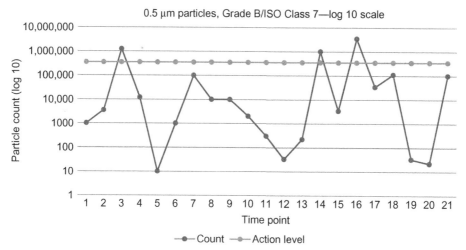

■ **FIG. 5** 0.5 μm particle counts plotted and converted to log base 10, data from a Grade B cleanroom.

- The use of graphs and tables. This allows the trend of one area to be compared with another and for informed questions to be asked.
- Each test should be reported separately. Multiline graphs and the use of more than one scale on a graph is generally confusing.
- Focus on each filling room or main operation separately. It is often useful to compare different areas, but it is confusing to attempt this on one graph.
- Include all of the available data. It is important to select the time period over which the data should be collected and plotted (typically this will be monthly, quarterly, yearly or, occasionally, over a longer term). Once a time period has been selected data must never be excluded.
- Include alert and action limits on graphs. A trend can sometimes be misleading. It is important to understand how a trend relates to the monitoring levels applied.
- Include appropriate information with tables and graphs. This helps to identify patterns and possible reasons for a given trend. Such information includes:
  - Locations;
  - Dates;
  - Times;
  - Identification results;
  - Changes to room design;
  - Operation of new equipment;

    o Shift or personnel changes;

    o Seasons;

    o HVAC problems (e.g., an increase in temperature).

INVESTIGATING OUT OF TREND

The degree of investigations into adverse trends should be commensurate with results of the impact assessment. For example, isolation of objectionable species recovered from a "clean" product contact surface would be more important than if it came from a surface some distance from the product.

Should the results of the investigation indicate that a root cause analysis is required a Corrective Action Preventative Action (CAPA) can be used. Such CAPA should be defined in terms of biocontamination impact to the safety and efficacy of the product. The efficacy of any corrective/preventive actions should be verified.

Management of microbiological results from risk zones should take the following factors into account:

- Types of result to be collected;
- Necessary information;
- Methods to process the collected results (e.g., statistical procedures, correlation analysis, artificial intelligence, etc.);
- Grouping of results to focus on important trends and deviations, that is, data stratification;
- Method by which the results will be expressed (e.g., qualitatively, quantitatively, graphically, numerically) and the units of measurement that will be used;
- Robustness of, and potential problems posed by, the analytical methods;
- Trend analysis;
- Control charting;
- Estimation, interpretation, and reporting of results.

Looking at numerical data is different to a comparison to microorganisms. To obtain semireliable estimates of microbiological contamination gathered, the following variables can be considered:

- Sampling—adequate number and homogeneity of the sample material and accuracy of dilution of the samples, if appropriate;
- Composition of the viable organism spectrum involved; its variability with time and the effect of stress and injury on survival and recovery;

- Results originating from different sampling sites in risk zones and other controlled zones;
- Culturing techniques and the methodology of counting;
- Selection of method of analysis and relationship between direct and indirect testing.

Examining the patterns of microorganisms in an environmental niche is not straightforward and reliable modeling of a microbial community composition is possible only if microbes show repeatable responses to extrinsic forcing (Bissett, Brown, Siciliano, Thrall, & Holyoak, 2013). In this context, several environmental stressors act as a force that shapes microbial community composition. An example is with water left for long periods in cleanrooms; in such circumstances it can predicted that a certain microbial composition is more likely than not.

TRACKING MICROORGANISMS

A robust biocontamination control program will include accurate identification of selected microbial isolates. Assessing this information provides an archive of historical data that can be used to select environmental isolates for growth promotion and enable benchmarking and trending. In the latter context, assessing microbial profiles is useful for tracking and trending microbial populations throughout the facility. Having a detailed record of the numbers and species of bacteria and fungi isolated at different locations and times can quickly reveal changes and give early warning of developing problems or system failures. For instance, if higher-than-expected levels of a specific bacterial species are isolated in critical areas, it is often possible to track the same species to less strictly controlled areas and establish their source. An example here is with bacterial spores.

Moreover, analysis of the data can sometimes reveal the route by which contamination may be occurring, allowing control to be regained before a critical excursion occurs. Similarly, tracking and trending species associated with personnel may identify inadequate hygiene procedures at an early stage. Any deviations from the norm can thus become apparent.

For visually representing the types of microorganisms, often a simple pictorial representation will suffice. Consider, for example, a typical microbiota profile of a purified water system (Fig. 6).

Fig. 6 shows a breakdown by morphological type. In this type of water system, Gram-negative bacteria would be expected to represent the overwhelming majority of isolates.

Microbiota from purified water system

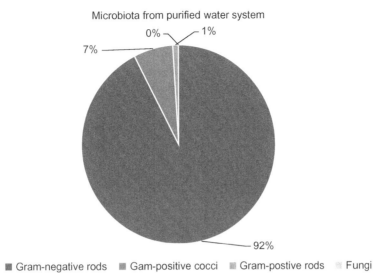

■ Gram-negative rods ■ Gam-positive cocci ■ Gram-postive rods ▨ Fungi

■ **FIG. 6** Example morphological data from a water system.

Exit suit gown plates for aseptic processing area

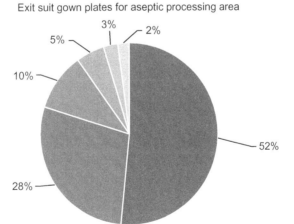

■ *Staphylococcus* sp. ■ *Micrococcus* sp. ■ *Kocuria* sp. ■ *Corynebacterium* sp. ▨ Fungi ▨ *Bacillus* sp.

■ **FIG. 7** Microbial profile from personnel exit suit contact plates.

The level of detail can be increased, in order to track species of concern. Consider, for example, in Fig. 7, exit suit gown plates relating to an aseptic processing area.

In this case the concern would be with high levels of fungi or *Bacillus* species, and whether these have altered over time.

ALERT AND ACTION LEVELS

Alert and action levels can be set as numerical values or as proportions of data (such as the proportion of data that records zero count and the proportion that does not). Generally the guidance documents from regulators prefer numerical values.

Action and alert levels should be set for each product/manufacturing process commensurate with the impact assessment. For some activities, the action level is the same as that recommended in a guidance document or standard. For example, for cleanroom monitoring in sterile facilities the action level is often set. Here alert levels need to be set by the user; moreover, for other activities, such as processing in nonsterile environments, both the alert and action level needs to be set.

All user calculated levels need to be reviewed periodically to ensure that the rationale for setting these levels is still correct. In some cases, the action and alert levels may be the same level, such as when the environment monitoring is checking for the absence of a species/group/family of microorganisms.

Setting Alert and Action Levels

In many circumstances, it is inappropriate to directly calculate control limits with a mean plus two or three standard deviations to represent the center and spread of the data (Novick, Zhao, & Yang, 2017). Instead alternative approaches should be adopted such as the percentile cutoff approach or the use of negative exponential distribution.

In selecting percentile cutoff values, typically, the warning level is set at the 90th or 95th percentile, and the action level set at the 95th or 99th percentile. Thus if the 90th percentile is selected, this means that any result above the 90th percentile is 90% higher than values typically collected over the past year (or whatever the data selection period was).

For higher count data (such as active air sample counts at Grade D), either standard deviations (if there is normal distribution) or negative exponential distribution (for skewed data) can be deployed employed. Unlike the percentile cutoff approach, this technique uses the mean count and observes the spread (or variance) of the different observations. Alternatively, gamma distribution can be used, which, in many ways is a continuous version of the negative binomial distribution for much larger counts where the probability of equaling a specific count is quite small (theoretically zero) (Gordon, Goverde, Pazdan, & Roesti, 2015).

DATA INTEGRITY

Data and integrity, relating to both raw data and metadata ("data about data" such as time of sampling) are critical components of ensuring the reliability of microbiological results. This means that the variations around data need to be understood and that the data-generating systems need to be well controlled. This book does not have the space to discuss data integrity issues for microbiology (there are papers available that do so) (Sandle, 2016); however, it is worth emphasizing the guiding principles.

The FDA first described the acronym ALCOA for data integrity, which refers to attributable, legible, contemporaneous, original, and accurate; this has subsequently been expanded to ALCOA-plus, which adds on enduring "truth"; available, "easy or possible to get or use or present or ready to use"; and accessible, "able to be reached or approached or able to be used or obtained."

One way to assess data integrity robustness, according to Ratan, is to use the "5 Whys" technique (Rattan, 2018):

The main question for the industry is to answer the 5 W's (Fig. 3). The FDA Data Integrity and Compliance with cGMP discusses these 5 W's:

1. What?
   a. What is raw data?
   b. What is metadata?
   c. What is audit trail?
   d. What were the user access rights (administrators versus users)?
   e. What was changed (old versus new values)?
2. When (date and time stamp)?
   a. When was the change made and by whom?
   b. When was the training done?
   c. When was the data processed?
3. Who?
   a. Who owns the data?
   b. Who made the change and when?
   c. Who reviewed the audit trails or change?
   d. Who generated the data?
4. Where?
   a. Where was the change made?
   b. Where and when did the data get archived?
5. Why?
   a. Why was the change made?

Data integrity improvements not only require understanding method limitations, an adherence to sound principles, improvements also require training, awareness, and an open and transparent.

SUMMARY

As this chapter has demonstrated, assessment of microbial data generated in relation to the biocontamination control program has a subjective element. This affects the ability of the microbiologist to engage in objective decision making. There are choices to be made in response to data distributions and with selecting the optimal tools to use in order to display data appropriately.

Generally charting is the best approach to adopt in order to convey a message about control status. Control charts, as a means of simple trend analysis, provide visual aids to interpretation of data that are more readily understood than are tables of data values. They identify when a process went out of control so that appropriate remedial action can be taken before "out of control" equates to "out of specification" with a subsequent manufacturing crisis.

REFERENCES

Bissett, A., Brown, M. V., Siciliano, S. D., Thrall, P. H., & Holyoak, M. (2013). Microbial community responses to anthropogenically induced environmental change: towards a systems approach. *Ecology Letters*, *16*(Suppl 1), 128–139. https://doi.org/10.1111/ele.12109.

Caputo, R. A., & Huffman, A. (2004). Environmental monitoring: data trending using a frequency model. *PDA Journal of Pharmaceutical Science and Technology*, *58*(5), 254–260.

Chang, C. W., Hwang, Y. H., Grinshpun, S. A., Macher, J. M., & Willeke, K. (1994). Evaluation of counting error due to colony masking in bioaerosol sampling. *Applied and Environmental Microbiology*, *60*(10), 3732–3738.

Clark, H. F., Geldreich, E. E., Jeter, H. L., & Karbler, P. W. (1951). The membrane filter in sanitary bacteriology. *Public Health Reports*, *66*(30), 951–997.

Eisenhart, C., & Wilson, P. W. (1943). Statistical methods and control in bacteriology. *Bacteriological Reviews*, *7*(57), 137.

Gordon, O., Goverde, M., Pazdan, J., & Roesti, D. (2015). Comparison of different calculation approaches for defining microbiological control levels based on historical data. *PDA Journal of Pharmaceutical Science and Technology*, *69*(3), 383–398.

Grigg, O. A., Farewell, V. T., & Spiegelhalter, D. J. (2003). The use of risk-adjusted CUSUM and RSPRT charts for monitoring in medical contexts. *Statistical Methods in Medical Research*, *12*(2), 147–170.

Hayes, G. D., Scallan, A. J., & Wong, J. H. F. (1997). Applying statistical process control to monitor and evaluate the hazard analysis critical control point hygiene data. *Food Control*, *8*, 173–176.

Hertroys, R., Van Vught, P. A., & Van De Donk, H. J. (1997). Moving towards an micro-biological environmental monitoring programme. *PDA Journal of Pharmaceutical Science and Technology*, *51*(1), 52–59.

Hussong, D., & Madsen, R. E. (2004). Analysis of environmental microbiology data from cleanroom samples. *Pharmaceutical Technology Aseptic Processing*, 10–15.

Jones, D., & Cundell, T. (2018). Method verification requirements for an advanced imaging system for microbial plate count enumeration. *PDA Journal of Pharmaceutical Science and Technology*, *72*(2), 199–212.

Kourti, T., & MacGregor, J. F. (1996). Multivariate SPC methods for process and product monitoring. *Journal of Quality Technology*, *28*(4), 409–428.

Lorowitz, W., Saxon, E., Sondossi, M., & Nakaova, K. (2005). Integrating statistics with a microbiology laboratory activity. *Microbiology Educcation*, *6*, 14–19.

McArthur, J., & Tuckfield, R. (2016). The role of statistical thinking in environmental microbiology. In M. Yates, C. Nakatsu, R. Miller, & S. Pillai (Eds.), *Manual of environmental microbiology* (4th ed., pp. 2.5.6-1–2.5.6-8). Washington, DC: ASM Press. https://doi.org/10.1128/9781555818821.ch2.5.6.

Novick, S. J., Zhao, W., & Yang, H. (2017). Setting alert and action limits in the presence of significant amount of censoring in data. *PDA Journal of Pharmaceutical Science and Technology*, *71*(1), 20–32.

Rattan, A. K. (2018). Data integrity: history, issues, and remediation of issues. *PDA Journal of Pharmaceutical Science and Technology*, *72*(2), 105–116.

Sandle, T. (2004). An approach for the reporting of microbiological results from water systems. *PDA Journal of Pharmaceutical Science and Technology*, *58*(4), 231–237.

Sandle, T. (2014). *Data review and analysis for pharmaceutical microbiology*. UK: Microbiology Solutions.

Sandle, T. (2016). Data integrity considerations for the pharmaceutical microbiology laboratory. *Journal of GXP Compliance*, *20*(6), 1–12.

Sokal, R. R., & Rohlf, F. J. (1995). *Biometry: The principles and practice of statistics in biological research* (pp. 411–422). New York: W.H. Freeman and Co.

Sutton, S. (2011). Accuracy of plate counts. *Journal of Validation Technology*, *17*(3), 42–48.

Tang, S. (1998). Microbial limits reviewed: the basis for unique Australian regulatory requirements for microbial quality of non-sterile pharmaceuticals. *PDA Journal of Pharmaceutical Science and Technology*, *52*(3), 100–109.

Tidswell, E. C., & Sandle, T. (2018). Microbiological test data—assuring data integrity. *PDA Journal of Pharmaceutical Science and Technology*, *72*(1), 2–14.

Wheeler, D. J., & Chambers, D. S. (1992). *Understanding statistical process control* (2 ed., p. 96). Knoxville, Tennessee: SPC Press.

Bioburden and Endotoxin Control in Pharmaceutical Processing

CHAPTER OUTLINE

Introduction   249
Gathering Information About Microbial Control   250
Microbial Risks During Manufacturing   251
Process Factors Affecting Contamination   253
Process Hold Times and Process Validation   254
Sterile Products Manufacturing   255
Testing Regimes   256
    Sampling   256
    Test Methods   257
    Monitoring Plan   258
Investigating Data Deviations   258
Summary   258
References   259

INTRODUCTION

Assessment of microbial and endotoxin levels in (and on) samples is an important part of pharmaceutical process control. Samples are drawn from intermediate product at defined stages (ideally based on risk assessment) and these allow for the microbial and endotoxin levels to be tracked from upstream processing to downstream processing (with an expectation that the microbial levels decrease, or at least remain unchanged provided they are below an acceptable action level). Microbial risks include bioburden and bacterial endotoxin. Bioburden assessment informs the manufacturer about both the expected microbial load of the product and the presence or absence of specific microorganisms, some of which might be classed as objectionable. Endotoxin informs about a risk involving a specific type of microorganism (Gram-negative bacteria) and the presence of a pyrogenic toxin that will be difficult if not impossible to eliminate.

Biocontamination Control for Pharmaceuticals and Healthcare. https://doi.org/10.1016/B978-0-12-814911-9.00015-8

Bioburden and endotoxin control form an essential part of the biocontamination control strategy (Sandle, 2012). This strategy will center on controlling the source of microorganisms and ensuring that conditions that promote microorganism survival, growth, and persistence are minimized. Specific aspects to consider as part of the biocontamination control strategy are discussed in this chapter. A routine testing strategy including alert levels and action levels is then developed. When out-of-limits events occur, investigations must be initiated. Hold conditions including time and temperature for a process should be validated to demonstrate control and prevention of potential microbial growth also need to be established. Test methods for both bioburden and endotoxin should be verified or validated as being acceptable. Pharmacopeial methods can be used or alternative rapid methods selected.

For aseptically filled products tighter standards are in place and European guidelines require a certain bioburden to be met at the point that a bulk product passes through a sterilizing grade filter. Due to the relatively low specification—of 10 cfu/100 mL—pharmaceutical manufacturers need to ensure that false positive results are avoided (as might arise from extraneous environmental contamination), given that false positives can result in batch rejection.

This chapter examines the importance of bioburden and endotoxin testing. Bioburden refers to the microbial content of a material (or on the surface) at a given point in time. This could be prior to sterilization or in relation to a process hold time. Bioburden refers to an estimation of the numbers of bacteria and fungi present in a liquid sample. With endotoxin, as Chapter 13 describes, the lipopolysaccharide component of the bacterial cell wall, found in abundance with Gram-negative bacteria and which can, at a certain threshold, elicit a pyrogenic response.

GATHERING INFORMATION ABOUT MICROBIAL CONTROL

The focus of intermediate product assessment is to inform about control. This allows the microbiologist to assess (Sandle, 2016):

- If levels of bioburden or bacterial endotoxin are higher at the start of the process (upstream samples) compared with later in the process (downstream samples).
- If parts of the process are considered to lead to bioburden reduction are effective.

- Whether additional process steps, such as water rinses, contribute to the bioburden.
- Where applicable, if additives to the process, such as formulation buffers, contribute to the bioburden and these are not filtered.

MICROBIAL RISKS DURING MANUFACTURING

Pharmaceutical preparations, especially biologic products, are at risk from microbial contamination in many stages. Such risks exist because biopharmaceuticals often include the types of carbon sources and other growth factors that favor microbial growth. Moreover, many of the types of microorganisms found within the environment including process areas can adapt and survive under a variety of conditions. Where microorganisms are capable of growth in conditions that favor cellular division, microbial contamination poses a significant risk to biologic products (Sandle, 2013).

The risk of microbial contamination arises from a variety of sources. These include the facility, equipment, process operations, raw materials, column resins, filter membranes, water, process gases, and personnel. These present areas where a breakdown in control can lead to microorganisms being present. Further weaknesses in control measures can lead to ingress of microorganisms into the product or formulated excipients.

There are many variables where contamination can occur. For example, open processing presents a greater contamination risk than closed processing. Open processing may be an individual event or may occur when a vessel is opened several times for mixing or addition of chemicals. The room environment and operator aseptic practices may also impact microbial risk. Whether microorganisms survive or proliferate is based on several physico-chemical factors. Thus the outcome, following microbial ingress, is either survival without growth, growth, or death. These outcomes are dependent upon product, process, time, and temperature. Some products and intermediates will be at more of a risk than others. For example, biopharmaceuticals or therapeutic protein products are derived from recombinant DNA and hybridoma technology; such materials are at a greater risk than inorganic additives. Chemicals added to the direct product, raw materials, media, buffer solutions, and in-process intermediates are also generally growth promoting.

Microorganisms need substances for energy generation and cellular biosynthesis. These are obtained from different growth sources. Many bacteria utilize carbon. Such organisms are divided into heterotrophs, which use organic molecules such as sugars, amino acids, fatty acids, organic acids, aromatic compounds, nitrogen bases, and other organic molecules for their source of carbon, and autotrophs which use inorganic molecules of carbon dioxide as their source of carbon. Other bacteria utilize nitrogen either alone or in addition to carbon. Other common nutritional requirements which bacteria utilize for growth include phosphorus, sulfur, potassium, magnesium, calcium, sodium, and iron. The actual nutritional types, quantities, and combinations will depend on the bacterial species (Raizada, 1971).

Bacterial growth individual cells divide in a process described as binary fission. Here two daughter cells arise from a single cell. The daughter cells are identical except for the occasional mutation. Exponential growth is a function of binary fission; this is because at each division there are two new cells. The time between divisions is called generation time—the time for the population to double. Generation times can range from minutes to several days depending on the species of bacteria. One of the fastest dividing bacteria is *Escherichia coli*, which can double every 15–20 min under ideal conditions (Andersen, von Meyenburg, 1980). Leading up to the beginning of growth is a lag phase; this time varies depending upon the physiological state of the organism and the growth conditions.

Bacterial growth does not go on indefinitely; there are factors that limit population growth. These factors are intraspecific competition for nutrients, which reduce as the culture ages and the accumulation of toxic metabolites. When these conditions occur, a stationary phase is reached when no growth occurs. If the depletion of nutrients or buildup of toxicity continues, cell death occurs.

The most frequently encountered pyrogen in pharmaceutical processing is endotoxin. Structurally lipopolysaccharides are part of the cell wall of Gram-negative bacteria. They are composed of a hydrophilic polysaccharide moiety, which is covalently linked to a hydrophobic lipid moiety. LPS from most species is composed of three distinct regions: the O-antigen region, a core oligosaccharide, and Lipid A (LipA). The lipid A is the most conserved part of endotoxin and is responsible for most of the biological activities of endotoxin (that is its pyrogenicity) (Ohno & Morrison, 1989).

The reason for the high prevalence of endotoxin in pharmaceutical facilities is a result of the use of large volumes of water in processing (water is a key ingredient to many products and it is also used for equipment rinsing.) The microorganisms found in association with water are Gram-negative bacteria (such as *Pseudomonads*). Although endotoxins are linked within the bacterial cell wall, they are continuously liberated into the environment. The release does not happen only with cell death but also during growth and division. Since bacteria can grow in nutrient poor media, such as water, saline, and buffers, endotoxins will be found at high levels in such environments (with the exception being highly purified forms of water like Water for Injections.) Other sources of pyrogens in pharmaceutical processing include solvents, drugs, additives apparatus used in manufacture, and containers. Primary sources are the water used as the solvent or in the processing; packaging components; the chemicals, raw materials or equipment used in the preparation of the product.

Aside from endotoxin, there are other forms of nonendotoxin microbial pyrogens. The degree to which these are prevalent in pharmaceutical environments (or rather prevalent at levels sufficient to trigger a pyrogenic response) is a point open to discussion. Aside from endotoxin, one important issue that pharmaceutical manufacturers of parenteral drugs need to consider is the risk posed by pyrogens of microbial origin that are not related to lipopolysaccharide. This requires a risk assessment, examining manufacturing process steps. Nonetheless, this author contends that although such nonendotoxin pyrogens are theoretically present, the risks that they pose are low for most processes. This is primarily because considerable quantities of nonendotoxin microbial material are required to elicit a pyrogenic response. For example, while staphylococcal enterotoxin is considered a "potent" pyrogen, a concentration of $1\,\mu g/Kg$ is required to elicit a pyrogenic response in the pyrogen test. When compared to endotoxin (threshold pyrogenic dose of 0.5 EU ($\sim$0.05 ng/kg), the difference is 20,000 fold. Thus the likelihood of sufficient staphylococci contaminating a drug produced, under cGMP conditions, to elicit a pyrogenic response is remote (Sandle, 2015a).

PROCESS FACTORS AFFECTING CONTAMINATION

Certain process factors can affect growth should contamination occur. Headspace ratio, for example, can be important. Increased headspace combined with agitation in a hold vessel can increase product oxygenation throughout the hold period. This may favor bacteria that prefer aerobic conditions. With temperature, there are some conditions that are more favorable to microbial growth than others. The temperature will depend upon the type of bacteria. Bacteria that grow optimally under different conditions are commonly divided into:

- Psychrophiles—low temperature optima $<15°C$.
- Mesophiles—midrange temperature optima $25–40°C$.
- Thermophiles—high temperature optima $40–80°C$.
- Hyperthermophiles—very high temperature optima $>80°C$.

Given that cleanroom contamination originates primarily from people, then mesophilic bacteria and fungi pose the biggest risk. This means that processes occurring at room temperature are at a greater theoretical risk. Other factors influencing the likelihood of microbial growth include pH. Most microorganisms prefer to grow between pH 5 and 9, with an optima at a neutral pH of 7. A further factor is oxygen, with many aerobic bacteria (which will be the most common) preferring aerobic conditions. Water activity is also important, where increasing dryness means fewer species of bacteria can grow or survive.

Product, process, time, and temperature should not be viewed as discrete factors. These factors often need to be combined since one factor in conjunction with another may lead to a different risk outcome. For example, one type of growth-promoting product held at 2–8°C would be at a lower risk due to this temperature inhibiting the growth of most microorganisms than the same product held for the same time period at 30–35°C.

PROCESS HOLD TIMES AND PROCESS VALIDATION

Due to the potential for microbial growth, pharmaceutical manufacturers typically conduct studies to define acceptable hold times for process intermediates (Grund & Sofer, 2007). These studies are based on the microbiological examination of in-process production samples. Microorganisms need substances for energy generation and cellular biosynthesis and certain parts of the process can encourage microbial growth; the possibility for growth becomes greater where process hold times occur. Process factors affecting contamination include headspace ratio, temperature, pH, oxygen, and water activity (Thillaivinayagalingam & Newcombe, 2011). Assessment of hold times should form part of the biocontamination control strategy.

The hold conditions (including both time and temperature) for a process should be validated to demonstrate control and prevention of potential microbial growth. These times should relate to the intermediate product and to any buffers or prepared ingredients intended to be added into the product. The validation plan should consider which time point sampling in relation to the process is required. Here the objective should be at the end of the hold time. According to Clontz: "Typically as part of a product hold-time validation study, bioburden/microbial limit testing is performed at time zero and then at the end of the storage period" (Clontz, 2013). Furthermore, it is important that the sample taken for testing is representative of the product and that it is homogenous. For this latter reason, some organizations elect to undertake hold time assessment in conjunction with mixing studies (Sandle, 2015b).

In evaluating results, any observed variability between time zero (T) and the maximum hold time evaluated (T) should be assessed. The most important aspect is with any rise in bioburden above either the action level or an acceptance threshold which may be a certain increase in bioburden, such as 50%. In undertaking validation, not every buffer or excipient will require testing although it is good practice to assess each intermediate product stage. With buffers, it may be possible to group similar buffers together. Adopting such a matrix approach can save time, although care needs to be taken with the grouping. It is important to consider the active ingredients to determine if they are potentially growth promoting. This will include sugars, which will promote the growth of many microorganisms, and inherently antimicrobial such as hydrochloric acid. Samples presented for validation should be materials obtained from production-scale batches and held at set temperatures and times as defined in process definitions.

STERILE PRODUCTS MANUFACTURING

The most important sample in relation to aseptically filled products is the sample taken of the bulk product prior to final filtration. Final filtration involves passing the bulk through a 0.2 μm sterilizing grade filter, into a sterile vessel. After mixing, the sterile homogenous bulk is aseptically filled. With filtration, the Parenteral Drug Association guidance document "Sterilizing Filtration of Liquids" published as Technical Report No. 26, defines sterilizing filtration as "the process of removing all micro-organisms, excluding viruses, from a fluid stream" (Yang, Li, & Chang, 2013).

Although there is no comparable limit in the United States, within Europe a maximal limit is in place for aseptically filled products at the point before the bulk passes through the sterilizing filter. With this, a CPMP Note for Guidance on Manufacture of the Finished Dosage Form has a section relating to the appropriate bioburden level of the bulk solution prior to sterilization by filtration, for products distributed in the European Union. This reads: "For sterilization by filtration the maximum acceptable bioburden prior to the filtration must be stated in the application. In most situations NMT 10 cfu's/100 mL will be acceptable, depending on the volume to be filtered in relation to the diameter of the filter (CPMP, n.d.)."

The U.S. FDA guidelines on aseptic filling states that a suitable limit must be set: "Manufacturing process controls should be designed to minimize the bioburden in the unfiltered product. In addition to increasing the challenge to the sterilizing filter, bioburden can contribute impurities (e.g., endotoxin) to, and lead to degradation of, the drug product. A prefiltration bioburden limit should be established (FDA, n.d.)." However, no actual value is specified. The origin of the CPMP limit appears to have a relationship with the recommended microbial count for bulk WFI (not >10 cfu/100 mL), and with consideration of the standard sterilizing filter rating of the retention of 107 colony forming units of the challenge microorganism *Brevundimonas diminuta* per cm^2 of the filter surface (based on a 0.2 μm filter pore size).

TESTING REGIMES

Once all controls are in place, the microbiologist will need to determine a test regime describing samples selected for testing and which types of tests required. Tests required will be bioburden testing and, in some cases, endotoxin analysis. Appropriate alert and action limits should be in place for specific process steps. It is expected that a bioburden reduction occurs throughout the process for sterile products. For example, the reduction in bioburden could be 500 cfu/mL for the start of the process, moving to 100 cfu/mL for mid-stage formulation, to 10 cfu/mL for later process, and finally <1 cfu/mL at the point of final filtration for aseptically filled products. With endotoxin, the limit prescribed will be based on risk. However, a limit similar to that used for pharmaceutical grade water (typically 0.25 EU/mL) will often be suitable. These limits could serve as action levels.

The establishment of alert levels is also important. The levels can be defined as follows:

- *Alert Level*: A level that, when exceeded, indicates a process may have drifted from its normal operating condition. Alert levels constitute a warning, but do not necessarily warrant corrective action.
- *Action Level*: A level that, when exceeded, indicates a process has drifted from its normal operating range. A response to such an excursion should involve a documented investigation and corrective action.

When setting alert and action limits, it is good practice to:

- Base levels on historical data
- Perform continued trend analysis and data evaluation to determine if the established levels remain appropriate.
- Watch for periodic spikes, even if averages stay within levels.

Sampling

Consideration should be given to sample containers, which are sterile with no leaching or inhibitory substances. Containers used for endotoxin sampling must be also pyrogen free and made of a material that does not interfere with the recovery of endotoxin (e.g., glass, polystyrene). Sample handling using aseptic technique is also important, as are the storage conditions (samples placed in 2–8°C within a validated process time), and the assigned expiry time which should also be validated.

The sampling process can be improved using single-use technology (Samavedam, Goldstein, & Schieche, 2006). The conventional way to sample the bulk product for bioburden is to withdraw a quantity of the material from a holding vessel, using a valve or syringe, and to transfer this to a sterile sampling container. This process, which is operator dependent and involves multiple steps, poses a risk of adventitious contamination and thus of a false positive result being reported which, at a sufficiently high bioburden, could lead to product rejection. Due to the integral nature, the use of single-use, sterile biocontainer bags allows the sample to be taken in a way which eliminates the possibility of external or operator contamination triggering a false positive result.

Test Methods

The sample test method for bioburden must be established and undertaken consistently. This is based on the total microbial count, which is typically a test for aerobic, mesophilic organisms unless any special testing is required (such as for anaerobic bacteria or bacteria requiring special growth conditions). Samples should be mixed in a standardized way prior to testing. Membrane filtration using a 100 mL sample or pour plates using a 1 mL sample are the most common total microbial count techniques deployed for bioburden testing (Sutton, 2011). It is commonplace to select a general-purpose agar such as soybean casein digest medium (SCDM) for testing and to incubate samples between 20 and 35°C (Sandle, Skinner, & Yeandle, 2013).

When established methods are verified, the sample must be shown to not be inhibitory to microbial growth so that a false negative result is avoided. This may involve challenging portions of the sample with a suitable panel of microorganisms with challenge inoculums of <100 cfu. The test panel should be made up from microorganisms traceable to a recognized culture collection; the panel can be enhanced with environmental isolates. The culture media used and incubation conditions (time and temperature) must be appropriate.

Regarding endotoxin testing, pharmacopeial methods can be used (those described in Chapter 13). With qualifying the test, the sample must be shown not to cause inhibition or enhancement based on an endotoxin challenge. When dilution is required, the Maximum Valid Dilution (MVD) must not be exceeded based on the relationship between the endotoxin limit and the end point of the standard curve or lysate sensitivity (Upton & Sandle, 2012).

Monitoring Plan

A comprehensive in-process sampling and testing plan is needed for the monitoring of the manufacturing processes. With sample selection, testing will apply to held intermediate product, and here representative samples should be taken at the end of the hold period. The process validation section later considers the notion of representativeness. In addition to the product, excipients and formulated buffers should also be considered for testing.

INVESTIGATING DATA DEVIATIONS

When conducting out-of-limits investigations, the following can be considered:

- Numbers and types of routine bioburden trends (product and environment)
- Identification of recovered microorganisms
- Evaluation of microorganism for resistance to the sterilization process
- Production personnel impact (e.g., proper training or new personnel)
- Manufacturing process changes
- Sampling and testing procedures changes
- Evaluation of laboratory controls and monitors
- Additional testing
- Cleaning and disinfection of production areas
- Any modifications to the sampling plan or changes to operator techniques.
- Any raw materials and supplier changes
- Origin of contamination, such as water source contamination or from incoming materials.

The previous list is not intended to be exhaustive.

SUMMARY

This chapter has looked at bioburden and endotoxin testing during pharmaceutical processing. These represent key components of the biocontamination control strategy. The biocontamination control strategy will, in turn, inform about process control. Any results relating to a process hold that are out of limits should be investigated. A drift in trends where counts are rising should prompt a review of the initial assessment. An investigation must consider the product impact and the origin of the contamination. Once the likely origin is established, preventative measures should be implemented.

The chapter has also considered the implications of the process hold times on microbial growth during pharmaceutical manufacturing. Microbiological risk exists—especially with biological products. If microbial contamination occurs where microorganisms enter a product in sufficient numbers and if the process hold time is long enough, the process hold time may be problematic.

REFERENCES

Andersen, K. B., & von Meyenburg, K. (1980). Are growth rates of *Escherichia coli* in batch cultures limited by respiration? *Journal of Bacteriology, 144*(1), 114–123.

Clontz, L. (2013). *Microbial limit and bioburden tests: validation approaches and global requirements* (p. 49). Boca Raton, FL: CRC Press.

CPMP The European Agency for the Evaluation of Medicinal Products Committee for Proprietary Medicinal Products (CPMP) Note for Guidance on Manufacturing of the Finished Dosage Form, CPMP/QWP/486/95.

FDA. Guidance for industry sterile drug products produced by aseptic processing—current good manufacturing practice, FDA, Bethesda, MD.

Grund, E., & Sofer, G. (2007). Validation of process chromatograph. In J. Agalloco, & F. Carleton (Eds.), *Validation of pharmaceutical processes* (3rd ed., p. 477). Boca Raton, FL: CRC Press.

Ohno, N., & Morrison, D. C. (1989). Lipopolysaccharide interaction with lysozyme: binding of lipopolysaccharide to lysozyme and inhibition of lysozyme enzymatic activity. *The Journal of Biological Chemistry, 264*, 4434–4441.

Raizada, M. M. (1971 Jul). Singh role of carbon and nitrogen sources in bacterial growth and sporulation. *Applied Microbiology, 22*(1), 131–132.

Samavedam, R., Goldstein, A., & Schieche, D. (2006). Implementation of disposables: validation and other considerations. *American Pharmaceutical Review, 9*, 46–51.

Sandle, T. (2012). Review of FDA warning letters for microbial bioburden issues (2001 – 2011). *Pharma Times, 44*(12), 29–30.

Sandle, T. (2013). Contamination control risk assessment. In: R. E. Masden, & J. Moldenhauer (Eds.), *Vol. 1. Contamination control in healthcare product manufacturing* (pp. 423–474). River Grove, IL: DHI Publishing.

Sandle, T. (2015a). Assessing non-endotoxin microbial pyrogens in relation in pharmaceutical processing. *Journal of GXP Compliance, 19*(1). Mar 2015 (2015a). http://www.ivtnetwork.com/article/assessing-non-endotoxin-microbial-pyrogens-relation-pharmaceutical-processing.

Sandle, T. (2015b). Assessing process hold times for microbial risks: bioburden and endotoxin. *Journal of GXP Compliance, 19*(3), 1–9. Oct 2015.

Sandle, T. (2016). Improving microbiological assurance for bioburden tests. *European Pharmaceutical Review, 21*(3), 41–44.

Sandle, T., Skinner, K., & Yeandle, E. (2013). Optimal conditions for the recovery of bio-burden from pharmaceutical processes: a case study. *European Journal of Parenteral and Pharmaceutical Sciences, 18*(3), 84–91.

Sutton, S. (2011). Accuracy of plate counts. *Journal of Validation Technology, 17*(3), 42–46.

Thillaivinayagalingam, P., & Newcombe, A. R. (2011). Validation of intermediate hold times. *Bioprocess International, 9*(4), 52–57.

Upton, A. and Sandle, T. Best practices for the bacterial endotoxin test: a guide to the LAL assay, Pharmaceutical Microbiology Interest Group: Stanstead Abbotts, 2012.

Yang, H., Li, N., & Chang, S. (2013). A risk-based approach to setting sterile filtration bioburden limits. *PDA J Pharm Sci Technol, 67*(6), 601–609.

Risk Assessment and Investigation for Environmental Monitoring

CHAPTER OUTLINE

Introduction   261
Introducing Quality Risk Management   263
Applying Risk Assessment to Environmental Monitoring   265
   Intrinsic Hazards   266
   Extrinsic Hazards   266
Using Risk to Construct the Environmental Monitoring Program   267
   Frequencies of Monitoring   267
Risk Assessment Tools   268
Hazard Analysis Critical Control Points (HACCP)   270
Failure Modes and Effects Analysis   273
   The FMEA Exercise   274
Numerical Approaches to Risk Assessment   275
Risks Associated With Conducting Environmental Monitoring   280
Out-of-Limits Investigations   281
Root Causes   283
Summary   284
References   284

INTRODUCTION

Environmental monitoring, as Chapter 10 discusses, describes the microbiological testing undertaken in order to detect changing trends of microbial count and microbiota within cleanroom environments. It is not the same as environmental control and monitoring is, ideally, targeted where the control is weakest. The results from environmental monitoring obtained provide information about the performance of the physical design of the room (most notably the HVAC system) and the performance of the people, equipment, and cleaning operations within the cleanroom. The sites where microorganisms

Biocontamination Control for Pharmaceuticals and Healthcare. https://doi.org/10.1016/B978-0-12-814911-9.00016-X

are recovered also allow for assessment to be made about the potential impact upon critical parts of the process or the potential risk to the product.

In the best approach to environmental monitoring is embedded with a focus on risk assessment, as part of wider quality risk management. Risk methodologies like HACCP provide examples of a systematic, proactive, and preventative tool to identify, assess, and prevent or reduce potential risks that can occur at specific steps in a process (Sandle, 2016).

Risk assessment is, however, not something "new." Many of the approaches merely formalize many of the activities that microbiologists have been undertaking for years. Nevertheless, a formalized approach is what many regulators now expect to see. There are some advantages as well in forcing microbiologists to move away from the laboratory bench and to work with other staff, as such risk assessments generally require a multidisciplinary approach to risk assessment.

A good risk assessment is one that uses sound science as part of the decision making. It should be a systematic and have a structured process, although not too rigid a structure to the extent that key concepts are overlooked. The process needs to be transparent and inclusive, regularly reviewed, and able to respond to changes (fitting in with continual improvement philosophies) (McGivern & Fischer, 2012).

Central to risk assessment in the context of this book is control of microbial contamination. To achieve this there needs to be (Sandle, 2018):

- Appropriate written procedures, designed to prevent objectionable microorganisms in drug products not required to be sterile need to be established and followed.
- Appropriate written procedures, designed to prevent microbiological contamination of drug products purporting to be sterile need to be established and followed. Such procedures should include validation of any sterilization process.

The most significant biocontamination risks arise from personnel (in a sense an operator working in a controlled environment is a "contamination generator"). Due to the limitations with environmental monitoring, as discussed at various junctures in this book (as relating to quantification of methods and sample times, for example), a significant focus of risk assessment must be with minimizing or removing personnel interaction with pharmaceutical ingredients and products. The ultimate objective of sterile product manufacturing, for example, is with removing personnel from any direct interaction, such as through the use of barrier technology.

INTRODUCING QUALITY RISK MANAGEMENT

The use of risk management for environmental monitoring, and for looking at wider processes of cleanroom management or specific activities like aseptic filling, is linked to a wider process called "quality risk management." Quality risk management is a systematic process for the assessment, control, communication, and review of risks to the quality of the medicinal product. It can be applied both proactively and retrospectively. Quality risk management has been promoted by European medicines inspectors and by the FDA as key to current GMPs (Sandle & Lamba, 2012).

Since the mid-2000s quality risk management has played a major part in the design and modification of pharmaceutical production. Risk management has always been an intrinsic part of the world of pharmaceutical and health-care—with the decisive calculation of benefit–risk for each medicine serving as the ultimate determinant for drug and patient safety. A significant change happened when the ICH (International Conference on Harmonisation) published a document called ICH Q9 (which was later "adopted" by the FDA and as Annex 20 of the EU GMP Guide) (ICH, 2006).

ICH Q9 is concerned with risk assessment methodologies. In ICH Q9 three key definitions are outlined. These help to contextualize what is meant by "risks":

- *Risk*: "The combination of the probability of occurrence of harm and the severity of that harm"
- *Harm*: "Damage to health, including the damage that can occur from loss of product quality or availability"
- Hazard: "The potential source of harm," one that either exists or does not exist (it is the assessment of risk that quantified or qualifies a hazard).

What is of concern with hazards are consequences; these are the potential outcomes resulting from a hazard when it occurs. Consequences shape risks, based on the potential severity of the hazard and the likelihood or probability that the hazard will cause something to occur. This may be a simple "risk" or feeling, or with one risk compared another or against a benchmark, when expressed qualitatively, as low, medium, or high; or semiquantitatively as a number.

Thus risk and hazard form the following relationship (Okrent, 1980):

$$\text{Risk} = \text{Hazard} \times \frac{\text{Vulnerability (or severity)}}{\text{Capacity (or likelihood)}}$$

So risk is an expression of the probability that a given hazard will cause harm. Here a hazard will pose low risk if the likelihood of its exposure is minimized.

Risk Management, in the context of this book, is fundamentally about understanding what is most important for the control of product quality and then focusing resources on managing and controlling these things to ensure that risks are reduced and contained. Before risks can be managed, or controlled, they need to be assessed.

Two important points to remember for any risk assessment are as follows:

1. There is no such thing as "zero risk" and therefore a decision is required as to what is "acceptable risk."
2. Risk Assessment is not an exact science—different people will have a different perspective on the same hazard.

Consequently, whichever tool is used, it is important that a team approach is taken utilizing an agreed set of definitions (and if required, numerical scores).

Whichever tool is used, risk assessment involves:

- Identifying hazards,
- Analyzing the risk associated with each hazard,
- Evaluating how significant the risks are.

Moreover, however, the outcomes are dressed up in terms of statements or numbers, the outcome is that either:

- The risk is acceptable;
- The risk is unacceptable.

The outcome of the assessment can then be used to determine appropriate control strategies to reduce the risk to a level that is deemed acceptable. These strategies are typically focused on reducing the probability of a risk occurring and/or increasing the probability of it being detected.

There are various examples of best practice for undertaking risk assessment. When doing so, it is important to clearly identify the process being assessed and what it is attempting to achieve, that is what the harm/risk is and what the impact could be on the patient. Risk assessment should always:

- Be based on systematic identifications of possible risk factors.
- Take full account of current scientific knowledge.
- Be conducted by people with experience in the risk assessment process and the process being risk assessed.
- Use factual evidence supported by expert assessment to reach conclusions
- Do not include any unjustified assumptions.

- Identify all reasonably expected risks—simply and clearly, along with a factual assessment and mitigation where required.
- Be documented to an appropriate level and controlled/approved.
- Ultimately be linked to the protection of the patient.
- Should contain objective risk mitigation plan.

Furthermore, there should be risk assessment procedure in place at each organization, and ideally a procedure especially written for addressing assessments of biocontamination concerns (Sutton, 2010b).

APPLYING RISK ASSESSMENT TO ENVIRONMENTAL MONITORING

The two key points for the microbiologist to demonstrate to a regulator are: firstly, that they have a well-defined environmental monitoring program in place, and, secondly, that any adverse results that may be generated from it are considered by way of risk assessment. One problem is the general lack of published material that relates specifically to the pharmaceutical industry on this subject and the industry has been slow to develop its own methodologies. Most approaches are "borrowed" from the food or engineering industries (Sutton, 2010a).

This unit generally draws on examples from aseptic filling. However, most of the applications can be applied with little modification to nonsterile manufacturing.

There are different stages toward which risk assessments can be directed (Ruzante, Whiting, Dennis, & Buchanan, 2013):

- Prospective analysis of process designs (which is considered before the commencement of any project, such as the purchase of a new filling machine or modification to a cleanroom);
- Comparative analysis of current processes (where a risk assessment model is applied to examine current manufacturing steps);
- Identification of process improvements;
- Optimization of the environmental monitoring process;
- Determination of worst-case conditions;
- Assistance is batch release.

Risk assessment involves the identification of hazards. These can be divided into (Whyte & Eaton, 2004a):

a. Intrinsic hazards;
b. Extrinsic hazards.

To draw on a sporting analogy, an example of an extrinsic hazard is with coaching. This would be the coach not completing a warm up or stretching with the players or showing them the wrong technique, which then could cause you to have an injury. An example of an intrinsic hazard is with nutrition. If we do not have the right diet and nutrition you might not get the right amount of energy we need to perform, you might not get enough fat/insulation you need to keep warm, and your bones might not become stronger and you might not recover from injury as quick.

Intrinsic Hazards

Intrinsic hazards represent those integral or inherent elements of processes or systems that have the potential to affect products quality. Often, these are associated with failure of plant, process, or systems and are discrete and singular events. This would include the natural microbial load of the products or an active pharmaceutical ingredient. These tend to be more "constant" than extrinsic hazards.

Extrinsic Hazards

Extrinsic hazards are entities that are not an integral characteristic of the product or process. An example would be the bioburden present on personnel or microorganisms resident in a water source that enters an item of equipment. The risk from extrinsic hazards is arguably greater than that from intrinsic hazards.

The risk from extrinsic hazards involves the following steps:

- Risk of ingress;
- Risk of accessing;
- Risk of contaminating;
- Risk of being retained.

Of the sources of microbial contamination (discussed in this module), personnel and water can be considered as primary risks, and surfaces and air as secondary risks. Where each is present there is the opportunity for product ingress, as illustrated in Fig. 1.

The events that need to occur for contamination to take place are as follows:

- Direct surface-to-surface transfer (such as, by personnel directly touching the product or contaminated water entering the process);
- Airborne transfer.

There are also a variety of different approaches that can be taken to performing risk assessment. Due to the vast number of techniques, we can only look

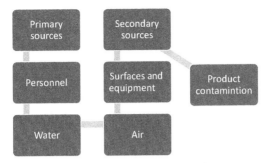

■ **FIG. 1** Primary and secondary sources of contamination and routes of contamination ingress.

at some of these and illustrate some of the approaches being taken in the pharmaceutical industry. This chapter uses several examples, which are mostly drawn from a sterile drug manufacturing facility and focuses mostly on aseptic filling. However, the concepts and tools are applicable to the environmental monitoring of other types of manufacture.

USING RISK TO CONSTRUCT THE ENVIRONMENTAL MONITORING PROGRAM

Chapter 10 discussed the construction of an environmental monitoring program. To enhance the program, risk assessment can be used, as the chapter demonstrates. Examples include:

- Deciding how often to monitor different types of cleanrooms
- The use of risk assessment tools to design the environmental monitoring program
- The use of numerical approach to risk assess data using a case study of excursion.

These are looked at briefly here.

Frequencies of Monitoring

Risk factors that help to determine monitoring frequencies include:

- Giving a higher weighting to a more "dirty" activity performed in an adjacent room to a clean activity, even if the clean activity represents later processing.
- Giving higher weighting to areas that have a higher level of personnel transit (given that people are the main microbiological contamination source). This may include corridors and changing rooms.
- Routes of transfer.

- Areas which receive incoming goods.
- Component preparation.
- Duration of activity (such as a lower criticality for a 30-min process compared to a 6-h operation).
- Having higher frequencies of monitoring in warm or ambient areas opposed to cold rooms.
- Having higher frequencies of monitoring to areas with water/sinks than dry ambient areas.
- Having higher frequencies for open processing or open plant assembly compared to processing which is open momentarily or to closed processing (where product risk exposure time is examined).
- Intensifying monitoring toward final formulation/purification/secondary packaging/product filling.

The previously listed can be assessed and weighted using risk scoring and then sorted against different monitoring frequencies using risk ranking and risk filtering (Haimes, Kaplan, & Lambert, 2002).

The decisions for each cleanroom should be reviewed at regular intervals. This may invoke changes to a rooms status (and hence the monitoring frequency) or to changes for different sample types within the room. For example, it maybe, that after reviewing data for 1 year, that surface samples produce higher results than air samples for a series of rooms. In this event that the user wishes to vary the frequency of monitoring and take surface samples more often than air samples. There would also be an increased focus on cleaning and disinfection practices and frequencies based on such data (Sandle, 2014).

Within the monitoring program it is also possible to vary the frequency of monitoring of surfaces within respect to an assessment of the air. This is because air samples are direct indicator of the quality of the process and assign a level of control to the process, whereas surface samples indicate cleaning and disinfection. If the results of surface samples are generally satisfactory, as indicated by trend analysis, then either the number of samples or the frequency at which they are taken can be reduced. If subsequent data showed an increase in counts the monitoring frequency could easily be restored. Indeed, all types of monitoring frequencies may increase as part of an investigation as appropriate.

RISK ASSESSMENT TOOLS

More sophisticated approaches for selecting monitoring locations can be derived by risk assessment tools. These approaches include FMEA (failure mode and effects analysis), FTA (fault tree analysis), and HACCP (hazard analysis critical control points), all of which employ a scoring approach. There are other tools as well, such as those which rely on computational analysis including Monte Carlo modeling (Tidswell & McGarvey, 2006).

At present, no definitive method exists, and the various approaches differ in their process and degree of complexity involved. However, the two most commonly used appear to be HACCP (which originated in the food industry) and FMEA (which was developed for the engineering industry).

These various analytical tools are similar, in that they involve (Sandle, 2011):

- Constructing diagrams of work flows.
- Pinpointing areas of greatest risk.
- Examining potential sources of contamination.
- Deciding on the most appropriate sample methods.
- Helping to establish alert and action levels.
- Taking into account changes to the work process/seasonal activities.

The general assumption that the approaches make is that when hazards cannot be controlled, the risk of the hazard requires assessment. Numerical approaches generally approach this on the following basis:

$$\text{Risk} = \text{Severity of occurrence} \times \text{Probability of occurrence}$$

With aseptic manufacture, some microbiologists will argue that all viable microorganisms irrespective of the species or the number are potentially "severe" and thus the emphasis is shifted toward probability of occurrence (or the probability that one microorganism will gain access inside the product presentation).

For the risk to occur, there must be:

- A source for contamination (generally water, air, or personnel);
- A given amount of viable microorganisms;
- A circumstance, event, opportunity, and a mechanism by which the contamination can enter the process (this requires some type of complex and dynamic exchange to occur).

These risk assessment approaches are not only concerned with selecting environmental monitoring locations. They integrate the monitoring system with a complete review of operations within the cleanroom to ensure those facilities, operations, and practices are also satisfactory. The approaches recognize a risk, rate the level of the risk, and then set out a plan to minimize, control, and monitor the risk. The monitoring of the risk will help to determine the frequency, locations for, and level of environmental monitoring.

Risks can be assessed by breaking down the process into a series of steps. For example:

1. The contribution of the facility (cleanroom environment) to the risk;
2. Preparation of equipment;
3. Transfer of equipment;
4. Setup of equipment;
5. Bioburden of excipients;
6. Bioburden from the previous manufacturing stage in the intermediate product;
7. Personnel interventions.

Such risks are compounded by the complexity of each risk. This can include:

- The amount of equipment transferred;
- The equipment setup complexity;
- The complexity of the room design (e.g., an area designed to control powder will have additional airflow considerations);
- Number of personnel involved;
- Personnel entry and exit;
- The number of personnel interventions;
- Material entry and exit;
- Material supply;
- Processing of consumables;
- Waste collection and disposal;
- Maintenance operations;
- Environmental conditions: time, temperature, humidity;
- Surface contamination levels;
- Function of the room HVAC.

In theory, it is personnel who represent the greatest variable.

HAZARD ANALYSIS CRITICAL CONTROL POINTS (HACCP)

HACCP is probably the most useful of the risk assessment tools for environmental monitoring. The HACCP concept was developed in the 1960s by the Pillsbury Company, while working with NASA and the US Army Laboratories to provide safe food for space expeditions. The system of HACCP evolved from these early approaches to understand and control food safety failures. HACCP came to be widely used by the food industry since the late 1970s and is now internationally recognized as the best system for ensuring food safety. In the 1990s, the system has begun to be adopted to examine pharmaceutical manufacturing.

The HACCP approach involves, in terms of core principles:

1. Identify hazards (contamination risks); methods to control the hazards, and assess their severity.
2. Determine critical control points (CCPs). CCPs are points in production and processing at which significant hazards can be controlled or eliminated.
   With appropriate measures at that point the risk can be:

- avoided
- eliminated
- or reduced to an acceptable level

3. Establish critical limits for each CCP. Each CCP must operate within specific parameters to ensure the hazard is being appropriately and effectively controlled.
4. Establish system to monitor control of the CCPs. Monitoring involves defining how the CCPs will be assessed, performing the monitoring at the appropriate time intervals, determining who will perform the monitoring and finally maintaining the proper monitoring records.
5. Establish the corrective action (when CCP is not under control). These can be both short- and long-term corrective actions. Appropriate records must be maintained.
6. Establish procedures for verification to confirm that the HACCP system is working effectively.
7. Establish documentation and reporting systems for all procedures. This includes all records required in the various parts of the HACCP plan, as well as other key records such as sanitation logs.

The most effective use of HACCP involves constructing process flow, and using these to identify contamination points and to use these information to attempt to reduce contamination and to determine monitoring locations. To identify sources of contamination, construct a risk diagram/diagrams. This will show sources and routes of contamination. Examples include:

- Areas adjacent to cleanroom/isolator (e.g., airlocks, changing rooms)
- Air supply
- Room air
- Surfaces
- People
- Machine
- Equipment

From these point, the microbiologist should assess the importance of these sources and if they are/are not hazards that need to be controlled. Examples include:

a. The amount of contamination on, or in, the source that is available for transfer.
b. Ease by which the contamination is dispersed or transferred.
c. The proximity of the source to the critical point where the product is exposed.
d. How easily the contamination can pass through the control method.

The use of a scoring method can be very helpful. Following this, the microbiologist should identify the methods that can be used to control these hazards. For example:

a. Air supply/HEPA filters
b. Dirty areas adjacent to cleanroom/isolator (including differential pressures; airflow movement)
c. Room air (air change rates; use of barriers)
d. Surfaces (sterilization; effectiveness of cleaning/disinfection procedures)
e. People (cleanroom clothing and gloves; room ventilation; training)
f. Machines and equipment (sterilization, effectiveness of cleaning, exhaust systems)

The next step is to determine valid sampling methods to monitor either the hazards or their control methods or both.

For example:

a. HEPA filter integrity tests
b. Air supply velocity, air change rates
c. Room pressure differentials
d. Particle counts
e. Air samplers; settle plates, contact plates, and so on.

The microbiologist should then establish a monitoring schedule with "alert" and "action" levels and corrective measures to be taken (for when these levels are exceeded). For example:

a. The greater the hazard, the greater the amount of monitoring required.
b. Trend analysis for alert and action levels: in or out of control.

The final phase involves verifying that the contamination control system is working effectively by reviewing key targets like product rejection rate, sampling results, control methods, and so on. These may need to be modified over time. For example:

a. System for data review
b. Examine filling trials
c. Audit
d. Reassess hazards, effectiveness of control systems, frequency of monitoring, appropriateness of alert and action levels.

At the end of the process, the user should establish and maintain documentation. For example:

a. Describe the steps being taken
b. Describe the monitoring procedures
c. Describe the reporting and review procedures

In addition, staff need to be trained in the process.

FAILURE MODES AND EFFECTS ANALYSIS

Failure modes and effects analysis (FMEA) contrasts with HACCP in that it attempts a quantitative approach. The risk tool follows a step-by-step approach, which is used for identifying all possible failures in a design, a manufacturing or assembly process, or a product or service. "Failure modes" means the ways, or modes, in which something might fail. FMEA schemes vary in their approach, scoring, and categorization. All approaches share in common a numerical approach. The example here, based on a sterility testing isolator, was to assign a score (from 1 to 5, in this case; other schemes use ranges of 1 to 10) to each of the following categories:

- Severity
- Occurrence
- Detection

Where:

- Severity is the consequence of a failure
- Occurrence is the likelihood of the failure happening (based on past experience)
- Detect is based on the monitoring systems in place and on how likely a failure can be detected.

By asking a series of questions of each main part of the isolator system. Such questions included:

1. What is the function of the equipment? How are its performance requirements?
2. How can it fail to fulfill these functions?
3. What can cause each failure?
4. What happens when each failure occurs?
5. How much does each failure matter? What are its consequences?
6. What can be done to predict or prevent each failure?
7. What should be done if a suitable proactive task cannot be found?

The scoring is 1 (very good) to 5 (very bad). Therefore a likelihood of high severity would be rated 5; high occurrence rated 5; but a good detection system would be rated 1. It should be noted that some microbiologists do not like the use of "detection" to be used in the scoring, seeing risk as simply an expression of severity and likelihood. The adoption of "detection" sometimes results in mitigating risk, through the scoring system. However, the risk can still remain and simply monitoring for a hazard, especially using insensitive environmental monitoring methods, can serve to obfuscate the extent of the risk to the product or patient.

Using the previous criteria a final FMEA score is produced:

$$\frac{x}{125}$$

This is derived from: severity score x occurrence score x detect score. The maximum score is 25, from: $5 \times 5 \times 5$.

Depending upon the score produced it can be decided whether further action is needed. There is no published guidance on what the score that dictates some form of action should be. Many users adopt a score of 27 as the cutoff value where action was required. This was based on 27 being the score derived when the mid-score is applied to all three categories (i.e., the numerical value "3" from severity (3) $\times$ occurrence (3) $\times$ detect (3)) and the supposition that if the mid-rating (or a higher number) was scored for all three categories then as a minimum the system should be examined in greater detail.

The FMEA Exercise

An example is reproduced as follows. It relates to a sterility testing isolator (Sandle, 2003).

EXAMINATION X: THE ISOLATOR ROOM
Description of critical area: The isolator is situated in an unclassified room. There is not requirement to place a sterility testing isolator in a classified room.

Table 1 Presenting the failure mode and assessing severity

Process step	Failure mode	Significance of failure	Severity of consequence (score)
Loading isolators presanitization/ performing sterility testing	That contamination from the room could enter transfer or main isolators	Reduced efficiency of transfer isolator sanitization/ contamination inside main isolator	3

FMEA schematic, as per Table 1.

The calculated FMEA score is:

$$\text{FMEA score}: \quad 3 \times 1 \times 1 \quad = \quad 3$$

Analysis: There is no problem considered from the room environment. Entry to the room is controlled; the sanitization cycle has been challenged with a level of microorganisms far greater than would ever be found in the environment (spores *of Geobacillus stearothermophilus*); all items entering the isolator are sanitized (using a chlorine dioxide based sporicidal disinfectant) and the isolator itself is an effective positive pressure barrier to the outside (at $>15\,\text{Pa}$).

As detailed earlier, environmental monitoring is performed inside the isolator during testing. This monitoring, which has an action level of 1 cfu, is designed to detect any potential contamination inside the isolator environment (Table 2).

NUMERICAL APPROACHES TO RISK ASSESSMENT

There are different approaches, other than FMEA, for assigning a level of risk through the use numbers, and many of these approaches are complementary to HACCP. This section examines the assessment of risks after an activity has taken place and the data is being examined. Examples of individual out-of-limits results and data sets relating to an operation are examined, using examples from an aseptic filling process. Numerical approaches are useful in applying a level of consistency between one decision and another.

The following section details some methods that can be used to quantify the risk of contamination in pharmaceutical cleanrooms. The models outlined are based on the work performed by Whyte and Eaton (Whyte & Eaton, 2004b; Whyte & Eaton, 2004c).

Table 2 Assessing occurrence and detection factors

Measures to detect failure	Occurrence (score)	Detection systems	Detection (score)
Would be shown from reduced evaporation rate for isolator sanitization/poor environmental monitoring results in main isolator/ potential sterility test failures/ sanitization cycle has been validated using BIs of 106 spores	1	Isolator room is monitored monthly for viables and particles/staff wear over-shoes on entry/Dycem mat in place/entry to room has controlled access/ environmental monitoring performed inside main isolator/ isolators are at positive pressure to the room and air is HEPA filtered	1

EXAMPLE 1: ESTIMATING THE RISK TO PRODUCT USING SETTLE PLATE COUNTS

The method applies to the assessment of settle plates at the point of fill, under the Grade A/ISO Class 5 zone. It allows an estimate of the probable contamination rate to the product as derived from the following equation:

$$\text{Contamination rate } (\%) = \text{Settle plate count} \times \frac{\text{Area of product}}{\text{Area of Petri} - \text{dish}}$$
$$\times \frac{\text{Time product exposed}}{\text{Time settle plates exposed}} \times 100$$

The fixed value is the area of the Petri dish, which for a 90-mm plate, is $64 \, \text{cm}^2$.

A worked example illustrates the use of the equation:

a. Area of Petri dish $= 64 \, \text{cm}^2$.
b. Settle plate count $= 1 \, \text{cfu}$.
c. Neck area of product $= 1 \, \text{cm}^2$.
d. Exposure time of product $= 1 \, \text{min}$
e. Exposure time of settle plate $= 240 \, \text{min}$

By inserting these example values into the equation:

$$1 \times \frac{1}{64} \times \frac{1}{240} = 0.000065 \times 100 = 0.0065\%$$

The formula can also be applied to the monitoring of product filtration activities when "1" is entered as a constant for neck area of product.

A rate of below 0.03% is considered to be a *low* risk. There is no available "guide" as to what percentage constitutes which level of risk. The 0.03% figure is based on the PDA survey of Aseptic Filling practices (2002) where it is common in the pharmaceutical industry to allow 0.03% of broth bottles in a media simulation trial to exhibit growth at a "warning level" (where $0.03\% = 1/3000$, with 3000 being the average size of a media fill). An "action level" is often set as 3/3000 bottles or 0.1%. This would constitute a *high* risk. Logically the range between 0.03 and 0.1 would be a *medium* risk.

Therefore risk categories would be, where the "risk" is the risk of microorganisms detected on a settle plate, with a probability of <0.1%, depositing in the neck of bottles when the bottles are exposed in a unidirectional airflow, as presented in Table 3.

Table 3 Expressions of settle plate contamination risk

Percentage	Risk
<0.03%	Low
>0.03%–0.09%	Medium
≥0.1%	High

EXAMPLE 2: FINGER PLATE ASSESSMENT

The formula can readily be applied to operations that relate to Grade A/ISO Class 5 operations, for example: filtration connection, vessel to filling machine connection, the filling activity, and loading a freeze-dryer. Where the operator is only present in the Grade B/ISO Class 7 room and has no impact on the Grade A/ISO Class 5 operation this is automatically considered to be low risk if there are no other special factors. The reader should note that low risk does not imply no action or assessment. However, it aims the conceptualizing of the result in terms of the probable risk to the batch.

The following formula is used:

Microbial count × Location × Method of intervention × Duration of operation

where:
    Microbial count = count in cfu for the plate.
    Location = area of the filling machine, or other location, which the plate relates to.

Method = whether the hand directly touched part of the filling machine or if utensils were used.
Duration = length of the activity in seconds.

The location and methods require weighting, as per Tables 4 to 6.

Table 4 Weighting by location

Location	Rating	Reason
General part of machine not close to filling zone	0.5	Data from airflow patterns suggests very low risk of contamination movement into the unidirectional airstream over the filling zone.
Off-load	0.5	Off-load areas are present for all filling machines. The bottles/vials are partially stoppered and utensils are normally used. The likelihood of contamination is considered to be low.
On-load	1	On-load areas are present for all filling machines. The bottles/vials are not stoppered and although utensils are normally used. The likelihood of contamination is higher than for off-load.
Stopper bowl	1.5	Stopper bowls are present for filling machines. A direct intervention into the bowl could result in microorganisms being deposited onto stoppers. The risk of this is considered higher than on-load or off-load activities, although such an intervention is rare.
Freeze-dryer loading	1.5	This is a direct intervention Grade A/ISO Class 5 activity. However, vials/bottles are partially stoppered and are contained with cassettes.
Point-of-fill: air sample placement	2	The placement of an air sampler does not involve the touching of any filling equipment (such as needles, balances, etc.) However, as a direct intervention into the Grade A/ISO Class 5 zone it is a higher risk than those parts of the filling machine previously examined.
Filtration transfer	2	The connection of a vessel for the purposes of transferring a product into the Aseptic Filling Suite requires human intervention and aseptic technique. If this process becomes contaminated this could affect the product. The time taken to perform the connection is

Table 4 Weighting by location *Continued*

Location	Rating	Reason
		normally very short (under 30 s), which reduces the risk.
Machine connection	2.5	The connection of a vessel to the filling machine requires human intervention and aseptic technique. If the transfer line is contaminated this could cause contamination to the product.
Point-of-fill: intervention	2.5	A direct intervention where filling needles are readjusted, for example, is the highest risk rating. Counts associated with such activities require detailed examination.

Table 5 Weighting by method

Method	Rating	Reason
Using forceps	0.5	The operative does not directly touch the machine and utensils used are sterile.
Hand	1	The operative directly touches the machine, thereby creating a greater risk. However, it is procedure to sanitize hands prior to undertaking the operation.

Table 6 Weighing by duration

Method	Rating	Reason
<30 s	0.5	The length of the intervention is considered minimal.
30 s–120 s	1	The intervention is at the average time taken (such as derived from the average time taken for media simulation trials).
Plus 120 s	1.5	The intervention has taken longer than average.

Worked Example

A finger plate with a count of 1 cfu for an activity at point of fill, using forceps, that lasts for 1 min.

Microbial count × Location × Method of intervention × Duration of operation

$$1 \times 2.5 \times 0.5 \times 1 = 1.25$$

The score produced can be examined for the following risk assessment:

Score	Risk
1–3	Low
4–8	Medium
9+	High

These risk ratings are based, in part, on the worked example. Based on historical data over the past 6 months, the highest record example of a Grade A/ISO Class 5 intervention finger plate is a count of 2 cfu using forceps to retrieve a fallen vial and lasting for >120 s. This would have given a score of 7.5, which fell within the medium risk category.

Other Examples

Other approaches can be produced, such as for surface sample assessment. A suitable formula would be:

$$\text{Microbial count} \times \text{Risk factor A} \times \text{Risk factor B} \times \text{Risk factor C}$$

where:

Risk Factor A = proximity to critical area
Risk Factor B = ease of dispersion of microorganisms
Risk Factor C = effectiveness of control measure

Similarly, the same approach can be used to examine active air samples. Here, the formulae associated with these are difficult to calculate in practice because all information is not often available and assessment of variables like impaction speed is not readily calculable. An example could be:

$$\text{Airborne microbial count} \left(\text{cfu/m}^3\right)$$
$$\times \text{Deposition velocity of microorganisms from air} \left(\text{cm/s}\right)$$
$$\times \text{Area of product exposed} \left(\text{cm}^2\right) \times \text{Time of exposure} \left(\text{s}\right).$$

RISKS ASSOCIATED WITH CONDUCTING ENVIRONMENTAL MONITORING

As well as environmental monitoring providing some information about risks, there are risks associated with the activity itself. These can be summarized as (Agalloco & Akers, 2005; Agalloco & Akers, 2006; Agalloco & Akers, 2007; Whyte & Eaton, 2004c) follows:

- Environmental monitoring of any form must not subject the product to increased risk of contamination. Sometimes no monitoring is preferable, especially if monitoring increases the risk of contamination for sterile materials.

- Monitoring can be subject to adventitious contamination pre- and postsampling that is unrelated to the environment, material, or surface being sampled.
- The results of environmental monitoring should neither be overemphasized (due to method limitations, as discussed in Chapter 6); nor should the resulting data be subject to overinterpretation (refer to Chapter 14).
- Environmental monitoring cannot recover all microorganisms present in an environment, nor on a surface
- Recovery of low numbers of microorganisms in occupied cleanrooms above properly assessed action levels should be rare, but not unusual.
- With aseptic processing, environmental monitoring activities are interventional activities, and these should be subject to the similar constraints and expectations (such as being detailed procedures) as any other intervention.
- Further with aseptic processing, is not a secondary test for sterility assurance. Assurance is provided through the maintenance of environmental controls. Environmental monitoring results cannot be considered as "proof" of either sterility or nonsterility. The absence or presence of microorganisms in an environmental sample is not confirmation of asepsis nor is it indicative of process inadequacy.

OUT-OF-LIMITS INVESTIGATIONS

Excursions from action levels are predefined pattern with alert levels (such as three consecutive alerts or three alerts every 10 samples), or an upward trend on a control chart should be investigated. The terminology for such investigations varies. To many microbiologists the term "out of limits" (OOL) is preferable in many cases to "out of specification" because action and alert limits or levels are used for environmental monitoring rather that "limits." An alternative term is "microbiological data deviations" (Sandle, 2016).

Investigations may need to consider other aspects of microbiological testing, including:

- The results of water system tests (Total Viable Aerobic Count and Bacterial Endotoxin);
- Final product testing (sterility, pyrogen, abnormal toxicity, and Bacterial Endotoxin);
- Tests on intermediate product and the bulk solution (especially the prefinal filtration step in aseptic manufacturing);
- Tests on incoming raw materials and excipients in process manufacturing (using the Microbial Limits Test). Excipients can include

binders, disintegrants, diluents, lubricants, glidants, colorings, sweeteners, preservatives, suspending agents, and coatings.

There difficulties associated with resolving OOL results, such as:

- Microorganisms are ubiquitous and common contaminants
- Analyst contamination of the test is possible
- Microorganisms may not be homogeneously distributed in a sample
- Microbiological assays are subject to significant inherent variability.

A suitable process will go through the following steps, each of which will be documented:

1. Describe the out-of-limits event.
2. Examine trends.
3. Investigate the cause of the out-of-limits event.
4. Risk assess the impact of the result.
5. Set corrective action.
6. Set preventative action.
7. Conclude the investigation.

It is likely that this process will lead to further questions being required. For example, when investigating the impact of the particle counts, an assessment of the impact of the counts upon the activity is required. In terms of aseptic filling the risk assessment may include consideration of the status of the product. For such a risk assessment it is important to examine other available data, such as:

- If cleanroom particles showed a series of excursions, how does this compare to data from the filling clean zone?
- What were the results of the viable environmental monitoring?
- Do the times of the particle excursions coincide with any special causes, such as machine break down and line clearing?

After consideration of the risk it is important to formulate corrective and preventative actions (CAPA). Corrective actions relate to either things that can be done at the time or if any additional testing or monitoring can be performed. This may include a particle count being noticed during an operation (from an alarm or beacon on a counter) and an activity being halted, and corrective measures taken. Or, the impact of particle counts may be reassessed through the conducting of an airflow (or smoke) pattern to note air direction and turbulence.

Preventative actions are concerned with how to prevent the event from happening again. This may involve the redesigning of an activity; the retraining of operators or major repairs to equipment and machinery. Senior management should endorse the conclusions.

ROOT CAUSES

Root cause analysis is a key part of risk assessment. Reviewing causes can be useful as a look-back when conducting proactive risk assessment, and it is often a necessary feature of reactive risk assessments in order to assess what went wrong and why, and in building-in corrective and preventative actions. Root causes can be divided into common and special causes. Hence to filter out things that could potentially often happen to things that only happen due to specific or unusual events, the terms common causes and special causes are sometimes used. These represent their origins in the early days of quality control. These are two distinct types of variation in a process. Common causes are the usual, historical, quantifiable variation in a system, whereas special causes are unusual, not previously observed, and nonquantifiable variations (Sandle, 2016).

Examples of common causes include poorly written standard operating procedures, poor equipment design, inadequate equipment maintenance, calibration errors, and so on. Examples of special causes include computer crashes, power surges, staff absences, and so on.

With root cause analysis, knowledge and understanding of the risk enables the appropriate action to be taken to mitigate the risk. Some advantages with this are as follows:

- It prevents recurrence through Risk Reduction actions focused on root cause and not symptom effects.
- It demonstrates full understanding of the root cause and related events.
- It structures interrelated events.
- It provides a record.

Some disadvantages are that it can be:

- Retrospective and reactive,
- Assumptions may be taken leading to incorrect identification of the root cause,
- Training and knowledge is required to apply root cause analysis effectively.

Basic steps to application of root cause analysis irrespective of the tool used are as follows:

1. Define the risk to be reduced. This is the output of the risk evaluation.
2. Define potential root causes for this risk to occur.
3. Define which root causes if removed will prevent or reduce the risk.
4. Implement risk reduction measures. This addresses the root causes.
5. Document and observe the effect of implementing the risk reduction measures.
6. Review and repeat as required.

SUMMARY

This chapter set out to provide an overview of hazards and risk outcomes in relation to biocontamination control. The subject area is vast, and the chapter can only examine some examples; these are designed to illustrate that risk assessment can often be useful. There are, nonetheless, several pitfalls and challenges to operating risk assessments.

The primary message is that risk assessment needs to be thought through as to the purpose of the exercise, the form (including the risk model) adopted, and the appropriate scientific-based method to determine the outcome. At the end of this, the identified risks need to be acted upon. It is important that attempts are made to mitigate risks before "detection" (i.e., lots of environmental monitoring is undertaken). Even when such monitoring is performed, the metrological limitations and small sample sizes need to be considered.

Further points with biocontamination control risk assessments are that they should ideally be proactive: spotting problems before they occur rather than overly reactive. There is, of course, a place for reactive assessments in the context of out-of-limits investigations. Furthermore, risk assessments should be based on sound science.

REFERENCES

Agalloco, J., & Akers, J. (2005). Risk analysis for aseptic processing: The Akers-Agalloco method. *Pharmaceutical Technology*, *29*(11), 74–88.

Agalloco, J., & Akers, J. (2006). Simplified risk analysis for aseptic processing: The Akers-Agalloco method. *Pharmaceutical Technology*, *30*(7), 60–76.

Agalloco, J., & Akers, J. (2007). The truth about interventions in aseptic processing. *Pharmaceutical Technology*, *31*(5), S8–11.

Haimes, Y. Y., Kaplan, S., & Lambert, J. H. (2002). Risk filtering, ranking, and management framework using hierarchical holographic modeling. *Risk Analysis*, *22*(2), 383–397.

ICH Q9. Quality risk management, international council for harmonisation of technical requirements for pharmaceuticals for human use, ICH, Geneva, Switzerland, 2006.

McGivern, G., & Fischer, M. D. (2012). Reactivity and reactions to regulatory transparency in medicine, psychotherapy and counseling. *Social Science & Medicine*, *74*(3), 289–296.

Okrent, D. (1980). Comment on societal risk. *Science*, *208*(4442), 372–375.

Ruzante, J. M., Whiting, R. C., Dennis, S. B., & Buchanan, R. L. (2013). Microbial risk assessment. In M. P. Doyle, & E. L. Buchanan (Eds.), *Food microbiology: Fundamentals and Frontiers* (pp. 1023–1037). Washington, DC: ASM Press.

Sandle, T. (2003). The use of a risk assessment in the pharmaceutical industry—The application of FMEA to a sterility testing isolator: A case study. *European Journal of Parenteral and Pharmaceutical Sciences*, *8*(2), 43–49.

Sandle, T. (2011). Risk management in pharmaceutical microbiology. In M. R. Saghee, T. Sandle, & E. C. Tidswell (Eds.), *Microbiology and sterility assurance in pharmaceuticals and medical devices* (pp. 553–588). New Delhi: Business Horizons.

Sandle, T. (2014). *Data review and analysis for pharmaceutical microbiology.* UK: Microbiology Solutions. ISBN: 9781492235217.

Sandle, T. (2016). *Risk assessment and management for healthcare manufacturing: Practical tips and case studies. (2016).* Bethesda, MD: PDA/DHI.

Sandle, T. (2018). Risk management library. In *Vol. 4. Practical approaches to risk assessment and management problem solving: Tips and case studies.* River Grove, IL: PDA/DHI.

Sandle, T., & Lamba, S. S. (2012). Effectively incorporating quality risk management into quality systems. In M. R. Saghee (Ed.), *Achieving quality and compliance excellence in pharmaceuticals: A master class GMP guide* (pp. 89–128). New Delhi: Business Horizons.

Sutton, S. (2010a). The environmental monitoring program in a GMP environment. *Journal of GXP Compliance, 14*(3), 22–30.

Sutton, S. (2010b). The importance of a strong SOP system in the QC microbiology lab. *Journal of GXP Compliance, 14*(2), 44–52.

Tidswell, E. C., & McGarvey, B. (2006). Quantitative risk modelling in aseptic manufacture. *PDA Journal of Pharmaceutical Science and Technology, 60*(5), 267–283.

Whyte, W., & Eaton, T. (2004a). Microbiological contamination models for use in risk assessment during pharmaceutical production. *European Journal of Parenteral and Pharmaceutical Sciences, 9*(1).

Whyte, W., & Eaton, T. (2004b). Assessing microbial risk to patients from aseptically manufactured pharmaceuticals. *European Journal of Parenteral and Pharmaceutical Sciences, 9*(3), 71–79.

Whyte, W., & Eaton, T. (2004c). Microbiological risk assessment in pharmaceutical cleanrooms. *European Journal of Parenteral and Pharmaceutical Sciences, 9*(1), 16–23.

Chapter 17

Assessing, Controlling, and Removing Contamination Risks From the Process

CHAPTER OUTLINE

Introduction   288
Quality by Design   288
Cleanroom Design   289
Equipment Design and Use   291
Cleaning and Disinfection   292
   Cleaning   292
   Disinfectants   292
   Types of Disinfectant and Activity   293
   Selection of Disinfectants   296
   Disinfectant Qualification   298
Control of Personnel and Contamination Transfer Risks   299
Cleaning Validation   301
Process Hold Times   302
Sterilization and Biodecontamination   302
   Moist Heat   303
   Dry Heat   304
   Radiation   304
   Gas   305
   Sterilizing Grade Filtration   305
   PUPSIT   306
Biodecontamination   306
Sterile Products: Aseptic Processing and Terminal Sterilization   307
   Single-Use Sterile Disposable Technology   308
Nonsterile Products: Preservative Efficacy   309
Primary and Secondary Packaging   311
Risk Assessment   311
Conclusion   311
References   312

Biocontamination Control for Pharmaceuticals and Healthcare. https://doi.org/10.1016/B978-0-12-814911-9.00017-1

INTRODUCTION

When designing a biocontamination control strategy (as discussed in Chapter 4), there are some key factors to take into consideration. These are designing process systems and controlled environments to avoid contamination, monitoring process systems to detect contamination, and reacting to contamination events and putting proactive measures in place. Each of these requires a risk-based approach (O'Donnell & Greene, 2006). As this book as discussed, control is *fundamenta inconcussa*, that is, the design of process systems and control of the environment is where maximal effort should be placed. The role of monitoring is to be reserved as a tool to verify control, and the system of control should be periodically assessed through the use of proactive measures.

Further with monitoring, looking at the totality of the monitoring data is of great importance. This means adopting a holistic approach, such as inferring what environmental monitoring from Grade C/ISO Class 8 areas informs you about Grade B/ISO Class 7 areas, and so on, and by drawing inferences from trends. Where patterns are seen away from direct product risks there is a possibility that these microbial risks could affect the product at a point in time; therefore, risk mitigation should be implemented.

This chapter draws together various themes discussed in the book and considers focal points for assessing, controlling, and removing contamination from the pharmaceutical process. The focus on quality by design is fundamental to the biocontamination control strategy. In doing so, it is necessary to cross-refer to some of the other chapters in the book. Here content will not be repeated, and the reader is encouraged to cross-refer to important design points that have already been made.

QUALITY BY DESIGN

Quality by Design is a concept that requires quality considerations to be considered and implemented at the initial design stage, in relation to products, services, and processes. This GMP-centric approach is recommended since many quality crises and problems arise as a result of the way in which quality was planned (or not) at the outset. Hence, quality by design is a systematic approach to developing a product or process that begins with the predefined objective of product and process understanding, and of process control. Essentially this means managing sources of potential variability by getting things "right first time" (Korakianiti & Rekkas, 2011).

The use of risk assessment, to pinpoint areas of risk, has been drawn into many Quality by Design processes. In particular, this is central to the aforementioned FDA report "Pharmaceutical quality for the 21st century: a risk-based approach" (FDA, 2007). Notably the FDA encourages the application of quality by design, especially for new drug applications (Riley & Li, 2011).

Here, FDA empathizes that quality should be built into a product or process with an understanding of what is involved at the beginning, this includes knowledge of the risks involved in manufacturing the product and how best to mitigate those risks. ICH Q9 also makes reference to the importance of quality by design (ICH, 2006). Through this process are identified, explained, and managed by appropriate measures. Analytical science and laboratory testing also play an important part in the identification and monitoring process.

The main elements of quality by design are (Lionberger, Lee, Lee, Raw, & Yu, 2008) as follows:

- Defining clinical design space. The concept of clinical design space can be used to quantify the clinical experience with a product.
- Defining product design space. The concept of design space can also be extended to quantify product quality. Similar to the clinical design space, the product design space could be represented as a multidimensional design space with each critical quality attribute serving as a dimension.
- Defining process design space. The concept of process design space is perhaps the most well understood of all three in the pharmaceutical and biotech industry. Once the acceptable variability in critical quality attributes has been established in the form of the product design space, process characterization studies can be used to define the acceptable variability in process parameters.

The use of the term "design space" refers to the combination and interaction of inputs (such as materials) and process parameters, with each coming together to ensure product quality.

CLEANROOM DESIGN

As this book has emphasized, environmental monitoring is inappropriate to assess weaknesses in facility design (the methods are too insensitive and the sample sizes a meniscal) (Sandle, 2011). This leads to a reliance upon design, maintenance, and operation. To design the cleanroom, the following factors must be accounted for:

- Minimize clean space
- Correct cleanliness level

- Optimal air change rate
- Consider use of mini-environments
- Optimize ceiling coverage
- Consider cleanroom protocol and cleanliness class
- Minimize pressure drop (airflow resistance)
- Location of large air handlers—close to end use
- Adequate sizing and minimize length of ductwork
- Provide adequate space for low pressure drop airflow
- Low face velocity
- Use of variable speed fans
- Optimizing pressurization
- Consider airflow reduction when unoccupied
- Efficient components
- Face velocity
- Fan design
- Motor efficiency
- HEPA filters differential pressures (ΔP)
- Fan-filter efficiency
- Electrical systems that power air systems

An important means to minimize contamination is through effective design of the clean space, be that a classified cleanroom or controlled environment. While cleanrooms are discussed in Chapter 5, it is worth reiterating the four principles which apply to the control of airborne contamination in cleanrooms. These are as follows:

- *Filtration*: cleanrooms need to be designed so that most of the contamination in the air is filtered out.
- *Dilution*: cleanrooms need to be supplied with a sufficient volume of fresh air at regular intervals so that any contamination generated by people working in the room is at first diluted and then removed from the room. This is achieved by having a set number of air changes per hour. The minimum requirement is normally 20 air changes per hour (i.e., the room air volume is replaced every 3 min).
- *Directional airflow*: for ultraclean activities, undertaken in unidirectional airflow cabinets operating at EU and WHO Grade A (ISO Class 5), the air needs to move in a straight direction so that any contamination generated within the area is removed. This is achieved by having the air enter at a high velocity (normally at 0.45 meters per second ±20%).
- *Air movement*: The air within cleanrooms needs to keep moving so that any contamination remains suspended in the air rather than being allowed to settle onto surfaces. This is achieved by having unidirectional or turbulent airflow.

Many HVAC parameters can be assessed through continuous monitoring, providing audible alarms so that processes can be halted, and actions taken as necessary. The use of real-time monitoring is in keeping with process analytical technology (PAT) principles. The PAT approach involves defining the critical process parameters (CPPs) of the equipment used to make the product, which affect the critical quality attributes (CQAs) of the product and then controlling these CPPs within defined limits (Scott & Wilcock, 2006).

As part of biocontamination control it is important to specify the types if air handling systems and HEPA filters required and to ensure that the cleanroom is designed in appropriate way. Once established regular performance checking and annual calibration is required in order to maintain control. Even with good facility design, it is still possible for contamination to occur and affect the product, especially through weakness in the control of heating, ventilation, and air conditioning (HVAC) and associated HEPA filtration deficiencies; contamination associated with other utilities, such as water; or through the transfer of materials; poor personnel and gown controls; or with inadequate cleaning and disinfection.

Furthermore, with cleanrooms, the rooms should have smooth surfaces (with no cracks, crevices, or shedding), and be easily cleaned and disinfected (the importance of which is set out later).

EQUIPMENT DESIGN AND USE

With the design of equipment, all equipment should have smooth inert surfaces which are not additive or adsorptive, and installed in an area that is easily cleaned (cleaning validation is assessed later). If the equipment is difficult to clean, then it should only be considered for a dedicated purpose.

A further aspect with equipment is determining how it will be used (this is in keeping with earlier discussions about the use of process flow risk assessments, which can help inform with the environmental monitoring program). Here it is important to consider the sequence of operation, paying particular attention to the location of equipment, hold times, and removal of unnecessary traffic. Furthermore, to minimize risk of contamination and cross-contamination, it is necessary to dedicate the facility to the manufacture of a single formulation of product and to manufacture products in a campaign, with the appropriately qualified cleaning processes and checks performed in-between batches to minimize the amount of product changeovers.

Cleaned and dirty equipment should not cross paths and cleaned equipment should be held in a defined area where it will not be subject to recontamination. Cleaning Status labeling must be used on all equipment and materials used within the manufacturing facility.

CLEANING AND DISINFECTION

In order to achieve microbial control in cleanrooms and in other areas where the minimization of contamination is important, like laboratories, the use of defined cleaning techniques, together with the application of detergents and disinfectants, is of great importance. The use of such detergents and disinfectants is a step toward control of contamination; however, the use of cleaning solutions should not merely cover up poor practices. For pharmaceutical and healthcare facilities, two disinfectants of different modes of activity should be rotated. One of these disinfectants should be a sporicide (Sandle, 2012a).

Cleaning

Cleaning, in the context of cleanrooms, is the process to remove residues and "soil" from surfaces to the extent that they are visually clean. This involves defined methods of application and often the use of a detergent. Cleaning steps are often necessary prior to the application of a disinfectant for it is essential that a surface or item of equipment has been properly cleaned before the application of a disinfectant in order for the disinfectant to work efficiently.

Cleaning can arguably be seen as a form of disinfection in its own right as the cleaning process can remove or dilute microbial populations and many detergents have chemical additives that can "disinfect." A detergent is a chemical used to clean equipment or surfaces by removing unwanted matter (often referred to as "soil"). Detergents generally work by penetrating soiling and reducing the surface tension (which fixes the soil to the surface) to allow its removal. Detergents also contain differently charged ions that can cause microorganisms to repel each other. This repulsion causes the microorganisms to disassociate from the surface and become suspended. Suspended microorganisms are easier to remove from the surface by the rinsing effect of the detergent (or a subsequent water rinse) or to be destroyed by applying a disinfectant.

Disinfectants

A disinfectant is a chemical agent, from a very diverse group of products, which reduces the number of microorganisms present (normally on an inanimate object). There are various different types of disinfectant with different spectrums of activity and modes of action. Disinfectants have differing efficacies. Some are bacteriostatic, where the ability of the bacterial population to grow is halted. Here the disinfectant can cause selective and reversible changes to cells by interacting with nucleic acids, inhibiting enzymes or permeating into the cell wall. Once the disinfectant is removed from contact with bacteria cells, the surviving bacterial population could potentially grow. Other disinfectants are bactericidal in that they destroy bacterial cells through different mechanisms including structural damage to the cell, autolysis, cell lysis, and the leakage or coagulation of cytoplasm. The destruction of fungal spores is a property which a given disinfectant may or may not possess. The process of disinfection is performed using manual or mechanical (automated methods), such as, a clean-in-place (CIP) system used to process production equipment like vessels.

Within these groupings the spectrum of activity varies with some disinfectants being effective against vegetative Gram-positive and Gram-negative microorganisms only while others are effective against fungi. Some disinfectants are sporicidal in that they can cause the destruction of bacterial endospores. However, a chemical agent does not have to be sporicidal in order to be classed as a "disinfectant" or as a "biocide." The bacteriostatic, bactericidal, and sporicidal properties of a disinfectant are influenced by many variables, not least their active ingredients.

Types of Disinfectant and Activity

There are a number of different types of disinfectant with different modes of activity and of varying effectiveness against microorganisms. These different disinfectants also have varying modes of action against microbial cells due to their chemical diversity. Actions against the microbial cell include acting on the cell wall, the cytoplasmic membrane (where the matrix of phospholipids and enzymes provide various targets), and the cytoplasm. Some disinfectants, on entering the cell either by disruption of the membrane or through diffusion, then proceed to act on intracellular components. There are different approaches to the categorization and subdivision of disinfectants including grouping by chemical nature, mode of activity, or by microstatic and microcidal effects on microorganisms. This chapter discusses some of the more commonly used disinfectants employed in the pharmaceutical environment by categorizing them according to their chemical properties. The two principal categories used are the division into oxidizing and nonoxidizing chemicals (Sandle, 2012b).

Nonoxidizing Disinfectants

The majority of this group of disinfectants have specific modes of action against microorganisms but generally they have a lower spectrum of activity compared to oxidizing disinfectants (Denyer & Stewart, 1998). Examples include alcohols, which have an antibacterial action against vegetative cells. The effectiveness of alcohols against vegetative bacteria and fungi increases with their molecular weight (therefore ethanol is more effective than methanol and in turn isopropyl alcohols more effective than ethanol). Alcohols, where efficacy is increased with the presence of water, act on the bacterial cell wall by making it permeable. This can result in cytoplasm leakage, denaturation of protein, and eventual cell lysis (alcohols are one of the so-called membrane disrupters). The advantages of employing alcohols include a relatively low cost, little odor, and a quick evaporation. Furthermore, alcohols have a cleansing action. However, alcohols have a very poor action against spore formers and can only inhibit spore germination at best (McDonnell & Russell, 1999).

Another group are the aldehydes, which include long chain chemical compounds, such as formaldehyde and glutaraldehyde. Glutaraldehyde is a very effective disinfectant (and sterilant) through acting on cell wall proteins. Glutaraldehyde has a wide spectrum of activity and is effective against bacterial and fungal spores. However, glutaraldehyde is little used today due to health and safety concerns. Formaldehyde and o-Phthalaldehyde are slightly less effective due to a slower rate of reaction but possesses an equally wide spectrum of activity. Aldehydes have a nonspecific effect in the denaturing of bacterial cell proteins and can cause coagulation of cellular protein (Angelillo, Bianco, Nobile, & Pavia, 1998).

Amphoterics are acidic and have a relative wide spectrum of activity but are limited by their ability to damage endospores. Amphoterics are frequently used as surface disinfectants. An example is alkyl di(aminoethyl) glycine or derivatives. Acid anionics are weak acids with a relatively limited spectrum of activity and are very pH dependent. An example of this group is carboxylic acid. They are not effective against fungi or spore-forming bacteria. Their bactericidal properties arise from their ability to cause bacterial cell disruption through proton motive force where the balance of hydrogen across the cell is disrupted which, in turn, affects cellular division by disruption of oxidative phosphorylation.

Biguanides are polymers supplied in salt form, such as chlorhexidine, alexidine, or hydrochloride. Biguanides have a relatively wide spectrum of activity with the exception of killing endospores. The group are limited by only being truly effective at an alkaline pH and are rarely effective under acidic conditions. Biguanides affect the bacterial cell membrane, enter the cell through diffusion, and cause cell disruption and cytoplasm leakage. Phenols are produced from the fractionation of tar and are among the oldest scientifically evaluated disinfectants dating back to Robert Koch's evaluation of phenol's bactericidal effect against *Bacillus anthracis*. The commonly used phenolic is basic phenol (carbolic acid) although synthetic variants are being widely used. Phenol can be made more complex by the addition of halogens such as chlorine (the bis-phenols and halophenols) to make compounds like triclosan and chloroxylenol. Phenols are bactericidal and antifungal, but are not effective against spores. Some phenols cause bacterial cell disruption through proton motive force while others attack the cell wall and cause leakage of cellular components and protein denaturation (Bergan & Lystad, 1972).

Quaternary ammonium compounds (QACs) are cationic salts of organically substituted ammonium compounds and have a fairly broad range of activity against microorganisms, albeit more effective against Gram-positive bacterium at lower concentrations than Gram-negative bacteria. They are considerably less effective against spore formers. QACs are sometimes classified as surfactants. An example is benzalkonium chloride. QACs are the most widely used of the nonoxidizing disinfectants within the pharmaceutical industry. Their mode of action is on the cell membrane leading to cytoplasm leakage and cytoplasm coagulation through interaction with phospholipids.

Oxidizing Disinfectants

This group of disinfectants generally has nonspecific modes of action against microorganisms. They have a wider spectrum of activity than nonoxidizing disinfectants, with most types able to damage endospores, but they pose greater risks to human health. The group includes halogens, which are among the oldest identified disinfectants and include organic and inorganic varieties. They can be divided into chlorine releasing and iodophors. Both types have a broad spectrum of activity against a range of microorganisms and are normally effective sporicides. Examples of chlorine-releasing chemicals are sodium trichloroisocyanurate, sodium hypochlorite, and chlorinated trisodium phosphonate. Hypochlorites are one of the oldest commercial disinfectants. The mode of action of this group is not completely known.

The common biocides used as sporicides in cleanrooms include oxygen releasing compounds like peracetic acid and hydrogen peroxide. They are often used in the gaseous phase as surface sterilants for equipment. These peroxygens function by disrupting the cell wall causing cytoplasm leakage and denature bacterial cell enzymes through oxidation. These oxidizing agents have advantages in that they are clear and colorless, thereby avoiding staining, but they do present some health and safety concerns particularly in terms of causing respiratory difficulties to unprotected users (Sandle, 2014).

Selection of Disinfectants

A number of factors require consideration in order to select a disinfectant. These can be grouped into two areas: chemical properties (which have been discussed before) and factors relating to the performance of the chemical agent. These differing factors are discussed later. In the discussion it should be noted that the effectiveness of a disinfectant is related to a complex interaction between all the factors. In addition, certain regulatory or health and safety standards may apply to particular laboratories. The reader should consider these as appropriate.

Among the most important factors for consideration are explained in the following headings (Morton, Greenway, Gaylarde, & Surman, 1998; Sandle, 2016a).

Concentration

Disinfectants are manufactured or validated to be most efficacious at a set concentration range. The setting of this concentration range involves ascertaining the minimum inhibitory concentration (MIC). The MIC is the lowest concentration of the disinfectant that is shown to be bacteriostatic or bactericidal. The MIC is measured through kinetic studies of the dilution coefficient. Kinetic studies demonstrate the effect of a change in concentration against cell death rate over time. The higher a disinfectant's concentration exponent, the longer it will take to kill cells. For example, if a disinfectant with a set concentration exponent was diluted by a factor of 2, the time taken for it to kill cells comparatively would double.

Time

Time is an important factor in the application of disinfectants for two reasons: in relation to the contact time of the disinfectant and the expiry time of the disinfectant solution. Contact time is the time taken for the disinfectant to bind to the microorganism, traverse the cell wall, and to reach the specific target site for the disinfectants particular mode of action. Contact time is expressed generally for each disinfectant type at its optimal concentration range. The killing affect, for a constant concentration of a disinfectant, increases over time until the optimal contact time is established. In practical situations, however, many variables enter the equation like the type, concentration, and volume of the disinfectant; the nature of the microorganisms; the amount and kind of material present and likely to interfere; and the temperature of the disinfectant and the surface it is applied to.

Another aspect relating to time is the deterioration of a disinfectant solution over time. Therefore an expiry time limit for the disinfectant solution should be established through chemical testing. As a rule, fresh solutions of a disinfectant should be used for each application.

Number, Type, and Location of Microorganisms

Different species of microorganisms vary in their resistance to different disinfectants. These can be affected by the numbers of microorganisms present, their species, and the community with which they are bound to. With numbers, an antimicrobial agent, like a disinfectant, is considerably more effective against a low number of microorganisms than a higher number or a population with a greater cell density. Similarly, a disinfectant is more effective against a pure population than mixed grouping of microorganisms. A routine disinfectant procedure will be unlikely to kill all microorganisms present and a number will remain viable. Whether the surviving microorganisms multiply in sufficient number is dependent upon the condition in which the surviving population remains, the available nutrients, and the time between repeat applications of the disinfectant.

The type of microorganism is also of importance, different types of microorganism have varying levels of resistance to broad spectrum disinfectants. The increased resistance shown is primarily due to the cell membrane composition or type of protein coat.

The location of microorganisms influences the effectiveness of disinfectant treatment. Microorganisms in suspension are easier to kill than those affixed to surfaces. This is due to the mechanisms of microorganism attachment, such as bacteria fixing themselves using fimbriae or when a biofilm community develops. Such positioning impact upon the contact time required for the disinfectant to bind to the microorganism, cross the cell wall, and act at the required site.

Temperature and pH

Each disinfectant has an optimal pH and temperature at which it is most effective. If the temperature or pH is outside this optimal range, then the rate of reaction (log kill over time) is affected.

Generally, temperature influences the rate of reaction. Most disinfectants are more effective and kill a population faster at higher temperatures although many disinfectants, due to practical considerations, are manufactured to be used at ambient. Some disinfectants, particularly oxidizing agents like peracetic acid which has an optimal temperature of 40-50°C, and sporicidal agents like orthophthalaldehyde are more effective at temperatures elevated above ambient. Disinfectants which are sensitive to temperatures other than at ambient are normally assessed through the use of a temperature coefficient, or Q10 (which relates the increase in activity to a 10°C rise in temperature).

The effect of pH is important because it influences the ionic binding of a disinfectant to a bacterial cell wall thereby ensuring disinfectant molecules bind to a high number of microorganisms. Many disinfectants are more stable at a set pH range, for example, acid-based disinfectants can become less potent in alkaline conditions whereas a glutaraldehyde is more potent at a basic pH. The use of a disinfectant outside of its desired pH range results in reduced efficacy.

Amount of Organic and Other Interfering Substances

The presence of different substances on the surface or in the equipment requiring disinfection can affect the efficacy of the disinfectant in a variety of ways ranging from increasing the contact time to complete inactivation. In order for a disinfectant to be effective, it must come into contact with the microbial cell and be absorbed into it. If substances, such as oil, dirt, paper, or grease, act as a spatial barrier between the microbial cell and the disinfectant the efficacy of the disinfectant will be adversely affected. The presence of such substances ("soil") halts disinfectant efficacy by either reacting with the disinfectant or creating a barrier for the disinfectant. This effect is increased if the surface itself has defects and crevices which limit disinfectant penetration (Frank & Chmielewski, 2001).

Disinfectant Qualification

An important aspect of pharmaceutical microbiology is in the selection and evaluation of disinfectants. This process should be conducted through controlled experiments and undertaken through a disinfectant validation program (Vina, Rubio, & Sandle, 2011). There are standards that outline efficacy, from both Europe and the United States. Of the different standards, those that focus on surface testing are the most important. However, the key test of a disinfectant is in the field, as assessed through an evaluation of surface environmental monitoring.

CONTROL OF PERSONNEL AND CONTAMINATION TRANSFER RISKS

Control of personnel relates to practicing good gown control and following cleanroom behaviors related to good behaviors, controlled movements, and glove sanitization. In relation to gowns, staff working in cleanrooms are required to wear special clothing designed for the clean environments. Such clothing is required because the human body creates its own microenvironment of potentially damaging particulate contamination. Since humans are essential to production situations, damage limitation through the use of purpose-designed cleanroom clothing has proved to be the most practical solution to the problem. The use of specialist clothing is now commonplace.

To be effective clothing must:

- form a particulate barrier for the human microenvironment,
- allow freedom of movement and be comfortable,
- address any specialist requirement, for example, static dissipation,
- avoid being a significant particulate contributor itself.

Cleanroom garments for aseptic processing areas normally consist of an under suit and over suit. The use of specially designed cleanroom under garments is not only for operator comfort, but these suits also aid the total filtration efficiency of the garment. The suit is used along with gloves, plus a mask, goggles, and a hood; here the term "garment system" is sometimes used. Garment systems are not "one unit" and typically are made up of the following articles (Ramstorp, 2011):

- Under suit
- Over suit
- Shoes or shoe covers, followed by cleanroom boots
- Cap and cap with integrated hair protection
- Beard protection (as necessary)
- A hood that covers the entire head, either integrated with the coverall or as a separate article
- Face mask
- Eye protection (goggles)
- Gloves

Cleanroom garments must meet specific protection criteria. This involves manufacturing the garments from special materials, following particular construction methods, and then tailored for individual styling. The gowns must be comfortable, easy to apply, and practical in use. The supplier of the cleanroom clothing should be subject to audit. The supplier should hold certification to demonstrate to customers that a laundry recognizes the relevant biocontamination hazards and has the necessary controls in place to reduce the likelihood or stop these hazards being present in the laundered textiles.

The cleanroom fabrics must contain the following features (Reinmüller, 2001):

a. Be low in particulate shedding.
b. Permit the body to breathe while trapping particles within the garment—the contaminant should be retained within the garment and not released into the surrounding atmosphere.
c. Be flexible enough for comfortable wearing.
d. Withstand repeated cleaning and sterilization cycles.
e. Meet any specific requirements like control of static.
f. Meet the opacity requirements.
g. Look and feel as good as possible.
h. Be cost effective

Working in clean environments demands knowledge, discipline, motivation, as well as a thorough understanding of contamination risks among all personnel involved. Each individual cleanroom should have its own documented rules and procedures. All personnel working in a cleanroom need to be trained in all the different techniques used in the cleanroom as well as the different operational systems that make the cleanroom work. Furthermore, inappropriate behavior should not be allowed within the cleanroom. The generation of contamination is proportional to activity. A person with head, arms, and body moving can generate about 1,000,000 particles $\geq 0.5\,\mu m/min$. A person who is walking can generate about 5,000,000 particles $\geq 0.5\,\mu m/min$. However, a person in motionless position can generate only 100,000 particles $\geq 0.5\,\mu m/min$ (Sandle & Vijayakumar, 2014).

As well as rules relating to people, controls must be in place in terms of occupancy levels. Only the necessary and limited number of persons should be allowed in a cleanroom at the same time. The more persons simultaneously present in a cleanroom, then the higher the contamination level will be (i.e., the higher concentration of particles in the air).

With contamination transfer, microorganisms are carried in airstreams until they are deposited on a surface. Unless they have recently been disinfected, most surfaces will have contamination on them. The risk arises when the contamination moves from a less critical to a critical location, so it follows that using clean utensils and having clean gloves is very important to minimize contamination transfer.

CLEANING VALIDATION

Cleaning validation is about obtaining a level of assurance that a cleaning process has removed residues and contaminants from a piece of equipment or machinery (Agalloco, 1992). Residues may be microorganisms; active pharmaceutical ingredients; other process chemicals, such as buffers; cleaning agents themselves (such as detergents); or microbiological culture media (in relation to aseptic process simulations). Pharmaceutical and healthcare manufacturer need to have the confidence about the effectiveness of the cleaning process and the consistency at which cleaning is applied. As with any other type of validation, the "validation" aspect refers to providing documented evidence that that the acceptance criteria have been met.

Cleaning is assessed based on the level of residues that remain, either those directly found on the equipment or those indirectly contained within the final rinse after water has passed through or over the equipment. Whether the residues remaining have been reduced to a satisfactory low level is based on predetermined acceptance criteria. The levels need to be sufficiently low to ensure that the next product manufactured is not compromised by waste or contamination from the previous product (that is in ensuring that cross-contamination does not occur). An additional concern is with the microbial bioburden and, in relation to Water for Injections rinses, bacterial endotoxin levels. Important to the microbiological aspect are microorganisms themselves (a direct hazard) and the presence of residues that potentially provide a microbial growth source, should contamination be present or contamination occur during the hold period (an indirect hazard) (Sandle, 2013).

With equipment cleaning, this can be undertaken using an automated process (such as CIP, clean-in-place technologies) or manually (which often involves the physical removal of the equipment and its transport to a wash bay; sometimes called COP, clean-out-of-place). In general, manual cleaning should be avoided due to process and operator variability. Where manual cleaning cannot be avoided, due to technical limitations, robust controls need to be in place to ensure consistency.

To evaluate these microbiological risks a sound microbiological sampling plan is required. The emphasis on sampling is important since microorganisms cannot be introduced into the process. This is unlike a chemical assessment where equipment can be deliberately soiled with a residue to test out cleaning efficacy. Microbial controls should not be introduced into the cleaning process. This article assesses the risks from microorganisms and the cleaning requirements necessary to achieve microbial control (Sandle, 2017).

PROCESS HOLD TIMES

Various stages in the manufacturing process require hold stages during biopharmaceutical manufacturing. Hold times may be needed for product formulation reasons, equipment issues, or relating to personnel change-overs. The most common reason for these holds is for processing. When processes are held, there are a number of potential risks including chemical stability and microbiological growth (Sandle, Roberts, & Skinner, 2009).

Certain process factors can affect growth should contamination occur. These factors include available nutrients and time. Another factor is headspace ratio, where increased headspace combined with agitation in a hold vessel can increase product oxygenation throughout the hold period. This may favor bacteria that prefer aerobic conditions. A further factor is with temperature; here there are some conditions that are more favorable to microbial growth than others. The temperature effect will depend upon the type of bacteria present and their growth characteristics.

To assess these risks then hold time must be controlled and evaluated. Bioburden assessment informs the manufacturer about both the expected microbial load of the product and the presence or absence of specific microorganisms, some of which might be classed as objectionable. Endotoxin informs about a risk involving a specific type of microorganism (Gram-negative bacteria) and the presence of a pyrogenic toxin that will be difficult if not impossible to eliminate. Due to the potential for microbial growth, pharmaceutical manufacturers typically conduct studies to define acceptable hold times for process intermediates. These studies are based on the microbiological examination of in-process production samples and it is of importance that these hold times are addressed within a biocontamination strategy (Sandle, 2015).

STERILIZATION AND BIODECONTAMINATION

Sterilization processes eliminate, remove, kill, or deactivate all forms of life including fungi, bacteria, viruses, spore forms, prions, unicellular eukaryotic organisms, and so on, within a specified region like a surface or fluid. As it stands, a sterile item is one which has been freed from all viable microorganisms (but not necessarily microbial by-products and toxins). Sterilization is achieved through various means: heat, chemicals, irradiation, filtration, and so on. Sterilization is distinct from disinfection and other forms of biodecontamination, such as the application of hydrogen peroxide vapor for isolators.

In practice there is no definitive test available to absolutely demonstrate sterility—sterility can only be assessed in terms of probability. Sterility is a "negative" quality attribute—it is well known that to "prove a negative" is philosophically well-nigh impossible. No method exists whereby an item can be examined and be shown conclusively to be sterile. Nor does any method exist where a sample of items can be taken from a larger batch of items and be tested to show conclusively that the larger batch of items is sterile.

The expression of confidence in a process is termed the probability of a non-sterile unit (PNSU) or more commonly as the sterility assurance level (SAL). The level of assurance or SAL which is normally accepted as a compromise for "absolute" sterility is that after treatment, there should be no more than one chance in 1 million of an item remaining nonsterile—an SAL of 10^{-6}. Pharmaceutical manufacturers typically seek to develop an SAL to give a sterilization cycle designed to achieve a 12-log reduction, based on the challenge population of a biological indicator (Pflug & Odlaug, 1986). In practice, sterilization processes can be developed using scientific principles, experimentation, and extrapolation. Safety margins can be built in, and then as long as the technology used to deliver the sterilization treatment functions properly the resultant preparation will comply with the required SAL and be safe to release (Gilbert & Allison, 1996).

Some common methods of sterilization are briefly described as follows.

Moist Heat

The sterilization method of choice in the pharmaceutical industry is steam sterilization in autoclaves. Steam sterilization is widely used as a terminal process for drug products in glass ampoules, vials, syringes, and plastic containers. It is also used for sterilizing closures, filters, manufacturing equipment, and cleaning equipment, and so on. It is more widely used than any other method of sterilization.

Modern autoclaves are highly reliable, computer controlled, and allegedly fail-safe. In their complexity it is sometimes forgotten that fundamentally they are pressure cookers. Water boils at 100°C at atmospheric pressure; these boiling temperatures alter in relation to pressures above and below atmospheric pressure. At a steam overpressure of 1 atm., water boils at approximately 121°C. Therefore it is very important to ensure that all of the trapped air is removed from the autoclave before activation, as hot air is a very poor medium for achieving sterility (Lemieux, 2006).

The manner in which populations of microorganisms are inactivated at high temperatures in the presence of steam and in the absence of air has been thoroughly researched. At high temperatures and in the presence of moisture, as in steam sterilization, the energy input from the steam inactivates microorganisms by denaturation of intracellular proteins.

Sterilization of aqueous fluid loads is achieved by contact of the external surfaces of the product containers with good quality saturated steam, and then by heat transfer through the walls of the container to increase and maintain the temperature of the pharmaceutical preparation at the specified sterilization temperature. Sterilization of porous loads occurs by direct contact of the load items with good quality steam. The temperature in the load items is raised and maintained at the specified temperature by transfer of the latent heat of steam to the load items as it condenses on their surfaces.

Dry Heat

Dry heat is the only one of the commonly used large-scale sterilization processes that can be relied on to inactivate bacterial endotoxins (pyrogenic substances). Thermal inactivation of endotoxin is not as well understood as thermal inactivation of microorganisms. Interpretation of experimental data has been complicated by problems relating to analytical techniques, problems relating to different microbiological sources of endotoxin, problems relating to the chemical purity of endotoxin, problems relating to the "carrier" used in studies, and problems relating to perceived differences in reaction rates between convectional and radiant heat transfer.

The general form of endotoxin inactivation appears to follow Second-Order kinetics. At any particular temperature there is an initially rapid rate of reaction. This is followed by a slower, flatter "tail." To all intents and purposes only the first part of the inactivation curve can be considered to contribute to practical depyrogenating conditions. This means that at any particular temperature there is an upper bounding limit to the proportion of endotoxin that can be inactivated.

At temperatures around 100°C there is practically no evidence of endotoxin inactivation; at temperatures around 170°C the upper bounding limit of inactivation of endotoxin appears to be around two $\log_{10}$ reductions, requiring >24-h exposure to reduce a challenge of 1000 EU (endotoxin units) to no >10 EU (Ludwig & Avis, 1990).

Radiation

Irradiation, usually by gamma radiation from cobalt 60 sources. The process of gamma radiation is a form of ionization (electron disruption). Gamma radiation is one of the three types of natural radioactivity, the other two being alpha and beta radiation. Gamma radiation is in the form of electromagnetic rays, like X-rays or ultraviolet light, of a short (less than one-tenth of a nanometer), and thus energetic, wavelength. Gamma radiation is a physical means of sterilization or decontamination as the rays pass through the product being sterilized (or "irradiated"). In doing so, gamma radiation kills bacteria, where there is sufficient energy, at the molecular level by breaking down bacterial DNA and inhibiting bacterial division. The radioactive Cobalt 60 functions as the isotope source. High-energy photons are emitted from the Cobalt 60 to produce ionization (electron disruptions) throughout a product. The gamma process does not create residuals or impart radioactivity in processed products.

Gamma irradiation is fundamentally a very simple process although its technology may appear daunting. The sole determinant of sterility assurance is dose (measured as Kilograys (kGy)).

Gas

Ethylene oxide in the gaseous form is the most common form of gaseous sterilization. The gas infiltrates packages as well as products themselves to kill microorganisms that are left during production or packaging processes. Ethylene oxide breaks down into two components: Ethylene Chlorohydrin and Ethylene Glycol. It is a longer sterilization process than gamma irradiation.

Of the several methods of sterilization which rely on inactivation of microorganisms, ethylene oxide is the most difficult to control reproducibly. Historically, the amount of gas added was set to a particular weight. However, the evolution of the process has gradually gone to adding gas to a validated pressure (concentration of gas). Inactivation of microorganisms results from alkylating effects on sulfhydryl, amino, carboxyl, and hydroxyl groups within the cell. Lethal effects are through blockage of reactive sites on metabolically active molecules.

Sterilizing Grade Filtration

Filtration is a means of sterilizing fluids by removing, rather than inactivating, microorganisms. A sterilizing grade filter has a pore size of 0.22 μm or smaller. The sterilization of liquids is used extensively in aseptic manufacturing; sterilization of gases is used both in terminal sterilization and in aseptic manufacture. Most applications use cellulose esters, polyvinylidene fluoride, polytetrafluoroethylene, nylon, and other polymeric materials. The removal of microorganisms from fluids by passage through filters is very complex; sieving, or surface retention, is only one of a series of mechanisms that depend on interactions among the chemistry and surface characteristics of the membrane, the microorganisms, and the suspending fluid.

Sterile filtration of liquids and gases in pharmaceutical manufacture is almost always done using membrane filters—thin uniform porous sheets which are in older literature described as acting like screens or sieves that trap particles larger in size than the pores in the membranes. It is now known that sieving is only one of several mechanisms of particle retention that may occur in membrane filters. Other mechanisms include inertial impaction to the walls or surfaces of the pores and lodgment in crevices, "dead ends" and "cul-de-sacs" within the depth of the membrane.

The porosity quoted for filters is not obtained by physical measurement of the dimensions of the pores. It is done on the basis of the pressure which is required to displace liquid from the pores—essentially a bubble point value—coupled to a formula which takes account of the pressure required, the surface tension of the liquid, and the contact angle between the liquid and the surface of the pore. It assumes cylindrical pores, and then, to compensate for nonideality, every filter manufacturer incorporates a correction factor of his own derivation. The "bubble point test" is also one of several options that the regulators require all users of bacteria-retentive filters to apply to their filters before and after use.

PUPSIT

A number of regulatory guidelines recommend preuse integrity testing of critical sterilizing liquid filters for aseptic processing. Arguments for this requirement include the fact that filter manufacturers do not often have transport qualification and there can be insufficient control on any outsourced gamma sterilization of filter units.

Before sterilization, the preuse test affirms that a filter is installed properly and was not damaged during shipment or handling; and performing a preuse test after sterilization will detect any damage that could have occurred during the sterilization cycle. Theoretically, testing after sterilization minimizes risk (Jornitz & Meltzer, 2011).

BIODECONTAMINATION

The most widely used method of biodecontamination is the application of hydrogen peroxide in the vapor state. This is sometimes referred to as a sterilization method. However, it has no penetrative ability and thus a safer term is "biodecontamination." The inference of this is with activities like aseptic processing, if an isolator is subject to a hydrogen peroxide cycle then items which are required to be sterile, such as a stopper bowl, must be subject to a separate method of sterilization and aseptically transferred into the isolator.

Vaporized hydrogen peroxide (VHP) is a broad-spectrum antimicrobial with virucidal, bactericidal, fungicidal, and sporicidal activity. VHP is a relatively rapid sterilization technology. VHP is produced by the vaporization (at 120°C) of liquid hydrogen peroxide to give a mixture of VHP and water vapor. As a "dry" process, the concentration of VHP is maintained below a given condensation point, which is dependent on the area temperature. Its advantage over other gaseous technologies is that it decomposes to water and oxygen, which are relatively safe and so-termed residue free (Kokubo, Inoue, & Akers, 1998).

VHP processes also have prerequisites in terms of the physical properties of the items being treated: they must be relatively smooth, impervious to moisture, and be of a shape that permits all surfaces to be exposed to the sterilant.

STERILE PRODUCTS: ASEPTIC PROCESSING AND TERMINAL STERILIZATION

Broadly, there are two approaches to manufacture of sterile products, terminal sterilization, and aseptic manufacture. The regulatory bodies favor terminal sterilization, and in the development of new sterile dosage forms the regulators demand that a "decision tree" is followed whereby the new dosage must be proven to be unable to withstand various defined processes of terminal sterilization before it is allowed to be manufactured aseptically.

When the term terminal sterilization is used it means that the dosage form is hermetically sealed in its final container and then the entire container is sterilized with the seals intact. This is achieved using one of the sterilization methods described before. For aseptic manufacture, in contrast, the components of the containment system and the dosage form are all separately sterilized and then brought together and sealed shut using sterile equipment in a highly protected area using techniques and methods which are designed to minimize the possibility of anything becoming recontaminated. Thus the meaning of asepsis is the avoidance or elimination of all forms of contamination of a sterile "field."

The Sterility Assurance Limit concept, as described before, was developed for sterilization processes and it should be limited to that application. It cannot really be applied to aseptic manufacture. Instead sterility assurance is developed through good design and controls. The most important design philosophy is with keeping people out of Grade A/ISO Class 5 areas through the application of barrier technology, with restrictive access barrier systems

(RABS) or isolators (Tidswell, 2011). Isolators are theoretically the most effective contained spaces for aseptic process manufacture; here contamination control can be improved with more effective or automated sanitization leading to measurable (with biological indicators) bioburden reduction on material surfaces. While these technologies offer advantages, it should not be forgotten that no barrier operated as a manufacturing system with complex interfaces, human interactions can provide an "absolute" control to microbiological transfer.

The minimization of personnel interactions in critical zones represents an important contamination risk reduction step: restricting or eliminating operator interventions where there is risk of exposure to critical areas, surfaces, or sterile product. Where rapid microbiological methods are deployed (see Chapter 9), such as the spectrophotometric air counters that can distinguish between inert and biologic particles (Sandle, Leavy, & Rhodes, 2015), then more aseptic processing and control can be strengthened. The effectiveness of aseptic processing can be partly assessed through the operation of robust media simulation trials.

Single-Use Sterile Disposable Technology

Single-use disposable technologies (sometimes referred to as biodisposable technologies) are generally sterile, plastic disposable items implemented to replace traditional pharmaceutical processing items which require recycling, cleaning, and in-house sterilization. The items are generally sterilized using gamma irradiation.

Such technologies include tubing, capsule filters, single-use ion exchange membrane chromatography devices, single-use mixers, bioreactors, product holding sterile bags in place of stainless steel vessels (sterile fluid containment bags), connection devices, and sampling receptacles. To an extent, the biopharmaceutical and biotechnology sector has been behind the medical device sector and hospitals in the advent of disposable technologies (such as artificial cardiac valves, stents and other implants, balloon catheters, as wells as gloves and other clothing).

The advantages of single-use technology are that the technology eliminates the need for cleaning, eliminates the need for the pharmaceutical company to perform in-house sterilization, reduces the use of chemicals, reduces storage requirements, reduces process downtime and increases process flexibility, and avoids cross-contamination. However, single-use technology is still in its infancy and there are a number of validation steps which need to be undertaken before such technology is adopted by a pharmaceutical manufacturer. These include assessing any leachables or extractables which might arise when the product comes into contact with the single-use technology. The presence of extractables could lead to adulterated product or to the inhibition of any microbial contamination (Sandle & Saghee, 2011).

These types of devices are in keeping with the control philosophy of the transition from open to closed systems, use of fixed versus disposable systems, and the points at which humans interact with automation. Such systems are not immune to risk, and there remains a need to consider any aspect of the process where humans interact with machines, equipment, and product for there will remain an inherent risk of contamination and cross-contamination.

The dependability of this critical aseptic processing step improved with new filter materials, designs, and the adoption of filters to single-use process technology to a functionally closed unit operation.

NONSTERILE PRODUCTS: PRESERVATIVE EFFICACY

With nonsterile products, protection of the product from objectionable microorganisms is key to contamination control during manufacturing. To protect the product when it ends up in the hands of the consumer, the use of a preservative is important.

In terms of objectionable microorganisms, pharmaceutical manufacturers should draw up a risk-based list of organisms of concern, in relation to what could be present in the environment and what could pose a risk to specific types of products and the intended patient population for those products. The outcome of this assessment process means that an organism may be objectionable in all circumstances or it may be objectionable under a set of conditions or for a particular product portfolio in relation to a given population of patients. In drawing up a list of alternative test methods may be required.

For such an assessment, the criteria developed by Sutton prove useful (Sutton, 2012). Here, assessing whether a microorganism is objectionable requires the assessment of a number of factors. The foremost factor is whether the organism is or is not pathogenic. If the organism is classed as a pathogen and the route of infection is the same as the route of administration for the product, then the organism is likely to be objectionable. This approach:

- Ranks administration routes in order of microbiological risk to patient,
- Discusses water activity and self-preservation/micro growth,
- Discusses preservative system for multiuse products.

Included in Sutton's approach are the ways by which objectionable microorganisms trigger a risk to the product or have potential to cause patient harm include:

1. Affecting product stability.
2. Affecting the security of the container/closure system (i.e., for instance, the container adequately designed to retard access to the environment and to prevent contamination from the environment?)
3. Affecting the active ingredient.
4. Producing off odors, flavors, or undesirable metabolites.
5. Having the potential to grow and exceed the total aerobic count specification.
6. Possessing high virulence and a low infective dose.
7. Resistance to antimicrobial therapy.

Also needing to be taken into account are the manufacturing steps and other control measures, like approved supplier purchasing and cleaning and disinfection processes.

The addition of a preservative to a pharmaceutical formulation is primarily aimed at minimizing the dangers of infection to the patient and also to prevent spoilage of the product. As mentioned before preservative addition is not to overcome poor manufacturing practices. The Pharmaceutical formulation, its mode of administration, and use (single/multi-dose) will determine the level of preservation required. For example, tablets and capsules are unlikely to readily support growth and are usually taken orally into an unfavorable acidic environment and so are seldom preserved; however, multidose, water-based products may support growth, be administered in a number of ways, for example, topically, and be at risk to contamination depending upon how the product is handled by the user.

There are a range of preservatives available for use in pharmaceutical formulations, for example, benzyl alcohol, chlorobutanol, benzalkonium chloride, thimerosal, benzoates, methyl/propyl parabens, and so on. Although a preservative may be added to pharmaceutical product the exact performance of the formulation/preservative system in relation to the level and type of microbial contamination cannot be predicted and therefore it has to be determined empirically using a preservative efficacy test (PET) or challenge test.

PETs are performed during product development to demonstrate that the preservative system (as well as can be determined) will remain effective. Preservative levels can be accurately measured by chemical analysis, but this data does not take into consideration the impact of other chemical and physical attributes of the formulation which may influence preservative activity. Such influencing attributes could be:

- pH
- Presence of nonaqueous phase (partitioning of the preservative in the nonpolar phase)

- Adsorption to suspended solids (adsorption may reduce preservative concentration)
- Adsorption to packaging (plastics may adsorb the preservative)

PET involves inoculating standardized suspensions of bacteria and fungi into separate portions of the product to be tested and then measuring the survival of each organism over a period of 28 days. The product is adequately preserved if the reduction in the inoculated level of microbial population meets the acceptance criteria tabulated in each pharmacopeia (Sandle, 2016b).

PRIMARY AND SECONDARY PACKAGING

Packaging is important for protecting both sterile and nonsterile pharmaceutical products from contamination during storage, distribution, and use. The protection afforded by the primary container is of particular importance for sterile products given that sterility is an unnatural and transitory condition. A key concern is with direct contact between the operator's hands and starting materials, primary packaging materials, and intermediate or bulk product.

For a sterile pharmaceutical preparation to remain sterile it must be protected from the external nonsterile environment by isolation within a container which is impermeable to microorganisms. The sterile condition is placed at risk as soon as the container is breached to gain access to the preparation; this means the sterility of contents cannot be guaranteed in a permeable, a cracked, or an opened container. In this context the secondary and primary packaging acts as important barriers for product protection.

RISK ASSESSMENT

An embracing biocontamination control concept is with the use of proactive risk assessment. A defined risk assessment approach enables the elements presented in this chapter to be drawn together, so that areas of weakness can be detected and improvement measures implemented leading to improved process and facility design. Moreover, a proactive response to biocontamination risk escalation can assist with controlled interventions during operations to prevent risk of a contamination event. Chapter 16 describes the risk assessment process in more detail.

CONCLUSION

This chapter has outlined the importance of taking a holistic view of biocontamination risks across pharmaceutical and healthcare manufacturing, for both sterile and nonsterile pharmaceutical products. Understanding and control of critical quality attributes monitoring for deviation is a necessary requirement in risk management. The focus should not only be centered around the product formulation or filling but there is also a need to look at the "big picture" and to understand the impact and contamination risks from downstream facilities and processes. By taking a holistic view of measurable control systems and environmental monitoring data, manufacturers can be alerted to potential risks earlier and undertake risk escalation ideally before biocontamination events occur that have a direct product impact.

The chapter has also acted as a means to capture the elements that feed into the biocontamination control process which have not featured in other chapters. This includes good design principles, especially for the clean space, cleaning processes, and equipment. Also discussed was the importance of cleaning and disinfection, including the importance of sporicides, and the advantages of single-use sterile technologies. Specific factors for both sterile products (aseptically filled and terminally sterilized) and nonsterile products (microorganisms of concern and preservatives) have also been outlined.

To capture the interconnected theme of the chapter, the prevention of contamination arises from determining the causes of the contamination; then anticipating the effect and assessing the risk; then designing out the routes of contamination, focusing on mechanisms to prevent any ingress and egress; and then controlling the remaining contamination. Monitoring can be used to assess the effectiveness of the controls, and the scope of this monitoring should be far and wide, and put together to provide an overall picture across time.

REFERENCES

Agalloco, J. (1992). Points to consider in the validation of equipment cleaning procedures. *PDA Journal of Pharmaceutical Science and Technology, 46*(5), 163–168.

Angelillo, I. F., Bianco, A., Nobile, C. G. A., & Pavia, M. (1998). Evaluation of the efficacy of glutaraldehyde and peroxygen for disinfection of dental instruments. *Letters in Applied Microbiology, 27*, 292–296.

Bergan, T., & Lystad, A. (1972). Evaluation of disinfectant inactivators. *Acta Pathologica Microbiologica Scandinavica Section B, 80*, 507–510.

Denyer, S. P., & Stewart, G. S. A. B. (1998). Mechanisms of action of disinfectants. *International Biodeteriroration and Biodegradation, 41*, 261–268.

FDA (2007) Pharmaceutical quality for the 21st century a risk-based approach Progress report, Food and Drug Administration Rockville: MD.

Frank, J. F., & Chmielewski, R. (2001). Influence of surface finish on the cleanability of stainless steel. *Journal of Food Protection, 64*(8), 1178–1182.

Gilbert, P., & Allison, D. G. (1996). Redefining the 'sterility' of sterile products. *European Journal of Parenteral Sciences, 1*, 19–23.

ICH. Q9 Quality risk management, International Council for Harmonisation of Technical Requirements for Pharmaceuticals for Human Use, Geneva, Switzerland, 2006.

Jornitz, M. W., & Meltzer, T. H. (2011). Pre-use/poststerilization integrity testing of sterilizing grade filter: the need for risk assessment. *American Pharmaceutical Review*, *14*(5), 5–8.

Kokubo, M., Inoue, T., & Akers, J. (1998). Resistance of common environmental spores of the genus *Bacillus* to vapor hydrogen peroxide. *Journal of Pharmaceutical Science and Technology*, *52*, 228–231.

Korakianiti, E., & Rekkas, D. (2011). Statistical thinking and knowledge management for quality-driven design and manufacturing in pharmaceuticals. *Pharmaceutical Research*, *28*(7), 1465–1479.

Lemieux, P. (2006). Destruction of spores on building decontamination residue in a commercial autoclave. *Applied and Environmental Microbiology*, *72*(12), 687–7693.

Lionberger, R., Lee, S., Lee, L., Raw, A., & Yu, L. (2008). Quality by design: concepts for ANDAs. *The AAPS Journal*, *10*, 268–276.

Ludwig, J. D., & Avis, K. E. (1990). Dry heat inactivation of endotoxin on the surface of glass. *Journal of Parenteral Science and Technology*, *44*, 4–12.

McDonnell, G., & Russell, A. (1999). Antiseptics and disinfectants: activity, action and resistance. *Clinical Microbiology Reviews*, *12*(1), 147–179.

Morton, L. H. G., Greenway, D. L. A., Gaylarde, C. C., & Surman, S. B. (1998). Consideration of some implications of resistance of biofilms to biocides. *International Biodeterioration and Biodegradation*, *41*, 247–259.

O'Donnell, K., & Greene, A. (2006). A risk management solution designed to facilitate risk-based qualification, validation & change control activities within GMP and pharmaceutical regulatory compliance environments in the EU, Parts I & II. *Journal of GXP Compliance*, *10*(4), 1–8.

Pflug, I. J., & Odlaug, T. E. (1986). Biological indicators in the pharmaceutical and medical device industry. *Journal of Parenteral Science and Technology*, *40*, 242–248.

Ramstorp, M. (2011). Microbial contamination control in pharmaceutical manufacturing. In M. R. Saghee, T. Sandle, & E. Tidswell (Eds.), *Microbiology and sterility assurance in pharmaceuticals and medical devices* (pp. 615–701). New Delhi: Business Horizons.

Reinmüller, B. (2001). People as a contamination source-clothing systems. In *Dispersion and risk assessment of airborne contaminants in pharmaceutical cleanrooms* (pp. 54–77). Royal Institute of Technology, Building Services Engineering, Bulletin No. 56, Stockholm.

Riley, B. S., & Li, X. (2011). Quality by design and process analytical technologies for sterile products—where are we know? *AAPS PharmSciTech*, *12*(1), 114–118.

Sandle, T. (2011). Environmental monitoring. In M. R. Saghee, T. Sandle, & E. C. Tidswell (Eds.), *Microbiology and sterility assurance in pharmaceuticals and medical devices* (pp. 293–326). New Delhi: Business Horizons.

Sandle, T. (2012a). Application of disinfectants and detergents in the pharmaceutical sector. In Sandle, T. (2012). The CDC handbook: A guide to cleaning and disinfecting cleanrooms, Grosvenor House Publishing: Surrey, pp 168–197.

Sandle, T. (2012b). Cleaning and disinfection. In Sandle, T. (2012). The CDC handbook: A guide to cleaning and disinfecting cleanrooms, Grosvenor House Publishing: Surrey, pp 1–31.

Sandle, T. (2013). Contamination control risk assessment. In R. E. Masden, & J. Moldenhauer (Eds.), *Vol. 1. Contamination control in healthcare product manufacturing* (pp. 423–474). River Grove, IL: DHI Publishing.

Sandle, T. (2014). Selection and use of cleaning and disinfection agents in pharmaceutical manufacturing. In G. Handlon, & T. Sandle (Eds.), *Industrial pharmaceutical microbiology: Standards and controls* (pp. 9.1–9.32). Passfield: Euromed Communications.

Sandle, T. (2015). Assessing process hold times for microbial risks: bioburden and endotoxin. *Journal of GXP Compliance, 19*(3), 1–9.

Sandle, T. (2016a). Disinfectants in the pharmaceutical industry. In A. S. Cardoso, C. M. M. Almeida, T. C. Cordeiro, & V. J. Gaffney (Eds.), *Disinfectants: Properties, applications and effectiveness* (pp. 109–142). New York: Nova Science Publishers.

Sandle, T. (2016b). *Pharmaceutical microbiology: Essentials for quality assurance and quality control* (pp. 171–172). Cambridge: Woodhead Publishing.

Sandle, T. (2017). Microbiological aspects of cleaning validation. *Journal of GXP Compliance, 21*(5), 1–12.

Sandle, T., Leavy, C., & Rhodes, R. (2015). Assessing airborne contamination using a novel rapid microbiological method. *European Journal of Parenteral and Pharmaceutical Sciences, 19*(4), 131–142.

Sandle, T., Roberts, J., & Skinner, K. (2009). An examination of the sample hold times in the microbiological examination of water samples. *Pharmaceutical Microbiology Forum Newsletter, 15*(2), 2–7.

Sandle, T., & Saghee, M. R. (2011). Some considerations for the implementation of disposable technology and single-use systems in biopharmaceuticals. *Journal of Commercial Biotechnology, 17*(4), 319–329.

Sandle, T., & Vijayakumar, R. (2014). *Cleanroom microbiology* (pp. 451–488). Bethesda, MD: DHI/PDA.

Scott, B., & Wilcock, A. (2006). Process analytical technology in the pharmaceutical industry: a toolkit for continuous improvement. *PDA Journal of Pharmaceutical Science and Technology, 60*(1), 17–53.

Sutton, S. V. W. (2012). What is an "objectionable organism"? *American Pharmaceutical Review, 15*, 36–42.

Tidswell, E. (2011). Sterility. In M. R. Saghee, T. Sandle, & E. C. Tidswell (Eds.), *Microbiology and sterility assurance in pharmaceuticals and medical devices* (pp. 589–602). New Delhi: Business Horizons.

Vina, P., Rubio, S., & Sandle, T. (2011). Selection and validation of disinfectants. In M. R. Saghee, T. Sandle, & E. C. Tidswell (Eds.), *Microbiology and sterility assurance in pharmaceuticals and medical devices* (pp. 219–236). New Delhi: Business Horizons.

Chapter 18

The Human Factor and Biocontamination Control

CHAPTER OUTLINE

Introduction   315
The Human Risk Factor   316
The Human Microbiome   316
Implications for Biocontamination Control   321
Importance of Clothing   321
  Cleanroom Garments   322
Cleanroom Personnel Behavior   326
Training   331
Changing Into Cleanroom Garments   332
Materials Access   333
Personal Hygiene   334
Summary   336
References   337

INTRODUCTION

It is difficult to quantify the proportion of contamination found within a cleanroom that is traceable to people; some surveys, such as those of Hyde (1998) and Sandle (2011a), suggest contamination levels may be up to 80%. Certainly, then pattern of cleanroom microbiota attributable to people is significantly high (and within aseptic processing areas, accounting for almost all of the recovered contaminants). Chapter 12 profiled such contamination. When it is considered that the outer layer of human skin can host up to 1 million microorganisms per square centimeter this risk factor does not come as a total surprise.

While the activities of people feature strongly throughout this book, this chapter explores the "human factor" in greater detail. The chapter discusses staff gowning and personnel behavior in pharmaceutical cleanrooms.

Biocontamination Control for Pharmaceuticals and Healthcare. https://doi.org/10.1016/B978-0-12-814911-9.00018-3

Further, the chapter describes the basic training for all cleanroom staff, addressing activities such as cleanroom entry, the collection of environmental monitoring samples, as well as the understanding of personnel hygiene.

In terms of what can be done to control the "human factor," this chapter is foremost concerned with practicalities: how can people enter cleanrooms, and work in cleanrooms, in ways that minimize contamination risks?

THE HUMAN RISK FACTOR

The main risk is with cleanroom operators shedding skin cells, and a proportion of these skin cells will be carrying microbial cells released from the outer layer of the epidermis. Here research suggests that atypical person sheds 1,000,000,000 skin cells per day of a size $33 \times 44 \times 4\,\mu m$ (equivalent to a rate of 30,000–40,000 dead skin cells shed from the surface of the skin every minute), of which approximately 10% have microorganisms on them. There are, on average, four microorganisms per skin cell (Chen & Tsao, 2013).

THE HUMAN MICROBIOME

The human body is an intricate system that hosts trillions of microbial cells across the epithelial surface, and within the mouth and gut. These microorganisms play a role in human physiology and organ function, including digestion and immunity. The microorganisms also impact on the outside environment as they are shed from the skin or deposited through different orifices. This latter issue has important implications for cleanrooms, personnel, and gown control. This collection of organisms is referred to as a "microbiome." A microbiome is "the ecological community of commensal, symbiotic, and pathogenic microorganisms that literally share our body space" (Lederberg & McCray, 2001). The human microbiome (or human microbiota) is the aggregate of microorganisms (and their genetic interactions) that reside on the surface and in deep layers of skin, in the saliva and oral mucosa, in the conjunctiva, and in the gastrointestinal tracts.

Data pertaining to the numbers and complexity of these microorganisms has been enriched in recent years through the findings of the Human Microbiome Project (HMP). HMP is a United States National Institutes of Health initiative, which began in 2008. The project was set the goal of identifying and characterizing the microorganisms which are found in association with both healthy and diseased humans (the human microbiome). The project has altered the scientific understanding and perceptions in relation to how the microbial community carried on and within the human body interacts with host cells and the immune system; and the project is shaping medical opinion and understanding about health and disease. This is to the extent that Geeves and colleagues described the research outcome as leading to the compilation of "a comprehensive human-associated microbial censuses" (Geeves, Pop, & Hawthorne, 2012).

While the various human host–microbial cell interactions are of great interest and have implications for other aspects of pharmaceutical microbiology (including the effectivity of medicinal products) (Cundell, 2012), this chapter is largely concerned with the human microbiome of human skin since this represents a key contamination transfer mode in relation to personnel working in cleanrooms.

The outcomes of the HMP research have shown that there is a high population on, and a considerable diversity of microbial species across, the outer layer of the skin (with bacteria there are around 1000 species upon human skin from 19 phyla) (Gao, Tseng, Pei, & Blaser, 2007). Of these, most bacteria can be categorized into just four phyla: Actinobacteria (51.8%) (Actinobacteria are a group of Gram-positive bacteria with high guanine and cytosine content, such as *Micrococcus, Corynebacteria,* and *Propionibacteria*), Firmicutes (24.4%) (includes the genera *Clostridia* and *Bacillus*), Proteobacteria (16.5%) (a major phylum of bacteria, which includes a wide variety of pathogens, such as *Escherichia, Salmonella, Vibrio, Helicobacter,* and many other notable genera), and Bacteroidetes (6.3%) (the phylum Bacteroidetes is composed of three large classes of Gram-negative, non-spore-forming, anaerobic, and rod-shaped bacteria) (Grice, Kong, Renaud, & Young, 2008). Here the skin flora is different from regions inside the body, such as the gut, which is predominately made up of the Firmicutes and Bacteroidetes.

With the four phyla, the microbial diversity across the skin is not evenly distributed as the density and composition of the normal flora of the skin varies with anatomical local (Roth & James, 1988). The distribution of microorganisms varies by topography and there are three main ecological areas of the skin: sebaceous, moist, and dry. Examples of microbial divergence include *Propionibacteria* and *Staphylococci* species dominating the sebaceous areas (with a high oil content); with dry, calloused areas (arms and legs), Gram-positive cocci (primarily the Micrococcaceae) are found on the arms and legs and Gram-positive rods are found in high numbers on the torso; and with moist areas, Staphylococci and Corynebacteria are found together with some Gram-negative bacteria (Grice, Kong, Conlan, et al., 2009).

The reason that Gram-positive bacteria predominate across the skin is because the skin is generally a dry environment, and any fluids present on the surface generally have a high osmotic pressure. Thus Gram-positive bacteria (especially the Staphylococci and Micrococci) are better adapted for such environments, not least to being resistant to desiccation. Where other species occur this is due to variations in temperature and with areas of higher sweat production.

Additional reasons for the topographical variations relate to the physico-chemical properties of the skin. The pH of the skin, for example, varies between neutral and alkali. Another important variation is with temperature, for the skin temperature ranges between 25°C and 37°C (Chen & Tsao, 2013). Another cause of variation relates to the level of humidity. Here the dampest places are the groin region, the armpits, and between the toe webs. In these relatively moist areas proportionately higher numbers of Gram-negative rods are found, with *Acinetobacter* the dominant genus. There is also a variation with oxygen levels. The lower oxygen regions across the forehead and within hair follicles provide environments for anaerobic bacteria to colonize. A further factor is salinity, to which can be added the presence of chemical wastes such as urea and fatty acids. Furthermore, other microbes can produce toxic substances which can inhibit the growth of other microorganisms. Ecologically, sebaceous areas have a greater species richness compared with the moist and dry regions (Hanski et al., 2012).

Further topographical variations occur with fungi. The greatest fungal richness occurs on the feet, especially on the heels and on the toes, with the next most populous area being the head, neck, ears, and eyebrows. The most common fungal genera on the skin are: *Malassezia* (the dandruff causing yeast like fungus), *Penicillium*, and *Aspergillus* (Findley, Oh, Yang, Conlan, et al., 2013). Notably, a common fungus to cleanrooms—*Cladosporium*—is not associated with human skin—this fungus is more commonly associated with walls and faulty HVAC systems (Vijayakumar, Sandle, & Manoharan, 2012).

Thus the topography of the skin can be viewed as being made up of different ecological niches. Table 1 summarizes the physical properties of the skin in relation to microbial survival.

Table 2 looks at areas of the body in relation to different microbiota.

From Table 2, the common skin flora are usually nonpathogenic, and either commensals (which are not harmful to their host) or mutualistic (offer a benefit). However, in relation to pharmaceutical manufacturing, the presence of such organisms remains problematic. The potentially pathogenic *Staphylococcus aureus* is found on the face and hands in individuals who are nasal carriers. Such individuals may auto-inoculate themselves with the pathogen or spread it to other individuals or foods.

Table 1 Physical properties of skin and the effects on microorganisms

Factor	Effect
Temperature	Allows growth of mesophiles, prevents growth of thermophiles or psychrophiles
Low moisture	Prevents the growth of many species, especially Gram negatives
High osmolality	Prevents the growth of many species, especially Gram negatives
Low pH	Prevents the survival of many species
Oxygen concentration	Prevents survival and growth of anaerobes, except in hair follicles where oxygen concentration is low. Here, some anaerobes or microaerophiles will grow.
Nutrient availability	High

Table 2 Regions of the skin and the types of bacteria recovered

Region	Important environmental determinants	Effect on microbiota
Forehead	Many sebaceous glands	High population density. Dominated by *Propionibacteria* and some *Corynebacteria*. Main species: *P. acnes, P. granulosum, S. hominis, S. capitis, S. epidermidis, M. luteus, M. lylae, Koc. varians, C. minutissimum*
Scalp	High density of sebaceous glands; abundant hair traps moisture; a warm and moist environment	High numbers of propionibacteria, staphylococci and micrococci. Species include: *P. acnes, P. granulosum, S. hominis, S. capitis*
Axillae	Many sebaceous glands. Partially occluded, therefore increased moisture, temperature, and pH	High microbial density. High numbers of moisture requiring corynebacteria, fungi, and *Acinetobacter* spp. Main species: *P. acnes, P. avidum, C. minutissimum, C. xerosis, Brevibacterium* spp., *S. epidermidis, S. saprophyticus, S. aureus, M. luteus, E. coli, Klebsiella* spp., *Proteus* spp., *Enterobacter* spp., *Acinetobacter* spp.
Perineum	Occluded: increased moisture and temperature	High microbial density. High numbers of moisture requiring corynebacteria, fungi, and *Acinetobacter* spp. Main species: *S. epidermidis, S. hominis, S. aureus.* Occasional intestinal organisms
Toe webs	Occluded: increased moisture and temperature	High microbial density. High numbers of moisture requiring corynebacteria, brevibacteria, fungi, and *Acinetobacter* spp.
Arms and legs	Few sebaceous glands, dry regions	Low microbial density, mainly staphylococci and micrococci. Main species: *S. epidermidis, S. hominis, P. acnes, M. luteus, Koc. varians*
Hands	No sebaceous glands, exposed, low water content	Mainly *Staphylococci, Corynebacteria*; a few *Propionibacteria*.
Soles of feet	Absence of hair follicles and glands. High moisture due to shoes and socks	Species include: *S. hominis, S. haemolyticus, S. warneri, S. capitis, S. epidermidis, M. luteus, M. lylae*

Another observation is that the ratio of the microorganisms recovered from the skin is relatively evenly divided between the aerobic and the anaerobic. The aerobic microorganisms tend to live on the outermost layers of the skin and the anaerobic microorganisms live in the deeper layers of the skin and hair follicles. The high numbers of anaerobes (notably *Propionibacterium acnes*) raises a potential implication for environmental monitoring, which tends toward the screening for mesophilic aerobic bacteria (Burton & Engelkirk, 2004).

A further observation of interest is temporal, where longer term data indicates that the microbiome alters over time. Furthermore, the species associated with the skin fungi change more often than bacteria. Moreover, variation occurs not only across different body locations, but there is also some variation between individuals, with men carrying more microorganisms than women. A further complication to understanding the skin microbiota is that the human skin microbiome may not be stable and may change over time as a person ages (Costello et al., 2009).

Notably the high moisture content of the axilla, groin, and folds between the toes supports the activity and growth of relatively high densities of bacterial cells. High levels are also found on regions of the skin close to mucosal openings (like the mouth and eyes). Here there are some areas of the skin with higher moisture content, especially occluded regions where sweat does not easily evaporate (such as toe webs). Furthermore, with these occluded areas there are found larger densities of microorganisms when compared with dry areas.

In terms of population, the density of bacterial populations at most sites is relatively low, generally in hundreds or thousands per square centimeter. The highest numbers of microorganisms are isolated from the sweat gland. With the numbers of microorganisms located on a given area of the skin, the numbers present at any one time are limited. This can be explained by the use of two long-established laws relating to biology. These are (Gorban, Pokidysheva, Smirnova, & Tyukina, 2011):

- Liebig's "law of the minimum." This is a principle developed in agricultural science by Justus von Liebig. It states that growth is controlled not by the total of resources available, but by the scarcest resource. With microorganisms, this can be translated to microbial numbers being determined by the available nutrients present.
- Shelford's "law of tolerance." This law suggests that a population is subject to an ecological minimum, maximum, and optimum for any specific environmental factor or complex of factors. The range from minimum to maximum represents the limits of tolerance for the factor or complex. In relation to microorganisms, this means that nonnutritional factors govern growth, such as pH, humidity, and temperature.

Also, another limiting issue is that factors like skin shedding continually remove microorganisms. Hand washing is a second example of mechanical action, where the microbial population can change, particularly those microorganisms contained within sweat, oil, and other secretions.

IMPLICATIONS FOR BIOCONTAMINATION CONTROL

The understanding of the skin microbiome presents some implications for biocontamination control. These are:

a. Is environmental monitoring sufficient? This is explored more fully in Chapter 6, but it concerns whether the agars selected, incubation conditions, and times are suitable for the recovery of the organisms that personnel are likely to shed. Here no single culture medium or set of conditions can fully be expected to recover all isolates. All that can be expected is to optimize the environmental monitoring as best as possible and to focus efforts on contamination control—good personnel hygiene and effective gowning.

b. The understanding that there is a greater diversity of microorganisms carried on the skin and that these will be shed within the cleanroom environment arguably has implications for the disinfectants used within cleanrooms as part of the contamination control program. The question here is whether the test panel used to challenge disinfectants requires widening? The answer, in this author's opinion, is "yes."

c. Similar to disinfectant efficacy, there may also be implications for broadening the test panel used for media growth promotion. If this is accepted the question is should these be environmental isolates or type cultures. This would be based on those microorganisms that are representative of the skin microbiome, including a range of Gram-positive cocci; a Corynebacterium, and an *Acinetobacter* species.

d. The fourth consideration is with operator gowning for entry into cleanrooms. This relates to the question of whether gowning practices are adequate to exclude all microorganisms from the richest areas of the skin microbiome? This is a pertinent point given that most bacteria free floating in cleanroom air current are not free living but are instead the result of direct particle shedding of desquamated skin cells and subsequent resuspension of skin detritus in the air stream.

IMPORTANCE OF CLOTHING

Staff working in cleanrooms are required to wear special clothing designed for the clean environments. Such clothing is required because the human body creates its own microenvironment of potentially damaging particulate contamination. Since humans are essential to production situations, damage limitation through the use of purpose-designed cleanroom clothing has proved to be the most practical solution to the problem (together with the use of barrier technology). The use of specialist clothing is now commonplace.

To be effective clothing must:

- form a particulate barrier for the human microenvironment especially for the moister parts of the body,
- allow freedom of movement and be comfortable,
- have an outer gown to cover all parts of the body, including the forehead
- address any specialist requirement, for example, static dissipation,
- avoid being a significant particulate contributor itself.

In addition, the level of training required for operators in relation to gowning and the way that gowning qualification as conducted. Each organization must also assess for how long a cleanroom suit can be worn for (in relation to material integrity against operator perspiration). A further point is with how often gowns should be recycled (which involves washing and irradiation)? At some point the material fibers will weaken, thereby reducing the bacteria filter efficiency of the gown.

The gown and skin shedding issues prompt consideration of:

- High air change rates in changing areas,
- Gowning training procedures,
- The quality of cleanroom certified undergarments,
- Stipulating maximum times for wearing cleanroom suits,
- Rejecting suits for loss of integrity
- And covering the forehead

Cleanroom Garments

Cleanroom personnel must wear specialized garments to protect the environment and the workplace from the human contaminant. Cleanroom garments must meet specific protection criteria. This involves manufacturing the garments from special materials, following particular construction methods, and then tailored for individual styling. The gowns must be comfortable, easy to apply, and practical in use.

The cleanroom fabrics must contain the following features (Reinmüller, 2001):

a. Be low in particulate shedding.
b. Permit the body to breathe while trapping particles within the garment—the contaminant should be retained within the garment and not released into the surrounding atmosphere.
c. Be flexible enough for comfortable wearing.

d. Withstand repeated cleaning and sterilization cycles.

e. Meet any specific requirements like control of static.

f. Meet the opacity requirements.

g. Look and feel as good as possible.

h. Be cost effective

There are three broad categories of fabric used in the construction of cleanroom garments.

These are:

1. *Woven fabrics*—Woven or reusable fabrics are the most commonly used fabrics in cleanroom environments. As the name implies, they are woven on sophisticated looms from yarns of continuous filaments of polyester. The thickness of the yarn and filaments is important (the finer the yarn the tighter the weave can be made and the better the filtration), but also the pattern and tightness of the weave is important to reduce the pore size to a minimum. The use of continuous filament polyester means that there are few loose ends from which particles may be shed.

2. *Laminated or membrane fabrics*—Laminated fabrics, favored for some high grade microelectronic environments, are produced by bonding together two or more layers (often a combination of woven and nonwoven fabrics). Particle retention and vapor permeability are achieved by incorporating a membrane that will give the filtration required. The lamination is a critical process in the production of these materials. To work efficiently garments from these materials require optimum sealing at all openings, making production relatively expensive. These types of garments are not commonly used in the pharmaceutical sector.

3. *Disposable or limited life materials*—The most common of these nonwoven fabrics are from spun bonded olefin and polypropylene. Comprising a densely interlinked matt of fibers, these fabrics can provide good results for a limited period. Garments from such materials need to be processed and decontaminated before use in the cleanroom. Disposable or limited use garments are mainly used in those environments where protection of the wearer against potentially hazardous products is required. A typical example is an environment where toxic chemicals are used. Other applications for these garments are situations where the process would ruin reusable garments, such as working with certain inks, or where the wearer is on a one-off visit to the cleanroom. Widespread use is seldom cost effective but in low-frequency applications where a managed cleaning cycle is unwarranted or where there is a casual

requirement for units off the shelf, the disposal concept may prove perfectly viable.

Garments are designed to provide protection for the head, body, hands, and feet. In establishing a system for garment selection one must consider the broader aspects of cleanroom use: suitability of fabric, garment style, layers, the nature of the tasks involved, costs, and any regulatory or specific customer requirement.

The classification of the cleanroom will inevitably be the major factor in determining the degree of personnel protection required and thus the fundamental choice of garments. Factors which also need to be addressed include the provision of changing facilities, operating procedures, and the garment management system.

Table 3 gives some indications for the types of garments in relation to different classifications of controlled environments.

The type of clothing expected in the various grades of pharmaceutical cleanrooms is as follows:

- *EU GMP Grade D*: Hair and, where relevant, beard should be covered. A general protective suit and appropriate shoes or overshoes should be worn. Appropriate measures should be taken to avoid any contamination coming from outside the clean area.
- *EU GMP Grade C/ISO 14644 Class 8 in operation*: Hair and where relevant beard and mustache should be covered. A single- or two-piece trouser suit, gathered at the wrists and with high neck and appropriate shoes or overshoes should be worn. They should shed virtually no fibers or particulate matter.
- *Grade A/B/ISO Classes 5 and 7 (in operation)*: Headgear should totally enclose hair and, where relevant, beard and mustache; it should be tucked into the neck of the suit; a face mask should be worn to prevent

Table 3 Types of garments used in pharmaceutical cleanrooms

Classification	Body	Head	Feet	Hand
ISO Class 5	Cover all	Full hood mask if required (beard-cover)	Long over boots	Powder and lint free
ISO class 6	Cover all or coat	Hood or snood	Over boots or overshoes	Powder and lint free
ISO Class 7	Cover all or coat	Hat or cap	Overshoes	As required
ISO Class 8	Coat	Hat or cap	Overshoes	As required

the shedding of droplets. Appropriate sterilized, nonpowdered rubber or plastic gloves and sterilized or disinfected footwear should be worn. Trouser legs should be tucked inside the footwear and garment sleeves into the gloves. The protective clothing should shed virtually no fibers or particulate matter and retain particles shed by the body.

Grades A and B are broadly comparable with ISO 14644 Classes 5 and 7 areas (in operation).

Outdoor clothing should not be brought into changing rooms leading to Grade B and C rooms (ISO Classes 7 and 8, in operation). Fig. 1 shows can operator working in a Grade C/ISO Class 8 cleanroom. The operator is wearing a single suit, mask, gloves, and a head cover.

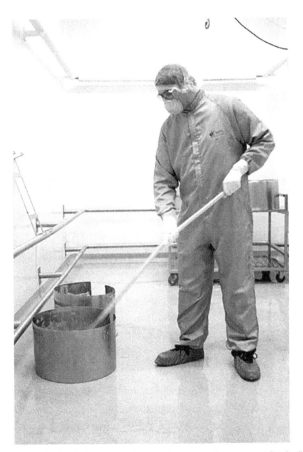

■ **FIG. 1** Operator cleaning the floor in a Grade C/ISO Class 7 area. *(Image courtesy Tim Sandle.)*

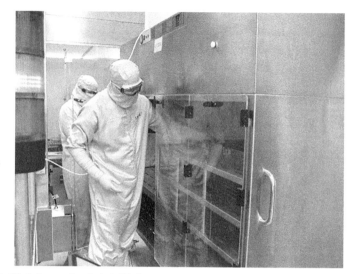

■ **FIG. 2** Operators in a Grade B (ISO Class 7 in operation) cleanroom. *(Image courtesy Tim Sandle.)*

For every worker in a Grade A/B area (ISO Classes 5 and 7 in operation), clean sterile (sterilized) protective garments should be provided for each work session. A time limit must be established for how long a gown can be worn for (each gown will have a finite capacity for maintaining integrity, especially as the operator perspires). Gloves should be regularly disinfected during operations. Masks and gloves should be changed at least for every working session. Fig. 2 illustrates operators working in a Grade B (ISO Class 7 in operation cleanroom). The operators are wearing gowns, boots, masks, hoods, and goggles.

CLEANROOM PERSONNEL BEHAVIOR

Working in clean environments demands knowledge, discipline, motivation, as well as a thorough understanding of contamination risks among all personnel involved. Each individual cleanroom should have its own documented rules and procedures. Despite the fact that each cleanroom can be said to be more or less unique, a number of more general rules exist (Ramstorp, 2011). These rules are (Sandle & Vijayakumar, 2014):

1. Only the necessary and limited number of persons should be allowed in a cleanroom at the same time. The more persons simultaneously present in a cleanroom, then the higher the contamination level will be (i.e., the higher concentration of particles in the air). This is particularly important in relation to changing rooms.

Thus in order to avoid heavy load of particles in connection with dressing and undressing for the cleanroom, together with performing other preparatory work before entering the cleanroom, it is important to establish the maximum number of persons that is allowed in changing rooms and air locks, respectively.

2. All personnel working in a cleanroom must be fully aware of their respective responsibility. They need to be trained in all the different techniques used in the cleanroom as well as the different operational systems that make the cleanroom work.

3. Only personnel having adequate training is allowed within the cleanroom. Persons needing access in order to perform minor and more specific activities, such as external service personnel, should only allowed into the cleanroom after briefing of the rules. Such personnel must be accompanied at all times. Ideally, major operations should take place during manufacturing shutdowns.

4. Training programs should ideally include visual assessment and microbiological assessment. The microbiological assessment varies, but can include the exposure of settle plates during the change process and the assessment of gown cleanliness through postuse suit contact plates.

5. Personnel must never bring any unauthorized material into the cleanroom. Only materials suited, as well as needed, for the production should be allowed to be taken into the cleanroom. Every item brought into the cleanroom must always be prepared prior to the intake, that is, cleaned, disinfected, and (or) sterilized, in order to not compromise the cleanliness of the cleanroom and the materials handled within.

6. The following items are normally not allowed to be brought into changing rooms, air locks, cleanrooms, as well as other controlled environments:
   a. Food or drink.
   b. Radios, mobile telephones, or other electronic equipment (except for devices purposefully designed for cleanroom use).
   c. Items manufactured from wood, rubber, paper (except for paper designed for use in cleanrooms), leather, cotton, or other types of natural materials.
   d. Lead pencils and rubbers, fiber-based felt pens, and pens of private nature.
   e. Other personal belongings.

7. All doors leading to the cleanroom, in as well as out from air locks, for personnel as well as material, together with different pass-through system, are not allowed to be left opened. Open doors give rise to over or under pressure, which in turn might result in uncontrolled air

movements and dispersion of contaminants within the cleanroom. All doors must have self-closing mechanisms.

8. Doors to airlocks and pass throughs, together with doors to local clean zones placed in cleanrooms, that is, a local filling zone, must always be opened and closed in a slow manner. Opening or closing a door with too high speed can lead to a situation in which air of lower cleanliness enters into spaces with higher cleanliness demands. Beneficially, doors can be supplied with dampers that control the speed by which doors are opened and (or) closed.

9. When entering through a door leading to an airlock, other doors should only be able to be opened after which the first one has been securely closed. In most cases different types of interlock systems are used of which some also have a time lapse before the next door can be opened and the airlock room air can, to a certain degree, be cleaned up by the ventilation air.

10. It should never be possible to enter a cleanroom without passing through an airlock. Moreover, there must be a defined robbing procedure. Used for entry of personnel, these airlocks are not only used for robbing procedures but also utilized as a buffer zone between a less clean, external area and the cleaner internal cleanroom area.

11. Personnel should not be allowed to use escape exits leading directly out of a cleanroom for normal entry and (or) exit. Escape exits are only intended in the case of emergency.

12. A cleanroom should always be maintained clean and in good order. Unnecessary, as well as old and obsolete, equipment should not be stored in a cleanroom unless it is clearly declared that the equipment must never be used. Cleanrooms with too much equipment will be more or less impossible to clean effective enough.

13. Personnel must not be allowed to touch critical products and (or) equipment with their naked hands. All critical work must be undertaken wearing gloves. In addition, for critical activities, such as aseptic processing, contact must be through the use of clean utensils such as tweezers, forceps, and so forth. All the devices and gloves used must fully comply with the cleanliness demands of the cleanroom itself and the work undertaken in the cleanroom, which means that they must be cleaned, disinfected or, with sterile filling activities, sterilized.

14. When carrying material within a cleanroom, such as products and (or) equipment, this must be performed in such a way that neither the carried gods nor the operator will be contaminated. It is good practice to not carry item so that it comes in contact with the cleanroom garment.

15. Inappropriate behavior should not be allowed within the cleanroom. The generation of contamination is proportional to activity. A person

with head, arms, and body moving can generate about 1,000,000 particles $\geq 0.5\,\mu m/min$. A person who is walking can generate about 5,000,000 particles $\geq 0.5\,\mu m/min$. However, a person in motionless position can generate only 100,000 particles $\geq 0.5\,\mu m/min$.

16. Personnel should reduce activities like talking, singing, whistling, coughing, sneezing, and so on, especially when being close to the handled products and (or) production equipment. The overall cleanliness of the cleanroom will have a major bearing on how much talking that is allowed: the higher the cleanroom grade, less talking that should occur. This rule must also be regarded even when using a protective mask. A protective mask has a much better effect when used for the protection of the wearer, that is, when breathing in. When taking a breath, the under pressure created will draw the mask closer to the face and most of the air entering will be filtered as compared to the opposite: when exhaling. During exhaling, coughing, and sneezing the over pressure created will force the mask to be expelled from the face whereby the air, to a major extent, will leave in an unfiltered state on the side and upwards and downwards.

17. A mouth protection must always be used in such a way that both mouth and nose are fully covered.

18. When sneezing and coughing the personnel should, if possible, turn away from their critical work, after which they should enter the last airlock to change the face mask according to stated procedures.

19. Persons entering a cleanroom must be fully aware of the cleanroom garment to be used. The cleaner cleanroom the more critical garment system and in what manner it is put on and worn. In the more critical cleanrooms, it is a normal procedure to certify the personnel in accordance with cleanroom robbing in order to control the contamination of the garment when put on.

20. Gowns used for aseptic processing areas must be sterile (typically by irradiation or gassing). With aseptic processing, personnel typically wear an under gown and an over gown.

21. Garments must be controlled and tracked. Any garment will have a maximum life, based on a set number of launderings and, where applicable, sterilization cycles. Tests are available that can assess the integrity of garment fabric and the particle generation from cleanroom gowns.

22. The personal hygiene of cleanroom personnel is of vital importance. In excess, some companies have additional rules which often are termed personnel hygiene. The most important issue in this context is the hand hygiene, but also the oral hygiene of operators is frequently addressed.

23. All equipment, ampoules, flaks, beakers, plastic tubing, sampling equipment, and so on, must always be cleaned, disinfected, and (or) sterilized according to prescribed procedures before taken into the cleanroom.

24. All communication between personnel within as well as outside of a cleanroom should be performed via dedicated system, like, intercom equipment, talk through, and so on.

25. Cosmetics, such as powder, rouge, eye liner, mascara, and lipstick, must be banned in cleanroom environments.

26. Jewelry, such as rings, watches, necklace, bracelet, earrings, and other items, together with all forms of visible piercing, is commonly not allowed in cleanrooms.

27. The personnel working in cleanrooms and other forms of controlled environments must be physically well. Diseases in the upper respiratory tract as well as stomach disorders can create problem in hygienic applications. If in any doubt a supervisor or occupational health professional should be contacted for guidance.

28. In relation, it is recommended that regular health checks are performed on personnel.

29. When carrying out aseptic handling or production a new, sterile cleanroom garment needs to be put on at every entry. Work undertaken in less clean environments routines has to be defined on how frequent the cleanroom garment is worn. A daily change is typical.

30. Materials or items dropped onto the floor must never be picked up and used directly. Every item used in a cleanroom must be cleaned according to detailed specifications, which in many cases means that a dropped item must be taken out of the cleanroom and cleaned in a step wise manner before taken back again.

31. When gowning for aseptic production it is good practice to use dressing gloves. These gloves should be powder free and clean enough, that is, sterile.

32. Barrier gloves (such as those connected to an isolator or RABS) should be changed on a regular basis. How often must be defined in a written instruction.

33. Barrier gloves, that is, rubber-based gloves, should be cleaned on a regular basis in order to reduce the possibility for cross-contamination. During aseptic production, for example, within the pharmaceutical industry where there is a demand of microbiological cleanliness, the gloves should be disinfected on a regular basis and used once per batch operation. The frequency by which this disinfection process should be undertaken must be stated in the instructions. Seventy percent ethanol or isopropyl alcohol is most commonly used for gloveport devices,

whereas automated biodecontamination will be in place with isolators (such as vapor hydrogen peroxide).

34. All alcohols used for disinfection purposes, such as 70% ethanol or isopropyl alcohol for glove sanitization or disinfectant solutions used for floors, must be sterile filtered before taken into a cleanroom with higher demands of cleanliness (Grade A and B areas/ISO 14644 Classes 5 and 7).

35. All cleaning equipment must only be used for the cleanroom in question or for the cleanroom suite of rooms, in order to minimize the possibility for cross-contamination.

36. Personnel must be aware not to touch the cleanroom garment in the changing area and in air locks.

37. Personnel must avoid rapid movements during gowning and when working in cleanrooms.

38. Tools for maintenance and setting of equipment must as far as possible be kept in the cleanroom and must not leave the room for use elsewhere. Special tools that are needed must be thoroughly cleaned, disinfected, and even sterilized prior to use in the cleanroom.

39. Mops and wipers that are to be used repeatedly, that is, that are washable and even sterilized, are only to be used a fixed number of times before discarded. Information of the life length, based on the number of washes and (or) sterilizing cycles, should be noted in the routines and instructions of the company. For Grade B/ISO 14644 Classes 5–7 cleanrooms, only single-use items should be used.

40. All handling of critical products and (or) components must be undertaken on clean surfaces and not at a low level (near the floor).

TRAINING

There is a general requirement for manufacturers to provide training in accordance with GMP for all personnel whose activities may affect the quality of the product. Pharmaceutical manufacturing sites have a broad spectrum of personnel in terms of education and experience. Typically only a minority of staff will have microbiological background knowledge. It is therefore important to provide appropriate levels of training to all relevant functions as part of the overall microbiological control arrangements (Sandle, 2014). The training of staff, including any contract staff, should emphasize the importance of their particular role in safeguarding the products made in the facility from contamination. In relation to the manufacture of nonsterile pharmaceutical products it is important to cover the following from a microbiological perspective.

All staff:

- Introduction to microorganisms and microbiological contamination control.
- Entry and exit of production facilities (including gowning).
- Personal hygiene training.

More specialized training, dependent on role:

- Environmental sampling, monitoring, and control.
- Microbiological risks associated with specific production tasks.
- Risk assessment and design of microbiological control features.
- Classified area/cleanroom practice (if required by facility/formulation).
- Statistical/data analysis.

Training must be documented and regularly reviewed. It is important that training is effective and competency should be assessed to demonstrate this. Training should be tailored on a facility-by-facility basis with an appreciation of the specific risks associated with the product formulations and facility design.

CHANGING INTO CLEANROOM GARMENTS

The best method of changing into cleanroom garments is one that minimizes contamination getting onto the outside of the garments. Therefore change areas can vary in design, but it *is* common to find them divided into three zones:

1. Prechange zone.
2. Changing zone.
3. Cleanroom entrance zone.

Access to the facility must be restricted to personnel who are fully trained and assessed as competent to work in that area, who are appropriately attired as described before gowning procedure (Sandle, 2017).

- All visitors should be accompanied at all times by fully trained personnel.
- Access is normally restricted by the use of an electronic access control system, or similar.
- Outside of changing rooms "tacky mats" or polymeric flooring can be positioned, to help reduce the level of particles carried on footwear.
- Personnel access must only be made via changing rooms. The changing room design contributes to the assurance of appropriate personnel access and microbial contamination control.

- Hand washing facilities should be included in the design of changing rooms and used prior to access to the production areas. It is useful to have a "step over" line or bench to define the boundaries of clothing requirements. An interlock may be appropriate in some facilities.
- The requirements for area entry must be written into procedures and it is usual to have pictures of correctly clothed personnel and mirrors to enable staff to check them before entry.
- A copy of the gowning procedure should be present in the changing room.
- The changing room should be provided with filtered air. Intermediate (bag) filters will typically be suitable for this purpose, though high efficiency particulate air (HEPA) filtration may be used. The air pressure should be negative with regards to the manufacturing area corridor, but positive relative to external adjacent areas.

MATERIALS ACCESS

Materials which may be transferred into the facility include active pharmaceutical ingredients, starting materials, in process materials, packaging components, consumables, and tools. These are all potential sources of microbial contamination and it is essential that suppliers and delivery process of these items are assured to ensure that quality is maintained. This is especially the case for materials of biological origin.

- Warehouses should be well ventilated, cool and low in humidity; materials should be checked regularly and used as quickly as possible especially in the case of herbal materials.
- Dispensing operations and traffic within a facility should minimize dust carryover and hence risk of cross-contamination of the production areas.
- Materials access must be via specified routes—generally via air locks, although certain items when justified may be introduced via the personnel changing rooms, for example, equipment for environmental monitoring.
- Wooden pallets and cardboard cartons should not be taken into manufacturing or packaging areas. Whenever possible, carts, pallet jacks, trolleys, and so on, should be dedicated to the production area.
- Active pharmaceutical ingredients, starting materials, and packaging components will have been dispensed for a specific job and should be provided in appropriate clean, sealed impermeable (e.g., plastic/stainless steel) containers.
- In-process materials and consumables should also be supplied in sealed, clean plastic bags and, if these are delivered in cardboard boxes, the

plastic bags should be removed from the boxes before being taken into the area.

- All containers taken into processing areas should be clean and dry. Tools have the potential to contaminate the equipment and product contact parts and their introduction to the facility needs to be appropriately controlled with consideration given to cleaning and sanitization requirements. Similarly, the introduction of new equipment and tooling into a production environment should be assessed and appropriate actions taken to ensure that contamination is not brought into the facility.

PERSONAL HYGIENE

Potentially harmful organisms could be transferred to a product by its direct contact with personnel. High standards of personal hygiene are therefore very important, especially where sterile products are being manufactured. Consequently, operatives should be free from communicable diseases and should have no open lesions on the exposed body surfaces. To ensure high standards of personal cleanliness, adequate hand washing facilities and protective garments, including headgear, must be provided.

The GMP contains information and requirements in relation to numbers of personnel and personnel hygiene. It is always important to limit the total number of persons to be present in a cleanroom at the same time. Direct contact between the materials and the operative's hands must be avoided; where necessary gloves should be worn. Staff should be trained in the principles of GMP and in the practice (and theory) of the tasks assigned to them.

This is why there is a requirement to keep all unauthorized personnel outside the cleanroom and why visual inspections as well as control of processes should be carried through windows from the outside of the cleanroom areas whenever possible. External personnel, such as those not actively involved in the cleanroom process and who have no specialist knowledge of cleanliness requirements, for example, building workers, service personnel, and so on, should be thoroughly briefed and informed before being allowed to enter a cleanroom. It is good practice that visitors should be accompanied by a member of staff who is familiar with all the rules concerning the cleanroom.

Personnel employed in the manufacture of sterile products should also receive basic training in microbiology. All other personnel, including those involved in cleaning, maintenance, and quality control should be trained on a regular basis, including hygiene and basic microbiology.

There is a general requirement for manufacturers to ensure hygiene programs are established, understood, and implemented. The programs should be adapted to the different needs of the facility and cover the following (Sandle & Sandle, 2013):

- Health,
- Hygiene,
- Clothing of personnel.

Typically, for nonsterile manufacture the hygiene program will include:

- Medical examination upon recruitment.

A procedure for the notification of health conditions that may affect product quality and subsequent actions to prevent contact with starting materials, primary packaging materials, and manufactured products by those personnel with:

- ○ Infectious disease,
- ○ Open lesions on any exposed part of body,
- ○ Shedding skin conditions, such as eczema or psoriasis, dermatitis and dandruff (skin scales may harbor objectionable microorganisms that may impact pharmaceutical products and patients),
- ○ Gastric upsets.

Furthermore (Sandle, 2011b):

- Steps should be taken to prevent direct contact between the operator's skin and any pharmaceutical product/product contact equipment
- The prohibition of eating, drinking, chewing or smoking, or the storage of food, drinks, smoking materials, or personal medication in the production or storage areas must be enforced.
- No cosmetics should be worn and facial hair must be covered.
- A requirement for personnel to wash their hands and legs before entering the manufacturing facility.

Effective hand hygiene relies on the use of an appropriate technique as much as on selection of the correct product. Inappropriate technique can lead to failure of hand hygiene measures to appropriately remove or kill microorganisms on hands, despite the superficial appearance of having complied with hand hygiene requirements.

Key factors in effective hand hygiene and maintaining skin integrity include:

- the duration of hand hygiene measures
- the exposure of all surfaces of hands and wrists to the preparation used
- the use of rubbing to create friction
- ensuring that hands are completely dry

The following types of hand hygiene techniques are followed in cleanrooms:

1. Hand washing with medicated soap and water (antiseptic handwash)
2. Hand rubbing

When decontaminating hands with an alcohol-based hand rub (i.e., antiseptic handrub), apply product to palm of one hand and rub hands together, covering all surfaces of hands, fingers, and wrists, until hands are dry (alcohol-based hand rubs are not to be used with water). The process typically takes between 30s and 1min. Follow the manufacturer's recommendations regarding the volume of product to use.

SUMMARY

This chapter has focused on the human factor in relation to controlled environments. The chapter has setout that people are the primary cause of contamination within cleanrooms, a fact informed by research into the human microbiome. The questions arising from the human microbiome project in relation biocontamination control are:

- Do environmental monitoring methods remain sufficient in light of Human Microbiome Project findings?
- Should cleanroom microbiologists be as concerned with anaerobic bacteria as they are with aerobic bacteria?
- Does the test panel used for disinfectant efficacy tests need to change?
- Similarly, does the culture media growth promotion panel need to alter?
- Can the Human Microbiome Project findings aid with the assessment of microbial data deviations?
- Are cleanroom gowning practices adequate?

Because of this, investment in training and reinforcing cleanroom behaviors is of great importance. This must go hand in hand with the use of the correct type of gown (and other associated cleanroom wear, including gloves, masks, head cover, and footwear) and practices designed to reduce contamination risks (like glove and hand disinfection). Each of these factors has been outlined in this chapter, with an emphasis upon providing points of practical use for the reader.

Much of the focus of the chapter has been upon training. This is because a significant factor in quality assurance of the production process is the qualification of personnel. Such training is not merely a matter of echoing the specific work content and guidelines on behavior, for specialist knowledge must also be conveyed und refreshed. Adopting some of the advice in this chapter can help with the control of people within cleanrooms and assist with the control of contamination and thus to minimize the risk to the product.

REFERENCES

Burton, G. R. W., & Engelkirk, P. G. (2004). *Microbiology for the health sciences* (pp. 254–256). Maryland: Lippincott Williams and Wilkins.

Chen, Y. E., & Tsao, H. (2013). The skin microbiome: current perspectives and future challenges. *Journal of the American Academy of Dermatology, 69*(1), 143–155.

Costello, E. K., Lauber, C. L., Hamady, M., Fierer, N., Gordon, J. I., & Knight, R. (2009). Bacterial community variation in human body habitats across space and time. *Science, 326,* 1694–1697.

Cundell, A. M. (2012). Implications of the Human Microbiome Project to pharmaceutical microbiology. In M. Griffinm, & D. Rever (Eds.), *Microbial identification: The key to a successful program* (pp. 399–406). Bethesda: MD: PDA/DHI.

Findley, K., Oh, J., Yang, J., Conlan, S., et al. (2013). Topographic diversity of fungal and bacterial communities in human skin. *Nature, 498*(7454), 367–370. https://doi.org/10.1038/nature12171.

Gao, Z., Tseng, C. H., Pei, Z., & Blaser, M. J. (2007). Molecular analysis of human forearm superficial skin bacterial biota. *Proceedings of the National Academy of Sciences, 104,* 2927–2932.

Geeves, D., Pop, M., & Hawthorne, C. (2012). Bioinfomatics for the human microbiome project. *PLoS Computational Biology, 8*(11).e1002779.

Gorban, A. N., Pokidysheva, L. I., Smirnova, E. V., & Tyukina, T. A. (2011). Law of the minimum paradoxes. *Bulletin of Mathematical Biology, 73*(9), 2013–2044.

Grice, E. A., Kong, H. H., Conlan, S., et al. (2009). Topographical and temporal diversity of the human skin microbiome. *Science, 324,* 1190–1192.

Grice, E. A., Kong, H. H., Renaud, G., & Young, A. C. (2008). A diversity profile of the human skin microbiota. *Genome Research, 18,* 1043–1050 (PMID: 18502944).

Hanski, I., Von Hertzen, L., Fyhrquist, N., Koskinen, K., Torppa, K., Laatikainen, T., et al. (2012). Environmental biodiversity, human microbiota, and allergy are interrelated. *Proceedings of the National Academy of Sciences, 109*(21), 8334–8339.

Hyde, W. (1998). Origin of bacteria in the clean room and their growth requirements. *PDA Journal of Science and Technology, 52,* 154–164.

Lederberg, J., & McCray, A. T. (2001). "Ome Sweet" Omics—a genealogical treasury of words. *Scientist, 15,* 8. E-publication(2001). http://lhncbc.nlm.nih.gov/files/archive/pub2001047.pdf.

Ramstorp, M. (2011). Microbial contamination control in pharmaceutical manufacturing. In M. R. Saghee, T. Sandle, & E. Tidswell (Eds.), *Microbiology and sterility assurance in pharmaceuticals and medical devices* (pp. 615–701). New Delhi: Business Horizons.

Reinmüller, B. (2001). People as a contamination source-clothing systems. In *Dispersion and risk assessment of airborne contaminants in pharmaceutical cleanrooms* (pp. 54–77) Royal Institute of Technology, Building Services Engineering, Bulletin No. 56, Stockholm.

Roth, R. R., & James, W. D. (1988). Microbial ecology of the skin. *Annual Review of Microbiology, 42,* 441–464.

Sandle, T. (2011a). A review of cleanroom microflora: types, trends, and patterns. *PDA Journal of Pharmaceutical Science and Technology, 65*(4), 392–403.

Sandle, T. (2011b). Keeping hands and surfaces clean. *Arab Medical Hygiene,* (3), 11–17.

Sandle, T. (2014). Best practices in microbiology laboratory training. In G. Handlon, & T. Sandle (Eds.), *Industrial pharmaceutical microbiology: Standards & controls* (pp. 2.1–2.24). Passfield, UK: Euromed Communications.

Sandle, T. (2017). The people factor: investigating the gown. *European Pharmaceutical Review, 22*(4), 23–26.

Sandle, T., & Sandle, J. (2013). An important aspect of healthcare: outlining the many considerations of infection control. *Arab Medical Hygiene, 2013*, 34–39 October.

Sandle, T., & Vijayakumar, R. (2014). *Cleanroom microbiology.* Bethesda, MD: DHI/PDA.

Vijayakumar, R., Sandle, T., & Manoharan, C. (2012). A review of fungal contamination in pharmaceutical products and phenotypic identification of contaminants by conventional methods. *European Journal of Parenteral and Pharmaceutical Sciences, 17*(1), 4–19.

Chapter 19

Biocontamination Deviation Management

CHAPTER OUTLINE

Introduction   339
Assessing Data Deviations: Terminology and Categories   341
Structuring the Investigation   342
Investigation of Laboratory Error   346
   Laboratory Controls   347
Assessing the Evidence   347
Impact Assessment   348
Concluding Investigations   352
Summary   353
References   354

INTRODUCTION

When alert or action levels are exceeded, or when an upward trend develops, it is necessary to undertake an investigation, assess the risk, and propose corrective and preventive actions in relation to the event. This is a regulatory expectation and it fits with the underlying philosophy of the biocontamination control strategy (as outlined in Chapter 4).

Conducting investigations into out-of-limits results can prove very challenging and often, especially with environmental monitoring, the outcome of an investigation is inconclusive. The difficulties associated with resolving microbial results are that:

- Microorganisms are ubiquitous in nature and common environmental contaminants;
- The technician has the potential to introduce contaminating microorganisms during sampling and/or testing;
- Microorganisms could not be homogeneously distributed within the sample or an environment or in water for pharmaceutical purposes. It is well established that microorganisms follow Poisson distribution in

Biocontamination Control for Pharmaceuticals and Healthcare. https://doi.org/10.1016/B978-0-12-814911-9.00019-5

water samples, for example, an effect which is considerably enhanced with low populations of microorganisms;

- Microbiological assays are subject to considerable inherent variability.

The investigation of an environmental monitoring level excursion should be covered by a Standard Operation Procedure (SOP) and formally documented. The SOP should contain decision tress to ensure that, where possible, the conclusions reached are consistent.

Have a structured approach is important, as is having undertaken a proactive risk assessment and understanding the nature of the contamination. This can save time in assessing the various factors that need to be considered when embarking on an investigation. Factors that contribute to bioburden contamination, for example, can be extensive (Lolas, 2014):

- Facility design and maintenance.
- Tools and utensils.
- Impact of adjacent areas.
- Seasonal effects.
- Process and cleaning water.
- Facility housekeeping/disinfection.
- Nonproduct contact equipment.
- Sterilization operation and validation.
- Product and material flow.
- Personnel gowns and hygiene.
- Personnel behaviors.
- Primary packaging components.
- Raw materials.
- Active pharmaceutical ingredients.
- Manufacturing and filling processes.
- Equipment cleaning and maintenance.
- Storage conditions.
- HVAC operation.
- Equipment design.
- Personnel flow.

Hence assessing some of these risks in advance can save time and help to contextualize the risk.

Before proceeding with a formal investigation (or simultaneously, if the issue is one of high risk and requires suspension of processing), a check should be made in the microbiology laboratory to ensure that the result is not due to "laboratory error" (FDA, 2014). Such considerations may include whether the sample was taken and handled correctly, if the correct culture media was used, if the equipment was within calibration date (such as an active air sampler), if the sample was incubated for the correct time and temperature, if there is any possibility of sample contamination, whether the result was read correctly and reported to the correct units of measurement.

This chapter describes some general approaches for conducting investigations and for documenting and assessing the results. This is supported by some examples of the investigation process in relation to biocontamination control.

ASSESSING DATA DEVIATIONS: TERMINOLOGY AND CATEGORIES

There are various terms used of microbiological results of concern:

- "Over action" or "over alert,"
- Upward trend,
- Out of trend,
- Out of specification,
- Out of limits,
- Aberrant result,
- Data deviation.

Whichever terms are deployed, they should be justified and defined, especially with what constitutes and "upward trend" or "out-of-trend" situation. With out of specification, this term is only really applicable to where a specification is stated in a pharmacopeial monograph (such as with the sterility test, microbial limits test, or with the antimicrobial effectiveness test); for most types of microbiological data, the term "out of limits" is generally preferred.

Aside from terminology, it is a long-standing regulatory expectation that results that equal or exceed a limit, as well as trends of concern, are investigated. The origins of this can be traced back to the first GMPs for the pharmaceutical industry which appeared in 1962 (as part of the U.S. Code of Federal Regulations) and later via the U.K. MCA Orange Guide, through the well-documented case of "United States vs. Barr Laboratories" in 1993 (and later FDA guidance issued in 2006) (FDA Guidance for Industry, 2006). Each of these has laid some general guidance, albeit not specifically microbiological, for addressing results that fall outside of an expected value or range. This guidance is in the form of a documented risk assessment and investigation.

The result obtained, where it does not meet the required value or range, will fall into one of three categories (Clontz, 2008):

1. It will be a laboratory error, such a cross-contamination during testing or from a breakdown of the test environment. Supporting data from negative controls can be useful here in determining that an error has occurred.
2. Non-process-related operator error. This could arise, for example, during processing where an activity of an operator leads to product contamination. A high count from environmental monitoring might signal such an event and a probability (or otherwise) of product contamination.
3. Process-related error, which is where microbial contamination is present in the product or intermediate product due to a control breakdown, such as use of a contamination material or contaminated water, or a breakdown or event that leads to an extended hold time.

STRUCTURING THE INVESTIGATION

OOL results must be documented and investigated to determine:

1. The description of the OOL event.
   The contamination event or upward trend should be clearly defined. In describing the event reference should be made to any similar incidents within a recent time frame.
2. Whether the OOL event was valid or invalid (this requires a consideration of laboratory error, see later).
3. The previous history of the OOL event and examination of trends.
   The contamination event should be placed in context by examining recent trends. This is especially important for environmental monitoring data for often individual results are of little significance and greater emphasis is placed on the direction that the data is taking.
4. Data collection.
   Often additional data is required to assess the impact of the contamination event. With environmental monitoring this often means additional samples taken from the same sample location and often from the same room in which the event occurred. Depending on the nature of the process, it may be necessary to take samples from adjacent rooms. As part of assigning a root cause, sampling is sometimes undertaken in the occupied and unoccupied states to distinguish between personnel, equipment, and air handling system causes. Data collection may also lead to a period of intensive monitoring (at an increased frequency) for a period of time.
   Data collection efficiency varies with sample type. Here the most variable of all is environmental monitoring data, since it is formed of

discontinuous measurements and a zero result in itself does not necessarily mean there were no microorganisms present. Furthermore, the techniques and methods are variable and microbial recoveries are medium and growth conditions dependent.

5. Investigation.

The purpose of the investigation is to determine the root cause of the incident. Even if the incident leads to a batch rejected, the investigation is necessary to determine the source of the contamination to prevent recurrence (corrective and preventative actions, as part of CAPA review) and to determine if the result is associated with other batches of the same drug product, other products (risk assessment is an important consideration), or reflects an ongoing concern with personnel practice or clean area environmental operations.

Investigations into contamination events should consider why the action level was exceeded and why the contamination event has occurred. This involves determining the source of the contamination. For this, invaluable data comes from understanding the microflora. The range of microorganisms found in the cleanroom environment can be subcategorized according to the source or their probable location. This can provide significant information when formulating corrective and preventative actions as resources can be directed to tackling the contamination source.

When undertaking investigations, there are a number of investigation tools which can be employed. These include flow charts, decision matrices, fishbone diagrams, contradiction tables, Failure Modes and Effects Analysis, and so on.

There are a number of areas which can be considered when investigating data, such as bioburden counts and environmental monitoring results (Sutton, 2010a):

- Check of cleaning and disinfection frequencies and methods.
- Bioburden of the water should be considered, especially if potable water is used. Gram-negative organisms are the most likely type of organism to be found in water.
- Residual water left on equipment and other surfaces can facilitate the growth of Gram-negative rods and other organisms.
- The in-use life of cleaning solutions once they have been removed from their original packaging needs to be checked.
- Check of HVAC parameters including air supply volume, air change rates, room pressure differentials, airflow patterns, leaks to HEPA filters.
- Review of utility monitoring data, such as compressed air and water.
- Examination of staff behavior and practices, including aseptic technique.

- Check of the number of people present in the clean area.
- Comparing the contamination incident with microorganisms recovered from other areas (such as determining if there is a link between a process area and changing room).
- Considering which types of equipment and consumables are introduced into the clean area.
- Noting equipment repairs, breakdowns, or problems with equipment operation.
- Linking any patterns with viable and particle monitoring data together.
- Examination of equipment as sources of contamination (such as equipment-generated particles).
- Visual observation of the process by QA staff, this may include checking for puddles of water on the floor, damage to fabric and personnel gowning.
- Noting any recent modifications to the room or to the process.

Looking for correlations in data can also be helpful, especially with environmental monitoring. The types of questions that can reveal patterns in data include (Pasquarellaf, Pitzurra, & Savino, 2000):

- What activities took place?
- Was there more activity?
- Was there construction?
- Were there any changes to cleaning? Cleaning agents? Media?
- Any changes to Suppliers? Laboratory Operations? Samplers?
- What did the other measures of environmental control look like?
    - Temperature
    - Humidity
    - Particles
    - Differential Pressure
    - Organisms recovered
- Any correlation to operators, rooms, tasks, and so on?

To be meaningful, the investigation should be thorough, timely, unbiased, well documented, and scientifically sound.

6. Risk assessment.

Risk assessment can be applied in two ways: to understand the impact of the contamination upon a room or process, and as part of the ongoing review to prevent the contamination from reoccurring.

In terms of assessing the impact upon the product or process, account should be taken of the level of contamination and the frequency of contamination events, the ease of dispersion, the ease of transfer of the contamination to the product, and the proximity of the contamination to the critical part of the process or product. Risks tend to increase if the product is exposed for a long period of time or if the frequency of contamination is high.

The use of risk assessment in the pharmaceutical industry is both an increasingly used tool and an expectation of regulatory authorities. Risk assessment forms part of the risk management program. Risk assessment tools and techniques can be applied to every aspect of pharmaceutical processing and for microbiological investigations. An important part of this application involves an understanding of the process. Although the microbiologist should be at the forefront of any investigation into a contamination event, there is a great advantage from the use of a multidisciplinary team.

With environmental monitoring, the most common risk assessment technique is hazard analysis and critical control point (HACCP) which is a risk assessment approach that addresses physical, chemical, and biological hazards. HACCP is designed so that key actions, known as critical control points (CCPs) can be taken to reduce or eliminate the risk of the hazards being realized. A typical risk assessment of a production process in a cleanroom might consist of:

- A route map (where the facility is drawn and the route indicated)
- Identification of hazards (which can be divided into biological, physical, equipment, transport and chemical). This will allow an assessment of existing control measures.
- Process flow.
- Assessment of environmental monitoring. This will determine if the activity is safe to proceed.

7. Root cause or most probable root cause determination.

The determination of the root cause is designed to provide the source of the contamination and an explanation as to why the contamination event happened. This is necessary in order to fully understand the problem and for assigning corrective and preventative actions. Often the process of assigning a root cause involves a process of elimination, working through an investigation checklist to determine what "is" or "is not" a potential problem. The final conclusion may be a "most probable" root cause based on no definitive cause but one which stands out following the elimination of all other potential issues.

8. Corrective actions and preventative actions.

Corrective and preventative actions are the consequences of the investigation and describe the actions taken which are designed to lead to an improvement of process and environmental quality.

Corrective actions relate to either things that can be done at the time or if any additional testing or monitoring can be performed. Preventative actions are designed to put in place measures to prevent the contamination event from reoccurring. Examples include:

- ○ Staff training.
- ○ Additional cleaning and disinfection.
- ○ Repairs to equipment.
- ○ Repairs to fabric.
- ○ Alterations to HVAC systems.
- ○ Changes to work practices and redesigning activities.
- ○ Further assessment of risk (such as conducting airflow studies).
- ○ Increased monitoring or review of monitoring locations.

9. Summary and conclusion.

It is important that all investigations have a clear and succinct summary which briefly describes the origin of the contamination, the risk upon the product and process, and the measures to prevent reoccurrence. Such summaries are useful for senior management and for showing to regulators.

Individual excursions and trends should be reported to senior management either directly or through summary reports (such as Quality Exception Reports). It is further recommended that completed investigations are independently reviewed.

INVESTIGATION OF LABORATORY ERROR

It is important to know that the results obtained are valid. As part of the examination of the biocontamination event the possibility of laboratory error should be considered. It can often be important to progress with a process impact assessment quickly, therefore the assessment of a laboratory error may run in parallel with a product or process investigation (e.g., when examining a sterility test or media simulation failure).

With laboratory error investigations, a potential stepwise framework is:

1. State the reason for the investigation
2. Summarize the procedure followed.
3. Describe the sequence of testing events.
4. Examine equipment and instruments, assess calibration and preventative maintenance.
5. Review raw data for discrepancies.
6. Review calculations, especially dilution adjustments.
7. Review the training status of the technician.
8. Undertake a historical review of results.
9. Review other tests, both tests on the same material and tests performed around the same time.
10. State any retesting undertaken.
11. Summarize the investigation.

12. State the risk.

13. Conclude.

According to Sutton, causes of laboratory error include (Sutton, 2010b):

- Incorrect mathematics
- Sample dilution series error
- Transcription error
- Clerical error
- Nonsensical microbial identification

Assessing each of the earlier factors is an important task of the laboratory supervisor or manager.

Laboratory Controls

To assist with laboratory error investigations, it is good practice to periodically trend laboratory data, and controls, and to review these on a regular basis. This will also include analysis of laboratory error, such as categorizing results into:

- Testing error
- Incubation error
- Equipment error or malfunction
- Media contamination
- Loss of environmental controls, and so on

Examples of controls might include is a negative control swab, where an unused swab is plated out at the same time as samples taken from an environmental monitoring session.

ASSESSING THE EVIDENCE

Once the out-of-limits result is reported, evidence should be collected. This includes the identification of the contaminating microorganism(s), since this will provide some clues as to the origin of the contamination (see later). Moreover, understanding the organisms can provide a basis of information for comparison of contamination sites found (Wu & Liu, 2007).

In addition, trend data relating to the process area should be reviewed. This helps to contextualize the extent of the contamination event. With trending, it is useful to look across multiple days, lots, and shifts. Personnel monitoring data should be reviewed and analyzed as part of this process. This is especially important where personnel perform specific tasks that could impact on the process or product. The examination should extent to personnel training records, including gowning (Jiminez, 2004).

Manufacturing records should also be reviewed, looking for deviations in processing or atypical events that may have led to a time delay (such as an increase to a product hold time). The extent of any bioburden reduction steps should also be noted. The manufacturing history can shed useful information, for instance, if a product line has experienced similar contamination problems in the past or any concerns with repeated equipment failures. Trending of data for utilities and the like, such as performance, aberrations, and the like can be additionally useful (McCullough & Moldenhauer, 2015).

When out-of-limits events occur in relation to the manufacturing environment other factors to consider include:

1. Compressed gases;
2. Room air;
3. Manufacturing equipment;
4. Monitoring/measuring devices;
5. Storage containers;
6. Number of persons present in zone;
7. Unprotected surfaces of personnel;
8. Personal attire;
9. Protective clothing;
10. Walls/ceilings;
11. Floors;
12. Doors;
13. Benches;
14. Chairs;
15. Air admitted from other sources;
16. Objectionable species should be carefully considered.

IMPACT ASSESSMENT

In cases of confirmed out-of-limits or out-of-specification results, the impact of the accepted result must be assessed. This relates to the product or batch under review and to any other batches or parts of the process that might be similarly affected. There is no book that will give the answer to the impact of finding say, 10cfu compared to 5cfu; the significance will rest with each company in terms of developing a risk assessment.

The general rules are that, with aseptic processing, all instances of contamination require investigation. With nonsterile processing, the investigation requires an assessment of product type, organism type, numbers, and so on, to assess the likelihood of the organisms surviving, proliferating, or dying off. The potential production of toxins also needs to be considered in relation to the organism type.

EXAMPLE 1: INVESTIGATING MICROORGANISMS RECOVERED FROM CLEANROOMS

Having such information can also be helpful in working out why, for instance, a microorganism normally associated with water appears in an area without a water source. This could, for example, be due to disinfectant residues where the active ingredient may evaporate faster than the water residues. In such circumstances, attention should also be paid to the possibility of disinfectant resistance arising with particular microorganisms. This can be examined, for instance, using the disinfectant efficacy tests using a high-level challenge of the microorganism and noting the log-reduction over the specified contact time (Eissa & 1st ed., n.d.).

Information about the microbial origin can lead down different investigative paths. For example, microorganisms typically associated with air could indicate a problem in the filtered air or the positive pressure cascade between rooms. As a result, suitable questions to ask here would include: has building work recently taken place? How well has it been contained? Further investigation may relate to the cleaning and disinfection undertaken, the procedures used, whether the chemicals used were approved and applied at the required frequencies.

There are also concerns regarding a microorganism's potential to survive in a process or to cause spoilage of the product (especially with regard to nonsterile manufacturing). This should be assessed by comparing the substances used by the microorganism for growth with the active ingredients and excipients used to formulate the product. Furthermore, an analysis of rapid identification system test results will provide an extensive list of compounds the microorganism can metabolize, or of carbohydrates utilized, and so on.

The information gained during the identification of the microorganism can be used to compare against product formulation to identify potential issues. Any microorganism can be considered objectionable if it has the potential to degrade the product's stability.

If a microorganism is linked to the process or product, the next logical step is to consider the potential for the microorganism to survive in the process. This can be assessed by taking into account the following factors (this list is not exhaustive):

- pH
- Salt concentrations
- Sugar concentrations
- Amount of water
- Temperature
- Time

Equally, such information can provide a degree of assurance that proliferation and survival of a contaminant is unlikely. Survival of microorganisms is generally lower under the following conditions:

- Low or high pH
- High salt concentrations (osmotic conditions)
- High sugar concentrations (osmotic conditions)
- Low presence of water
- High temperature (above 45°C)
- Low temperature (below 10°C)
- Freezing steps

However, these lists are dependent upon the species recovered. For some fastidious microorganisms, the conditions on the second list may be preferable. The range of microorganisms found in the environment can be subcategorized according to the source or their probable location. This can provide significant information when formulating corrective and preventative actions as resources can be directed to tackling the contamination source. Some examples are illustrated later (Jiminez, 2004).

Airborne Types

Microorganisms associated with the air, such as *Bacillus* spp., when isolated in high numbers or on frequent occasions, then this should lead to an investigation of the filtered air and positive pressures. A possible question to ask would include whether any refitting of the air handing system has recently taken place and how well was this contained?

In terms of corrective actions, with *Bacillus* spp., the application of a suitable sporicidal disinfectant should be considered. However, this would be a case of only dealing with symptom and not the cause. Greater control following HVAC works should be drawn up by local management.

Personnel Contamination

Where microorganisms that are commonly associated with personnel (or those that can be traced to personnel sampling), such as *Staphylococcus* spp. and *Micrococcus* spp., then actions related to personnel must be undertaken. This could include a review of gowning procedures or glove spraying during processing. A review of past personnel data can also be particularly revealing. One issue is that some managers are reluctant to discuss the results of personnel monitoring with operators. This can lead to problems continuing to present a risk to processing (Grice et al., 2008).

Water or Dampness

Microorganisms that are associated with wet areas or from water deposits, such as *Pseudomonas* spp., present a process risk (based on previous discussions of water as both a vector and a growth medium). The presence of such microorganisms suggests water contamination, where the failure to dry equipment to a satisfactory standard or the failure to adequately separate wet and dry equipment is a common cause in pharmaceutical manufacturing. Other issues include disinfectant residues or water levels. Poor finishes to cleanrooms are also a problem. For example, an area of plastic coated chipboard can trap water and provide a source for microbial survival and proliferation.

The microbiologist should perform comparative checks using the environmental isolates found in wet areas within the manufacturing environment alongside microbial isolates recovered from the pharmaceutical grade water system. This will provide an indication of the possible source of the contamination.

Product and Processing Factors

The characteristics of the product impact upon the survival of microbial growth should anything detected from the environment impact upon the manufacturing processes.

Spore-Bearing Microorganisms

The continued presence of endospore-forming bacteria can suggest that the application of sporicidal disinfectants is either insufficient in regularity or is being applied in an ineffective or inconsistent way. Disinfectant resistance is another consideration, although there remains little scientific support for this phenomena and inadequate cleaning remains more probable than the resistance mechanisms associated with bacterial resistance to antibiotics emerging.

EXAMPLE 2: CONSIDERING MICROBIAL IMPACT ON NONSTERILE PRODUCTS

Dedicating time to the detection and identification of microorganisms is a key part of any robust environmental monitoring program, especially in relation to the risks that might be presented to nonsterile products. Should a high number of specified or objectionable microorganisms be found, at the wrong time; or in higher numbers; or in inappropriate places; then product quality, cleanroom operation, or environmental control in general become cause for concern. Factors to be considered when performing an investigation include:

- Determination of whether the microorganism is part of the normally recognized microflora or a new entity. If it is a new entity, do the numbers recovered indicate a cause for concern?
- As the identification of the microorganism performed correctly?
- Has the microorganism been tested for susceptibility to the disinfectant (e.g., using the suspension test)?
- Was cleaning and disinfection undertaken using approved procedures and using approved chemicals, at the required frequencies?
- All equipment being used for cleaning and disinfection should be checked.
- As the disinfectant used for the correct contact time and the correct dilution?
- As the disinfectant within its expiry date?
- As there any possibility of contamination of the disinfectant solution?
- Does the disinfectant contain the proper concentration of the active ingredient?

- Were staff correctly following the cleaning and disinfectant procedures?
- Was ancillary equipment (e.g. mop heads, cloths) used properly?

The following factors are useful in assessing any microbial risk (Sandle, 2006):

Absolute Number of Microorganisms Seen

High numbers of nonpathogenic microorganisms may not pose a health hazard. However, they may affect product efficacy and/or physical/chemical stability. The presence of an unusually high number of organisms may also indicate a problem during the manufacturing process or an issue with a raw material. The high bacterial counts may indicate that the microorganisms are thriving in the product. If it is a preserved product then this could indicate that the preservative system is not functioning, or worse, that the preservative was missing or incorrectly formulated.

The Characteristics of the Microorganism

The characteristics of the microorganism can be determined by textbooks or library work, by internet searches, or a combination of all of these. To obtain a more thorough range of sources, searches should not be restricted to pharmaceutical data. Useful information from food, environmental, clinical, and perhaps cosmetic microbiology sources should be considered in addition to the pharmaceutical field.

The widespread use of genetic techniques, which are causing considerable changes in taxonomy, should be taken into account for the names of some organisms have undergone multiple changes. Thus one difficulty with a long review of microflora is the potential for the reclassification of microorganisms. (This is through the Committee on Systematics of Prokaryotes, who operate a list containing in excess of 22,000 names. For a microorganism name or new or a reclassified species to be accepted it has to be approved by the Judicial Commission of the International Association of Microbiological Societies and be accepted in an approved publication.) This difficulty notwithstanding, the national culture collections are a good source of synonyms and all name variants should be researched.

The numbers of microorganisms recovered do not address themselves to the question of objectionable or specified microorganisms. The presence of objectionable or specified microorganisms is of significance, primarily due to a possible risk to the products and due to their central concern to regulatory agencies.

CONCLUDING INVESTIGATIONS

There are different possible outcomes when concluding investigations, such as:

1. *Laboratory error*: In this instance, it may (as with a raw material) or may not (as with batch specific environmental monitoring) be possible to repeat the result, following the original result being declared invalid.

2. *Confirmed failure*: Where the result is valid, the out-of-limits or out-of-specification result is accepted. A product impact assessment will be required and the obtained result is considered as a manufacturing deviation.
3. *Inconclusive result*: Here the balance of probability should be toward the result being valid, and a manufacturing deviation assumed.

As part of ongoing reviews, it is useful to consider all of the microbial excursions that have occurred over a defined period (such as quarterly or annually), in order to look for patterns and to assess common causes. An example of this is a biocontamination oversight committee. This can feed into wider facility improvement and contamination reduction initiatives and programs. In addition, quality metrics can also be developed, such as targets for production managers in terms of assessing cleaning and disinfection effectiveness and improving environmental monitoring results.

SUMMARY

Good manufacturing practice (GMP), in providing the minimum standard that a medicines manufacturer must meet in their production processes, aims to ensure that products are of a consistent high quality, are appropriate to their intended use, and that they meet the requirements of the marketing authorization or product specification. Ensuring this involves the investigation of product related out-of-specification results and an assessment of associated out-of-limits results (such as from bioburden testing or environmental monitoring), together with an assessment of any upward or adverse trends.

Within this, data must be considered to ensure that the obtained result is not due to laboratory error. Typical issues to investigate include analyst error, performance of the test, analysis of the data, instrument error, reagent failure, and so on, as the chapter has discussed. If reason to doubt the accuracy of the result is identified, the test is invalidated (but data retained) and a new test may be performed, depending on the nature of the sample (for instance, a microbial limits test can be performed again but environmental monitoring cannot).

The majority of microbiological excursions will be valid and here an investigation needs to be performed, in order to verify microbial control or to consider the risk to a product. Here the investigation may be expanded to include areas like materials, equipment, processes, the controlled environment, and operators. In the case of environmental monitoring or in-process bioburden issues, additional testing may be executed to investigate hypotheses as to what might have gone wrong.

At the end of the investigation, the root cause must be established (or most probable root cause) and corrective and preventive action proposed. The conclusion to the investigation must consider impact on the product. As this chapter has described, this is not often straightforward. Nonetheless, as structured approach, drawing on scientifically sound assessments and data, can assist considerably in the assessment of microbial data excursions.

REFERENCES

Clontz, L. (2008). *Microbial limit and bioburden test: Validation approaches and global requirements* (2nd ed., p. 300). Boca Raton, RL CRC Press.

Eissa ME: Studies of microbial resistance against some disinfectants: Microbial distribution & biocidal resistance in pharmaceutical manufacturing facility. 1st ed. Saarbrücken: LAP Lamber Academic Publishing; 2014, pp 14–53.

FDA (2014) Pharmaceutical microbiology manual, Version 1.2, FDA, Bethesda, MD.

FDA Guidance for Industry (2006) Investigating out-of-specification (OOS) est results for pharmaceutical production, US Department for Health and Human Services, Food and Drug Administration, CDER and CBER, Bethesda, MD.

Grice, E. A., Kong, H. H., Renaud, G., Young, A. C., Bouffard, G. G., Blakesley, R. W., et al. (2008). A diversity profile of the human skin microbiota. *Genome Research, 18* (7), 1043–1050.

Jiminez, L. (2004). Microorganisms in the environment and their relevance to pharmaceutical processes. In L. Jiminez (Ed.), *Microbial contamination control in the pharmaceutical industry* (pp. 1–14). New York: Marcel Dekker.

Lolas, A. (2014). The role of microbiology in the design and development of pharmaceutical manufacturing processes. *Pharmaceutical Bioprocessing, 2*(2), 125–128.

McCullough, K., & Moldenhauer, J. (2015). In K. McCullough, & J. Moldenhauer (Eds.), *Introduction in microbial risk and investigations*. Bethesda, MD: Parenteral Drug Association (PDA) and Davis Heathcare International (DHI). Chapter 1.

Pasquarellaf, C., O. Pitzurra, O. Savino, A. (2000) The index of microbial air contamination, Journal of Hospital Infection, 46 (94): 241–256.

Sandle, T. (2006). Environmental monitoring risk assessment. *Journal of GXP Compliance, 10*(2), 54–73.

Sutton, S. (2010a). The environmental monitoring program in a GMP environment. *Journal of GXP Compliance, 14*(3), 23–30.

Sutton, S. (2010b). Laboratory investigations of microbiological data deviations (MDD). In S. Sutton (Ed.), *Laboratory design: Establishing the facility and management structure* (pp. 81–100). DHI Publishers.

Wu, G. F., & Liu, X. H. (2007). Characterization of predominant bacteria isolates from clean rooms in a pharmaceutical production unit. *Journal of Zhejiang University Science B, 8*(9), 666–672.

Index

Note: Page numbers followed by *f* indicate figures, *t* indicate tables, and *b* indicate boxes.

A

Acid anionics, 294
Actinobacteria, 317
Actinomycetes, 202
Action level, 339, 343
Active (volumetric) air samplers, 88–95, 89*f*
Adenosine triphosphate (ATP), 200
Aerotolerant organisms, 182
Agar
  blood, 109
  Columbia blood, 109
  nutrient, 107–108
  sabouraud dextrose agar (SDA), 108–109, 108*t*
  tryptone soya agar (TSDA), 105–107, 106*t*, 112
Air
  of gas, 189
  microbial contamination, 15–17
Airborne contamination, in cleanrooms, 290–291
Air samplers
  active (volumetric), 88–95, 89*f*
  efficiency, 92–93
  practical use of, 94
  surface, 91
Alert level, 339
Alternative microbiological method, 142, 144–145
Amphoterics, 294
Anaerobes
  facultative, 182
  obligate, 182–183
Anaerobic environmental monitoring, 182–183
Anaerobic microorganisms, 320
Aqueous fluid loads, sterilization of, 304
Aqueous granulation and drying, 13–14
Aseptic Filling Suite, 175
Aseptic processing, 180, 182
ATP. *See* Adenosine triphosphate (ATP)
Atrium, sterilizable microbiological, 91

B

Bacillus, 209
  B. anthracis, 294–295
  B. fusiformis, 208
  B. genus, 208
  B. infernus, 200–201
Bacteria
  endospores, 202
  endotoxin, 51, 192
  gram-negative, 202–203, 216–217
  gram-positive, 202–203, 317–318
  growth, 252
  spores, 22, 202
Bacterial endotoxins test (BET), 222
Bacterial retentive filter, 189
Barrier technology, 50–51
Behavior, cleanroom personnel, 326–331
BET. *See* Bacterial endotoxins test (BET)
Biguanides, 294–295
Bioburden, 250
  assessment, 249
  control, 250
Biocontaminant, definition, 47–48
Biocontamination
  control
    culture media for, 105–109
    implications for, 321
    ISO 14698, 39–40
  control strategy, 1–2, 48, 50–62, 288
    cleaning and disinfection, 58
    contamination control review cycle, 57*f*
    continuous improvement, 61–62
    control of utilities, 51–52
    data recording and handling, 61
    design of plant and process, 50
    equipment and facilities, 50–51
    in-process controls, 53
    monitoring systems, 58–60
    outsourced services, 54
    preventative maintenance, 58
    prevention, 60–61
    process risk assessment, 55–57
    process validation, 57–58
    product containers and closures, 54
    product development, 53
    raw materials control, 52–53
    regulatory expectations, 49–50
    training and control of personnel, 51
    vendor approval, 54
  definition, 1
  deviation management, 339–341
    data deviations, terminology and categories, 341–342
    evidence, assessing, 347–348
    impact assessment, 348–352, 351–352*b*
    investigations, 342–346, 352–353
    laboratory controls, 347
    laboratory error investigation, 346–347, 349–351*b*
Biodecontamination, 306–307
  sterilization and, 302–306
Biofilm, 219
  chlorination of, 202
  formation, 202
Biopharmaceuticals, 251
Biosafety cabinets, 66–67
Blood agar, 109
Blow-fill technology, 182
Buffers, 254–255, 258

C

CAPA. *See* Corrective action preventative action (CAPA)
CCPs. *See* Critical control points (CCPs)
Cell component analysis, 147
Centrifugal sampler, 91
CFRS, Food and Drug Administration (FDA), 13
cGMP. *See* Current Good Manufacturing Practice (cGMP)
Chlorination of biofilm, 202
CIP. *See* Clean-in-place (CIP)
Cleaning, 292
  and disinfection, 292–298
  validation, 301
Clean-in-place (CIP), 292–293, 301
Clean-out-of-place (COP), 301

Cleanroom, 65–67
  airborne contamination in, 290–291
  assessment of results, 77–79
  classification, 27–29, 33–34, 74–79,
    135–137
    air volumes to be sampled, 136–137
    number of locations, 135–136
    particle counters location, 136
    particle sizes, 135, 136t
    results assessment, 137
  and clean air devices, 66–67
  contamination control, 68–73
  design, 289–291
  in different operating states, 172–174
  disposable/limited life materials, 323
  environment, microbial survival,
    201–202
  fabrics, 300
  garments, 299–300, 322–326, 324t
    for aseptic processing, 299
    changing, 332–333
  HVAC systems, 73
  in-use, 172–173
  laminated/membrane fabrics, 323
  microbiota, 207–210, 315
  microorganisms, 69, 203–207
  newly built, 172
  operators, risk, 316
  particle counting in, 128f
  particles, 73–74
  personnel behavior, 326–331
  pharmaceutical, grades of, 324–325,
    325–326f
  staff working in, 321–322
  users, 135
  woven fabrics, 323
Clothing, importance of, 321–326
"Cold loving" microorganisms, 185
Columbia blood agar, 109
Committee for European Normalisation
  (CEN), 32
Compressed air sampling, 190
Compressed gas, 192
  microbial survival in, 189
  monitoring, 187–192
  sampling, 94–95
Compressor failure, 189
Contact plates, 98–99
Contamination control, cleanrooms, 68–73
Contamination risk
  particle counts and, 126–128
  transfer risks, 299–300

Controlled environment, 288, 290–291
Conventional microbiological method,
  141–143
COP. See Clean-out-of-place (COP)
Corrective Action Preventative Action
  (CAPA), 241
Corrective and preventive action (CAPA),
  50, 282
Corynebacterium species, 209
CPPs. See Critical process parameters
  (CPPs)
CQAs. See Critical quality attributes
  (CQAs)
Critical control points (CCPs), 174, 345
Critical process parameters (CPPs), 291
Critical quality attributes (CQAs), 291
Cryophiles, 184
Culture media
  for biocontamination control, 105–109
  definition, 104–105
  general-purpose, 112
  microbiological, 104
  quality control testing of, 109–110
  supply of, 105
Current Good Manufacturing Practice
  (cGMP), 40

D
Detection factors, 276t
Detergents, 292
Disinfectants, 292–293
  concentration, 296
  nonoxidizing, 294–295
  number, type, and location of
    microorganisms, 297
  organic and interfering substances,
    298
  oxidizing, 295–296
  qualification, 298
  selection of, 296–298
  temperature and pH, 297–298
  time, 296–297
  types and activity, 293–296
Disinfection, 6, 8
Dry heat, 304
Dry swabbing, 96

E
EMA. See European Medicines Agency
  (EMA)
Endospores, 202
  bacterial, 202

Endotoxin, 215, 252–253, 302
  bacterial, 51, 192
  control, 250
  levels, 249
  risks
    control, 217–218
    and water for injection (WFI),
      216–218
  thermal inactivation of, 304
Environmental controls, weaknesses with,
  21–22
Environmental monitoring, 7, 24, 79–80,
  83, 179, 261–262
  anaerobic, 182–183
  assessing cleaning and disinfection
    effectiveness, 174
  cleanrooms
    in different operating states, 172–174
    in-use, 172–173
    newly built, 172
  considerations, 173–174
  critical areas in aseptic filling, 163–165
  criticality factors, 165–167, 166t
  data review, 174–175
  design of, 160
  duration of monitoring, 168–169
  frequency of, 161–167, 164t
  incubation strategies for, 110–111
  locations for monitoring, 169–171
  methods, application, 84–85
  monitoring methods, 171–172
  parametric release, 179, 181f
    monitoring to support, 180–182
  for particulates, 175–176
  risk assessment to, 265–267
  risk-based approach to, 163–167
  risks associated with conducting,
    280–281
  staff training, 176
  Standard Operation Procedure (SOP),
    340
  time of monitoring, 167–168
  written program, 176–177
Environmental monitoring program, 2–3, 7,
  83–84, 159–160, 162–163
  using risk to construct the, 267–268
    frequencies of monitoring, 267–268
Environment, sterility test, 192–194
EPS. See Extra polymeric substance
  (EPS)
Equipment design and use, 291–292
Ethylene oxide, 305

EU GMP, 66
    Grade A/ISO 14644 Class 5
        environments, 130
    guidance, 28
        cleanroom grades, 28t
European Medicines Agency (EMA), 184
European Pharmacopoeia (Ph. Eur.), 148
European Regulations, 29
Excipients, 251, 255, 258
Exponential growth, 252
Extra polymeric substance (EPS), 202

F

Facultative anaerobes, 182
Facultative psychrophiles, 184–185
Failure mode and effects analysis (FMEA),
    24–25, 268–269, 273–275, 275t
Fault tree analysis (FTA), 268–269
FEMA. *See* Failure mode and effects
    analysis (FMEA)
Filter
    high efficiency particulate air, 126–127
    samplers, 92
Finger plate assessment, 277–280b,
    278–279t
Finger plates, 99
Flocked swabs, 96
Flocking, 96
Floor monitoring, 167
Food and Drug Administration (FDA), 30,
    184, 289
    aseptic processing microbial limits, 43t
    CFRS, 13
    Code of Federal Regulations, 30–31
Force, gravitational, 127–128
FTA. *See* Fault tree analysis (FTA)
Fungal spores, 16–17
Fungi, in pharmaceutical processing
    environments, 209

G

Gamma
    irradiation, 305
    radiation, 304–305
Garments, cleanroom, 322–326, 324t
    changing, 332–333
Gas, 305
    compressed, 192
    monitoring, compressed, 187–192
    sampling, compressed, 94–95
Glovebox, 68
Glutaraldehyde, 294

GMP. *See* Good manufacturing practice
    (GMP)
Good Distribution Practice, 57
Good manufacturing practice (GMP), 49,
    53, 353
    centric approach, 288
    deficiencies, 44
    guidance, 28
        cleanroom grades, 28t
    Regulations and Standards, 27
        assessment of results, 37–39
        current Good Manufacturing Practice
            (cGMP), 40
        documentation and record keeping, 45
        European Regulations, 29
        initial nonzero contamination rates, 43t
        International Regulations, 32–40
        ISO 13408, 32
        ISO 14644, 32–34
        ISO 14644-1, 33
        ISO 14698, 32
        issue of limits: competing standards,
            40–44, 41t
        location of particle counters within the
            cleanroom, 36
        North American Regulations, 30–31
        number of locations to be measured
            within cleanroom, 35–36
        particle sizes to be measurement,
            34–35
        synergy of US and European
            Regulations, 31–32
        volume of air to be sampled, 36
    requirements, 28, 42, 42t
Gordon' incubation study, 117
Gown, 321–322, 330, 332–333
    plate, 99
    and skin shedding issues, 322
Grade A (ISO 5) cleanroom environment,
    89
Gram-negative bacteria, 202–203, 209,
    216–217
Gram-negative rods, 318
Gram-positive bacteria, 202–203, 317–318
Gram-positive cocci, 207–208
Gram-positive microorganism, 207
Gram-positive rods, 202, 207–208
Gravitational forces, 127–128
Gravitational sedimentation, 127–128
Gravitational settling, 86
Growth promotion testing, 195, 196t
Guinet's incubation study, 119

H

HACCP. *See* Hazard analysis and critical
    control point (HACCP)
Hatches, 68
Hazard analysis and critical control point
    (HACCP), 24–25, 53, 55, 174, 262,
    268–273, 345
    risk assessment tool, 39
Healthcare products, 47–48
Heating ventilation and air conditioning
    (HVAC), 204, 291
    cleanrooms HVAC systems, 73
    functions, 73
    parameters, 291
HEPA. *See* High efficiency particulate air
    (HEPA)
High efficiency particulate air (HEPA)
    filtered airflow, 68
    filters, 70–71, 126–127, 291
High-energy photons, 304–305
HMP. *See* Human Microbiome Project
    (HMP)
Hold times, 302
Human microbiome, 316–321
Human Microbiome Project (HMP), 20,
    204, 316–317
Human risk factor, 316
Hypochlorites, 295

I

ICH. *See* International Conference on
    Harmonization (ICH)
ICH Q9, 263
Impinger, 92
Incubation, 119–120, 120t
    Gordon' incubation study, 117
    Guinet's incubation study, 119
    Marshall's incubation study,
        114–115
    and microbial recovery, 111–112
    Sage's incubation study, 117–118
    Sandle's incubation study, 115–117,
        116t
    strategies, 112–120
    studies to evaluate two-tiered, 114
    Symonds' incubation study, 118
    time, 120–121
Indicator organisms, 12
Internal company obstacles, 150–151
International Conference on Harmonization
    (ICH), 49

International Standards Organisation (ISO), 32
ISO 14644, 66, 74–75, 78
ISO 14698 biocontamination control, 39–40
In-use cleanrooms, 172–173
Irradiation, 304–305
gamma, 305
Isolators, 66–68, 307–308

J

Japanese Pharmacopoeia, 148–149

L

Laminated fabrics, 323
Laser particle counter, 128–129
Liebig's "law of the minimum", 320
Light scattering, 129
Light scattering airborne particle counter (LSAPC), 34
Limulus Amebocyte Lysate (LAL) test, 222
Lipid A (LipA), 252
Lipopolysaccharide, 216–217
LSAPC. *See* Light scattering airborne particle counter (LSAPC)

M

Marshall's incubation study, 114–115
Mass distribution, 131–132
MAT. *See* Monocyte activation test (MAT)
Materials access, 333–334
Maximum valid dilution (MVD), 257–258
Maxwell–Boltzmann distribution, 131–132
Maxwell speed distribution, 131–132
Membrane fabrics, 323
MEMS. *See* Micro-electrical-mechanical systems (MEMS)
MIC. *See* Minimum inhibitory concentration (MIC)
Microaerophiles, 182
Microbial adhesion, 170
Microbial carrying particles, 68, 125
Microbial cells, 200
Microbial contamination, 47–48
effective cleaning and disinfection, 23–24
facility repairs and maintenance, 22
remediation actives, 22
risk of, 251
sources, 15
air, 15–17
human body, 20–21
materials and surfaces, 18–20

water, 17–18
weaknesses with environmental controls, 21–22
Microbial control, 214, 250–251
program, 55
Microbial data, 226
alert and action levels, 244
setting, 244
control charts, 230–231, 236*f*, 239
common causes, 231
cumulative sum charts, 237–239, 238*f*
setting up, 233
Shewhart charts, 233–237
special causes, 231–233
data integrity, 245–246
deviation, terminology and categories, 341–342
distribution of, 227–229
frequency of trending, 239–241
histograms, 229–230
investigating out of trend, 241–242
statistical interpretation of, 225–226
tracking microorganisms, 242–243
trending, 229–239
variations, 226–229
Microbial ecology, in pharmaceutical environments, 201
Microbial flora, 201
Microbial identification, effect of survival strategy on, 202–203
Microbial recovery, temperatures of incubation and, 111–112
Microbial risks
control, to water systems, 218–219
during manufacturing, 251–253
Microbial species, 204
Microbial survival
in cleanroom environment, 201–202
in compressed gases, 189
Microbiological contamination, 11–12
Microbiological culture media, 104
Microbiological environmental monitoring, 177, 193
test controls, 194–195, 195*t*
Microbiological environmental program, 160
Microbiological monitoring methods, 39–40
Microbiological requirements, 190–192
Microbiological results
out of limits, 339–341, 347–348, 353
out of specification, 341, 348, 353

Microbiological test, 194–195
Microbiology laboratories, monitoring, 194, 194*t*
Microbiome, human, 316–321
Microbiota
cleanroom, 207–210
originating, proliferation, 13–14
Micro colonies, 202
Micro-electrical-mechanical systems (MEMS), 147–148
Microenvironment, 67
Microorganisms, 1, 6–7, 88–89, 251–252
in cleanrooms and origins, 203–207
air, 204
packaging materials, 206
personnel, 203–204
raw materials, 205–206
surfaces (equipment, walls and ceilings), 205
water, 207
cold loving, 185
compressed gas sampling for, 187
contamination of, 14
growth requirements of, 200–201
number, type, and location of, 297
objectionable, 222, 309
tracking, 242–243, 243*f*
types, 12–13
Minimum inhibitory concentration (MIC), 296
Mobile particle counters, 132
Moist heat, 303–304
Monitoring. *See also specific types of monitoring*
microbiology laboratories, 194, 194*t*
sterility test environments, 192–194
Monocyte activation test (MAT), 222
MVD. *See* Maximum valid dilution (MVD)

N

Nanaerobes, 182
Nonendotoxin microbial pyrogen, 253
Nonoxidizing disinfectants, 294–295
Nonsterile products, 12–13, 216
microbial impact on, 351–352*b*
pharmaceutical products, 29
preservative efficacy, 309–311
Nonviable particle counting, 125
Nucleic acid amplification, 147
Nutrient agar, 107–108
Nutritive properties test, 110
Nylon fibers, 96

O

Objectionable microorganisms, 12–13, 222, 309
Obligate anaerobes, 182–183
Obligate psychrophiles, 184
OOL investigations, 174
Optical spectroscopy methods, 147
Osmosis, reverse, 215
OUL. *See* Out-of-limits (OUL)
Out-of-limits (OUL)
   investigations, 281–282
   microbiological result, 339–341, 347–348, 353
Out of specification, microbiological result, 341, 348, 353
Oxidizing disinfectants, 295–296

P

Packaging, primary and secondary, 311
Parametric release, 179
   definition, 180
   key factors, 181*f*
   monitoring to support, 180–182
Parenteral Drug Association (PDA), 31
Particle
   cleanrooms, 73–74
   deposition rate, 127–128
   microbial carrying, 125
   size of, 126
Particle counter, 129
   flow rate, 129
   laser, 128–129
   limitations of, 130–131
   location, 136
   mobile, 132
   operational issues with, 131–133
   operation basics, 128–130
Particle counting, 126, 128–129
   in cleanroom, 128*f*
   for contaminants, 175
   and contamination risk, 126–128
   frequency of, 134–135
   limits setting, 133, 134*t*
   nonviable, 125
PAT. *See* Process analytical technology (PAT)
PDA. *See* Parenteral Drug Association (PDA)
Personal hygiene, 334–336
Personnel monitoring, 99
Pharmaceutical cleanroom, grades of, 324–325, 325–326*f*

Pharmaceutical environment, microbial ecology in, 201
Pharmaceutical Inspection Co-operation Scheme (PIC/S), 36
Pharmaceutical manufacturing, 52
   areas, 11–12
   risk management for, 49
   sterile and nonsterile products, 216
   water for injection (WFI), 215–216
   water in, 214–216
      potable, 214–215
      purified, 215
Pharmaceutical microbiology, developments with, 142–144
Pharmaceutical processing
   investigating data deviations, 258
   monitoring plan, 258
   process factors affecting contamination, 253–254
   process hold times and process validation, 254–255
   sampling, 256–257
   testing regimes, 256–258
   test methods, 257–258
Pharmaceutical products, 13, 47–48
Pharmaceutical quality system, 49
Pharmacopeial Forum, 30
Photons, high-energy, 304–305
Piping distribution systems, 189
PNSU. *See* Probability of a nonsterile unit (PNSU)
Poisson distribution, 228
Potable water, 214–215
Preservatives, 309–311
Probability of a nonsterile unit (PNSU), 303
Process analytical technology (PAT), 60, 142, 291
Product risk, assessing, 13–15
Proteins, psychrophile, 184
Pseudomonas aeruginosa, 222
Psychrophile, 184
   facultative, 184–185
   obligate, 184
   proteins, 184
Psychrophilic monitoring, 183–186
Pupsit, 306
Purified water, 213–215
Pyrogen
   nonendotoxin microbial, 253
   in pharmaceutical processing, 249, 252–253, 256–257

Q

QACs. *See* Quaternary ammonium compounds (QACs)
QMS. *See* Quality management system (QMS)
QRM. *See* Quality risk management (QRM)
Qualitative rapid method, 142
"Quality by Design"concept, 288–289
   elements of, 289
Quality control testing, 109–110
   of culture media, 109–110
Quality management system (QMS), 49
Quality risk management (QRM), 29, 49, 142, 263–265
Quaternary ammonium compounds (QACs), 295

R

RABS. *See* Restrictive access barrier systems (RABS)
Radiation, 304–305
   gamma, 304–305
Rapid microbiological method (RMM), 142–144, 221
   benefits of, 144–145
   cell component analysis, 147
   classes of, 146–148
   direct measurement, 146
   expectations from the vendor, 155
   growth-based methods, 146
   guidance for selecting, 148–155
   internal company obstacles, 150–151
   key considerations, 149–150
   micro-electrical-mechanical systems (MEMS), 147–148
   nucleic acid amplification, 147
   optical spectroscopy methods, 147
   regulatory acceptance of, 145–146
   training, 154–155
   transfer method, 154
   validation, 151–154
Reasoner's 2A medium (R2A), 220–221
Remediation actives, 22
Restrictive access barrier systems (RABS), 67, 307–308
Reverse osmosis, 215
Risk assessment, 7, 15, 262, 311
   to environmental monitoring, 265–267
      extrinsic hazards, 266–267, 267*f*
      intrinsic hazards, 266
   numerical approaches to, 275–280
   tools, 268–270

Risk factor, human, 316
Risk management, quality, 263–265
RMM. *See* Rapid microbiological method (RMM)
RODAC, 98
Root cause analysis, 283

S

Sabouraud dextrose agar (SDA), 108–109, 108*t*
SAL. *See* Sterility assurance level (SAL)
Sandle's incubation study, 115–117, 116*t*
SCDM. *See* Soybean casein digest medium (SCDM)
SDA. *See* Sabouraud dextrose agar (SDA)
Sedimentation, gravitational, 127–128
Settle plate, 85–88, 86*f*
    assessing suitability, 87–88
    counts, estimation, 276–277*b*, 277*t*
Shelford's "law of tolerance", 320
Sieve impactor, 91
Single-use sterile disposable technology, 308–309
Skin
    flora, 317
    microbiome, 321
    physical properties, 319*t*
    regions of, 319*t*
Slit-to-Agar Air Sampler (STA), 90
Soybean casein digest medium (SCDM), 257
Spores, 189
    bacterial, 202
    fungal, 16–17
    ingress of, 17
STA. *See* Slit-to-Agar Air Sampler (STA)
Standard Operation Procedure (SOP), environmental monitoring level, 340
Staphylococci, 208
Staphylococcus aureus, 204, 318

Steam sterilization, 303–304
Sterile products, 12, 216, 307–309
    manufacturing, 255–256
Sterility assurance level (SAL), 303
Sterility Assurance Limit concept, 307–308
Sterility test, 180–182
    environments, 192–194
Sterilizable microbiological atrium, 91
Sterilization
    of aqueous fluid loads, 304
    aseptic process, 307–309
    and biodecontamination, 302–306
    terminal, 307–309
Sterilizing grade filtration, 305–306
Surface air system sampler, 91
Surface contact plates, 98
Surface monitoring, 167
Surface sampling, 95–99
Swabbing, 96–97
    advantages, 97
    dry, 96
    qualification criteria for, 97–98
Symonds' incubation study, 118

T

Terminal sterilization, 307–309
Test controls, viable microbiological environmental monitoring, 194–195, 195*t*
Therapeutic protein products, 251
Thermophilic monitoring, 186–187
Training, 331–332
Tryptone soya agar (TSA), 105–107, 106*t*, 112, 193

U

UDAF devices, 67
Ultra-low penetration air (ULPA) filters, 70
Ultraviolet light (UV), 204

Undesirable (objectionable) microorganisms, 222
Unidirectional airflow (UDAF) devices, 66–67
US Pharmacopeia (USP), 148

V

Validation plan (VP), 153–154
Vaporized hydrogen peroxide (VHP), 307
Vectors, 12, 16–19
    of microorganisms, 15–16
VHP. *See* Vaporized hydrogen peroxide (VHP)
Viable but nonculturable (VNBC) microorganisms, 143
Viable microbiological environmental monitoring, 83–85
    test controls, 194–195, 195*t*
Viable monitoring, 161, 168–169
Viruses, 210

W

Water
    microbial contamination, 17–18
    in pharmaceutical manufacturing, 214–216
Water for injection (WFI), 213–216
    endotoxin risks and, 216–218
Water system
    contamination, 219–220
    microbial risks control, 218–219
    monitoring
        bacterial endotoxins test (BET), 222
        sample-related contamination, 223
        total aerobic viable counts, 220–221
        undesirable (objectionable) microorganisms, 222
WFI. *See* Water for injection (WFI)
World Health Organization, 66
Woven fabrics, 323

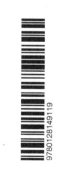